The Roots of the
Recovery Movement
in Psychiatry

The Roots of the Recovery Movement in Psychiatry

Lessons Learned

Larry Davidson

School of Medicine and Institution for Social and Policy Studies
Yale University, USA

Jaak Rakfeldt

Southern Connecticut State University and School of Medicine
Yale University, USA

John Strauss

School of Medicine, Yale University, USA

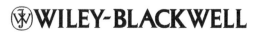

WILEY-BLACKWELL

A John Wiley & Sons, Ltd., Publication

Library of Congress Cataloguing-in-Publication Data

Davidson, Larry.
    The roots of the recovery movement in psychiatry : lessons learned /
Larry Davidson, Jaak Rakfeldt, John Strauss.
        p. ; cm.
    Includes bibliographical references and index.
    ISBN 978-0-470-77763-3 (cloth)
    1. Recovery movement–History. 2. Social psychiatry. 3. Community
psychiatry. 4. Humanistic psychotherapy. I. Rakfeldt, Jaak. II.
Strauss, John S. III. Title.
    [DNLM: 1. Community Mental Health Services–history. 2. History,
Modern 1601-. 3. Mental Disorders–rehabilitation. 4. Mentally Ill
Persons–history. WM 11.1 D252r 2009]
    RC455.D38 2009
    362.2′2–dc22
                                                2009038790

ISBN: 978-0-470-77763-3

A catalogue record for this book is available from the British Library.

Set in 10.5/12.75 Minion by Laserwords Private Limited, Chennai, India

This book is dedicated to my parents, Faye and Bernie Davidson, who gave me the opportunity and support to do what I wanted with my life. – LD

This book is dedicated to the memory of my parents, Miralda and Ilmar Rakfeldt, who inspired me through their capacity to retain love, warmth, compassion and a sense of humour, even after having confronted the tragic dislocations and vicissitudes of our refugee, immigrant life experiences. – JR

To my parents, Augusta and Walton Strauss, and to my kids, Jeff and Sarah. – JSS

Contents

Foreword

Since the issuance of the report of the President's New Freedom Commission on Mental Health in 2003, the challenge of transforming the nation's mental health system with the goal of recovery has been accepted by the mental health community with amazing enthusiasm. But while the concept of recovery has been generally accepted, there seems to be considerable divergence of opinion as to the meaning, and the implications, of the term 'recovery'. As someone who has personally been in recovery from schizophrenia throughout the past four decades, I find this an exciting time. Indeed, as I often say during the self-revelatory talks I sometimes give concerning recovery from schizophrenia, this is the best time in history to be a person with schizophrenia.

However, despite my enthusiasm for these exciting, recovery-oriented times, it seems clear to me that we must begin to wrestle with trying to get a better grasp on what is meant by the term recovery.

In this regard, I find this volume, *The Roots of the Recovery Movement in Psychiatry: Lessons Learned*, a most welcome, useful and timely contribution. It is particularly relevant for those interested in the evolving delivery of mental health care as it impacts persons with schizophrenia and other forms of serious mental illness.

The authors characterize their work as a conceptual, as opposed to an historical overview of the development of care for the mentally ill during the past few centuries. I would suggest, however, that this fine publication is both, with a special focus on those aspects of care which can be viewed as precursors to the recovery approach.

The authors survey the perspectives of those thinkers whom they view as being major contributors to advancing our care of the mentally ill, as we have evolved from a medical (disease) model, through a rehabilitation perspective, to our emerging recovery view of care. I found much about the authors' thesis appealing throughout the text, but I feel some aspects of this work are particularly noteworthy.

First, of the various figures the authors have chosen to review, none are characterized as being messianic deliverers of truth. All these progenitors of the current recovery movement are portrayed as being important contributors who might have been driving forces during their times. Nevertheless, all had views discordant not only with many in their own eras but also with each other. This point is charmingly brought to the fore in the concluding chapter. Here the major forerunners of the recovery movement engage in an imaginary dialogue along the lines of the old Steve Allen television show *The Meeting of the Minds*.

Second, throughout the text, primary attention is given to the person in recovery being first a human being, as opposed to an object of scientific or even social manipulations. Continual focus is directed to the importance of the personal perspective of the recovering individual, as opposed to his adherence to procrustean, ideologically driven models that have too often been the basis of treatment approaches in the past. As an example of this, I found particularly attractive how the authors bring home this point with the encouragement of, but not the usual 'word-police' insistence on, the use of 'person first' language.

Third, in their historical overviews, the authors for the most part focus on pragmatic approaches to care. I was very pleased to see both Adolf Meyer and Lev Vygotsky extensively portrayed, and characterized as being progenitors of occupational therapy, a field which deserves profound respect for its focus on 'purposeful work'. Many forget that occupational therapy had its professional beginning in the state psychiatric hospitals. Although today most occupational therapists are involved in what they cavalierly refer to as 'physis' (physical disorders), this publication may serve to remind our occupational therapy friends of their roots and hopefully nudge them back a little in that direction.

Finally, *Schizophrenia Bulletin* recently published an article in the March 2009 issue, co-authored by myself, Dr Ed Knight and Professor Elyn Saks. In that manuscript, we focussed on our definitions of recovery and those of seven other doctoral level persons, mostly psychiatrists and psychologists who are also in recovery from schizophrenia. Upon reading the personal tribulations of Dorothea Dix and others, who apparently experienced psychotic episodes, it was refreshing to be reminded that we are not the first mental health professionals with schizophrenia to be open about our conditions. Particularly poignant is the portrayal of Harry Stack Sullivan, who viewed his ongoing recovery from schizophrenia as a major motivating factor in his efforts to help others.

In summary, this well-written, interesting volume should serve to provide significant edification and enlightenment to anyone desirous of a better grounding in how we have arrived at these relatively halcyon days of transforming our approach to persons with serious mental illness from one focusing primarily on care to one where the primary goal is that of recovery.

Frederick J. Frese III, PhD

Acknowledgements

Much of this book was written during two sabbaticals; Jaak's from Southern Connecticut State University and Larry's from Yale University. We wish to acknowledge the long-standing mentorship and friendship we have both enjoyed from our co-author, John Strauss. Last, but certainly not least, we would both like to acknowledge our wives and children for standing by us through thick and thin. We hope that this book, in however small a measure, might contribute to improving mental health care in the future, so that when they, or their children, seek care from mental health practitioners, they will find it to be a welcoming, healing and confirming experience.

Finally, we thank Fiona Woods and the other staff of Wiley-Blackwell for their enthusiasm, wise counsel and ongoing pestering. They made sure that this book saw the light of day, long before the sun was getting ready to set.

Larry Davidson
Jaak Rakfeldt

1

Introduction

1.1 What is the recovery movement in psychiatry?

In 1999, the Surgeon General of the United States – the top physician for the
country – issued a first-ever *Report on Mental Health* (Department of Health and
Human Services, 1999). This 458-page tome included much important information
and many surprises, but to those of us who consider ourselves part of the recovery
movement, its most prominent feature came near the very end of the book with the
simple assertion that all mental health care should be 'consumer oriented and focused
on promoting recovery' (Department of Health and Human Services, 1999, p. 455).
To naïve readers, this statement may appear simply to be asserting the obvious, that
is if mental health services were not focused on promoting recovery, what else might
they be for? Or perhaps some readers will see this statement as indicating that mental
health care should just become more like general medical care, assuming more of the
'customer service' philosophy that has been spreading throughout medicine for the
last decade under the rubric of 'patient-centred' or 'person-centred' care (O'Brien,
1987; O'Brien and Lovett, 1992; Laine and Davidoff, 1996; Marrone, Hoff and Helm,
1997; O'Brien and O'Brien, 2000; O'Brien, 2002; Tondora *et al.*, 2005; McCormack
and McCance, 2006). The matter-of-fact tone with which this statement was made
could certainly support either of these interpretations.

But for those readers who are more familiar with the history of psychiatry, and
who are aware, in particular, of the history of the use of the term 'consumer'
within psychiatry, this statement means something entirely different. Its appearance
in a Surgeon General's report on mental health in fact heralded the beginning
of a new era in psychiatry, an era in which radical reforms are to be made in
how we understand and treat mental illnesses and, equally importantly, how we
understand and treat individuals living with mental illnesses. To those individuals
who considered themselves mental health 'consumers', and to those other advocates
of 'recovery' – a term we define below – who had been fighting a battle of values,
principles and ideas for over 30 years, this statement indicated that we had, at last,

The Roots of the Recovery Movement in Psychiatry   Larry Davidson, Jaak Rakfeldt, John Strauss
© 2010 John Wiley & Sons, Ltd

won a prolonged – if relatively bloodless – war. One of the many surprising things about this statement appearing in an official federal report in 1999, though, was that it was not at all clear yet what war precisely it was that we had won.

The following book represents one more attempt to help to define the nature of the war and the implications of its having been won for individuals with mental illnesses, their loved ones and the mental health practitioners, programme managers and system leaders who have the privilege of serving and supporting them. Perhaps it is not unusual for wars to be won before either party realizes all of what has been at stake and what exactly is to result from victory. The current wars in Iraq and Afghanistan certainly confirm this, but so do the American and French revolutions. So perhaps it is perfectly understandable that we now are in a position of having to establish, clarify and defend what it is that has been won in the process. Unlike the American and French revolutions, and the wars in Iraq and Afghanistan, however, this was a war that the vast majority of the public, including that segment of the public involved directly in mental health care, did not even know was being waged. It was for perhaps this reason in particular that the war's having already been won in 1999 came as such a surprise, at least to those of us who were not serving on the front line at the time.

Some readers will undoubtedly object to our use of the term 'war', as the mental health consumer and broader recovery movements have never involved use of force or other violent means. They have not even involved labor or hunger strikes, sit-ins, large-scale political rallies or other non-violent acts of resistance, although there have been occasional marches and the creation and dissemination of protest songs, folk ballads, inspirational poetry and manifestos. On the other hand, though, it is important to recognize that these movements were indeed in response to centuries of violence and bloodshed in which people with mental illnesses were stoned, burned at the stake, locked in cages, chained to posts and walls, confined to squalid and inhumane living conditions, insulin-shocked, hydro-shocked, electro-shocked and lobotomized.

Lest the reader think that these atrocities are all only in the distant past, or only continue to occur in the developing world, a recent report released by the US Medical Directors Council of the National Association of State Mental Health Program Directors suggests otherwise. Since the mid-1980s, there has been an increase, rather than a decrease, in the discrepancy in average lifespan between those with and those without a serious mental illness. While the discrepancy in lifespan was a 'mere' 12 years in 1986, it more than doubled to 25 years by 2006 (McCarrick et al., 1986; Colton and Manderscheid, 2006). That means that in 2006 in the United States people with serious mental illnesses died on average 25 years younger than their peers. This loss of one-third of their lifespan is due to a combination of factors, including higher rates of suicide and substance use; a lack of access to and/or inadequate treatment of medical conditions like diabetes, heart and respiratory diseases; and higher rates of preventable and modifiable risk factors, such as obesity, poor nutrition and lack of exercise. It is hard to imagine that a prosperous society would tolerate a loss of one-third of the expected lifespan in any other population of its own citizens, providing at least one clear and unequivocal indicator of the fact that stigma and discrimination continue to exist against individuals with mental illnesses – with concrete, tangible and appalling results.

The stigma experienced by and the discrimination against individuals with mental illnesses – while not carried out (any longer) through burnings at the stake, lobotomies or other violent means – thus remain nonetheless serious, life-or-death, matters. Add to this recognition of the huge numbers of individuals with serious mental illnesses currently being held in jails across the country for non-violent and petty crimes and one can begin to appreciate the need for radical reform. How did the Surgeon General's assertion that mental health care should be 'consumer oriented and focused on promoting recovery' intend to change this picture? What kind of transformation is required in mental health care – 'transformation' being the term chosen by the subsequent US President's New Freedom Commission on Mental Health to capture the degree of deep and substantive change required (Department of Health and Human Services, 2003) – and how is it to be achieved? To return to our metaphor, what war precisely is it that we have won and, perhaps even more importantly, what will we now need to do to establish and keep the peace?

We return briefly to the Surgeon General's landmark report. The sentence which follows the assertion quoted above reads: 'That is, the goal of services must not be limited to symptom reduction but should strive for restoration of a meaningful and productive life' (Department of Health and Human Services, 1999, p. 455). 'Recovery' for the person with the illness (the 'consumer') is thus defined as restoration of a meaningful and productive life. This is what the mental health consumer/survivor/ex-patient movement advocated, and this has been the overarching aim of the recovery movement: to afford people with serious mental illnesses the rights, opportunities and resources needed to lead meaningful and productive lives. The New Freedom Commission's final report which followed four years after release of the Surgeon General's report went several steps further, defining this life as involving living, learning, working (a somewhat puritanical list to which we have added the terms 'loving' and 'playing') and participating fully in community life, having as its vision 'a life in the community for everyone' (Department of Health and Human Services, 2003, p. 1).

At a minimum, this vision would suggest that individuals with serious mental illnesses should no longer be confined to hospitals or other institutional settings but should be free and enabled to live in the community alongside their non-disabled peers (Davidson, 2007a). The New Freedom Commission, and the Supreme Court's *Olmstead Decision* which was issued at almost the same time, stressed that this was a vision that should be accessible to everyone with a serious mental illness, no matter how disabled they may be or the nature of the supports they may require in order to live as independently as possible. It is rather an issue of (i) assisting the person in learning how to live with and manage his or her condition and (ii) identifying the services and supports needed to enable him or her to do so. The field of psychiatric rehabilitation will take on these related challenges and will develop approaches and strategies for instilling hope and encouraging the person to mobilize his or her remaining strengths and resources in order to gain mastery over the illness; identify, set, pursue and accomplish personal goals; and, in general, live a meaningful and satisfying life in the face of an ongoing, if not necessarily life-long, condition (Corrigan *et al.*, 2008).

Two major obstacles to adopting a disability model and addressing these challenges in relation to serious mental illnesses are recognition of the fact that we do not currently have a cure for these disorders (even though many people recover fully from them nonetheless; Davidson, Harding and Spaniol, 2005) and the need to move from an acute care to a disease, or recovery, management model. Although we may already tell people with serious mental illnesses that they have 'chronic' diseases for which they may have to take medication for the remainder of their lives – just as people with diabetes have to take insulin – we have not taken this model very seriously ourselves. We have not fully accepted that there currently is no cure for psychosis, and that there does not yet appear to be promise of one any time soon. Instead, we insist that people adhere to prescribed treatments, including medications which have limited effectiveness (i.e. not nearly as effective as insulin), and expect them to wait until their illness abates before they resume their lives, as if they are suffering from an acute illness. We do not expect people with diabetes to put their lives on hold until the illness resolves, because we know that as of today we have no way to resolve the illness. They are thus encouraged to pursue their own hopes, dreams and aspirations – learn how to play football, drive a car, go on dates and marry – managing their illness within the context of this life as best they can. This is the meaning of the term 'recovery' in relation to serious mental illnesses that is used in the Surgeon General's and New Freedom Commission's reports, and the meaning of the term articulated and promoted by the subsequent federal *Action Agenda*, in which we read that the magnitude of change that will be required to implement this vision of recovery is 'revolutionary' (Department of Health and Human Services, 2005, p. 18).

The following book is concerned primarily with identifying what is revolutionary about this use of the term recovery and what its transformative implications for mental health practice are. Is it possible for serious mental illnesses to be treated truly the same as other chronic medical conditions? Is it possible to imagine a world in which serious mental illnesses were as well accepted, almost invisible, a part of life as diabetes? Will it be possible to develop supports and prostheses that represent the equivalent of psychiatric wheelchairs or Braille to help people compensate for the more enduring and disabling aspects of these 'brain diseases'? Will we be able to afford people a personally meaningful and gratifying life in the communities of their choice while they continue to experience a serious mental illness? These are some of the questions that face the recovery movement in psychiatry, some of the questions that will have to be addressed in establishing, and keeping, the peace if we are to be successful in ushering in a truly new era in mental health, an era in which despair will be replaced by hope, demoralization and helplessness will be replaced by dedication and commitment and empty lives will be filled with both the joys and the sorrows of ordinary everydayness (Davidson *et al.*, 2005; Borg and Davidson, 2007).

While the answers to these questions remain far from certain, earnest efforts are being made every day to come up with innovative and creative solutions to the problems posed by mental illness. We consider this book one of those efforts. We hope that as a result of looking backwards we will be able to offer some useful directions for moving the recovery movement, and the broader field of psychiatry, forwards.

Because we are primarily looking backwards, a note on the language used in this book is unfortunately necessary. We believe strongly in, and adhere to, person-first language in our own work, including in our own writing in this volume. We thus refer to individuals with serious mental illnesses as people with serious mental illnesses, or people in recovery, rather than as 'the mentally ill' or any one of the historical epithets used to refer to such individuals (e.g. 'mental patients', 'schizophrenics', 'manic depressives', etc.). It is, as we will repeatedly stress, a foundation of the recovery movement to view people with serious mental illnesses as people first and foremost, and only secondarily as people who have happened to develop a mental illness. The illness or diagnosis can no longer be viewed as subsuming the person.

We cannot, however, change the past. And thus, when quoting from some of these historical figures, we have had to include their own language, despite the fact that it may very well be offensive to some readers. We agree that it is offensive. But we also think it important to include their original language rather than to purge it of these offensive terms. For one reason, it is important that we be reminded of how people with serious mental illnesses were viewed and treated in the past so that we not repeat these same mistakes. Second, it can be taken as a sign of the progress we have made thus far that we no longer refer to such individuals as 'maniacs', 'lunatics' or 'schizophrenics'. As here, when we use these terms in the text, we set them apart using single quotation marks to denote their historical significance and to remind the reader, if necessary, that these are now outdated terms of reference.

1.2 Rationale for the book

Why did we choose to write a book on the *roots* of the recovery movement in psychiatry? Especially for a movement so early in its evolution, and whose ultimate impact on the field is so far from certain, it may seem premature to be looking backwards and trying to discern its history. This is not that kind of history, however. We use the term 'roots' in a conceptual sense rather than in a historical one. In other words, this book is not a historical account of how the recovery movement actually came to be. There is a very simple answer to that question, which we and others have discussed elsewhere (Chamberlin, 1990; Deegan, 1992; Davidson *et al.*, 2009). For a more thorough and complex answer, we will all have to wait for the historians to take the long view of the role of this movement as a social, political and intellectual force in psychiatry; but many more years will need to pass before we will be able to look back on and determine that history. It will be a very different history, for example, should recovery represent no more than a temporary fad, going the way of phrenology in the nineteenth century or problems in living in the 1970s, as opposed to bringing about the transformation of care that it currently promises to achieve (Department of Health and Human Services, 2003; Department of Health and Human Services, 2005). We will leave that determination for others.

What, then, do we mean by the 'roots of recovery', and why are we interested in them? The answer to this question is not nearly as simple as the historical one, but it is one that we think cannot wait until the movement has come to its natural conclusion. In fact, we think that the answer to this question – if given clearly, persuasively and with ample illustrations of its concrete implications – may be able to contribute to the eventual success of this movement, and it is for this reason that we are offering this book now rather than waiting until the movement has attained greater maturity. Briefly stated, many of our presentations, workshops and trainings on recovery and recovery-oriented practice have been met with the response: 'But we are doing this already.' Granted, this response only comes from a select few participants each time; it typically comes from those participants who have the most invested in the current system and who hold considerable power and authority over any possible changes that might be made in the future. They are, more often than not, those individuals we are most concerned about reaching in a given system, those individuals who most need to grasp and appreciate the scope and magnitude of the transformation that is involved in re-orienting mental health services to promote resilience and recovery.

As we noted above, according to the President's New Freedom Commission on Mental Health, we are being called upon to 'fundamentally refashion' mental health care (Department of Health and Human Services, 2003, p. 5). According to the subsequent American federal *Action Agenda* that provides the blueprint for implementing the recommendations of the Commission:

> Mere reforms to the existing mental health system are insufficient . . .
> Applied to the task at hand, transformation represents a bold vision
> to change the very form and function of the mental health service
> delivery system . . . It implies profound change – not at the margins of
> a system, but at its very core . . . (Department of Health and Human
> Services, 2005, p. 5)

Parallel documents in Canada (Standing Senate Committee on Social Affairs, Science and Technology, 2006), New Zealand (Mental Health Commission, 1998) and the United Kingdom (Care Services Improvement Partnership, 2006) reflect similar sentiments. Clearly, the organizations and institutions endorsing the recovery vision and recommending that all mental health services be re-oriented to promote resilience and recovery do not think that we are 'doing it already'.

It is on this gap between a revolutionary vision for the future of mental health care and the current realities of everyday clinical and rehabilitative practice that this book will focus. When we have asked our sceptics in what ways they are already offering recovery-oriented mental health care or practising in ways that promote resilience and recovery, their responses usually land in one of several camps. They may, for example suggest that recovery is simply a throw back to the days of 'moral treatment', in which humane staff used gentle, supportive and primarily educational interventions to help the residents of their asylums get back on their feet and resume their normal routines and responsibilities, a time during which 'recovery' rates were estimated to be as high as 90%. Or they may suggest that being recovery-oriented refers to the active listening and other efforts that psychoanalytically oriented practitioners made to explore and understand the subjective experiences, or inner lives, of their patients in psychodynamic treatment within the context of long-term hospitalization. Here much attention was paid to developing respectful relationships in which the practitioner helped the person to identify and pursue his or her own goals, with adherents of this approach claiming also to have seen the successful resolution of many cases (Karon, 2008). In both of these examples, of course, what appears to be overlooked is that the care provided was institution-based and that it was extremely difficult to establish and lead 'a life in the community' – the vision of recovery put forth by the New Freedom Commission – when confined to a psychiatric hospital. This point is also ignored by people who point to the heyday of the large state hospitals as evidence of a time when people with serious mental illnesses were put to work as part of self-sustaining farms, work for which they, unfortunately, were never paid.

At the opposite end of the spectrum, others will suggest that we already treat people with serious mental illnesses the same way we treat people with other chronic medical illnesses, such as asthma or diabetes. They agree with the sentiments that mental illnesses are illnesses like any other, that they are treatable and that people can lives meaningful live in the face of them. Others will argue that we have been 'doing recovery' at least since 1976, with the emergence of the community support movement. This was the movement that introduced such advances in practice as assertive community treatment, self-help and peer support, family education and support and psychiatric rehabilitation. It is true, of course, that use of the term 'recovery' in relation to serious mental illnesses did develop in its contemporary form (i.e. as opposed to during the moral treatment era) within the context of this movement. In these two cases, though, what appears to be lost is the important if subtle distinction between recovery, which refers to what the person with the mental illness does, and recovery-oriented care, which refers to what practitioners provide in support of the person's recovery (Davidson et al., 2007). We will argue in the following that the recovery movement is first and foremost a civil rights movement by and for people with serious mental illnesses (Davidson, 2006; Davidson et al., 2006). It is only secondarily a movement which has implications for the way mental health practitioners practise. To the degree to which people associate recovery solely with how practitioners practise, they miss the critical and central role played by the person him- or herself. In this case, even if *we* (i.e. practitioners) do actually 'do it already', this is of little consolation if people with serious mental illnesses have yet to reclaim their lives as citizens of their community.

In the end, however, we are not as much interested in refuting these examples as we are in learning from them. It is not helpful simply to point out how people offering up these examples have missed important aspects of recovery-oriented care, such as the desire to live in the community rather than in the hospital or the right to be paid a decent wage for one's labor. What is more interesting is the way in which these examples were right about certain aspects of care, and what we can learn from these prior efforts. We could argue, for instance, that one thing that was common to all of these efforts was the recognition – as partial as it might have been – that people with serious mental illnesses remained people who had certain interests and capacities. If we agree with Patricia Deegan, an international leader of the recovery movement, that 'The concept of recovery is rooted in the simple yet profound realization that people who have been diagnosed with a mental illness are human beings' (Deegan, 1993, p. 8), then this insight was a core element of these earlier approaches that is shared by the contemporary notions of recovery and recovery-oriented care. Rather than argue that we are not proposing a return to moral treatment or to exploratory psychoanalytic treatment, it is useful to acknowledge that the recovery movement does share certain values, principles and perhaps even strategies with some of these approaches. We certainly understand that this is not the first time in the history of psychiatry that we have attempted to treat people with serious mental illnesses *as* people. What we take up in the following volume is what lessons have been learned by these previous attempts, and how these lessons can help us in our current efforts to get it right this time round.

It is useful to note, for example, that people with serious mental illnesses participated actively in music, art, exercise and educational activities when offered such opportunities within well-staffed and therapeutically oriented hospitals. It is also useful to note that even within largely custodial institutions people with serious mental illnesses were able to work with little, if any, support. It is equally useful to know that many more people can work with supports, and that work has an ameliorative effect on symptoms (Drake *et al.*, 1994; Drake *et al.*, 1999). Each of these camps thus has important information and experience to offer us as we continue to push the notions of recovery and recovery-oriented practice further. By 'roots', then, we mean to refer to those prior efforts that have been made within psychiatry to treat people with serious mental illnesses as people and to afford them the opportunity to lead decent and gratifying everyday lives, either in the absence or in the ongoing presence of the symptoms of the illness. We will point out along the way some of what might have been missed in the earlier efforts, and in this way hope to persuade our sceptics that there is still much work to do in 'achieving the promise' (Department of Health and Human Services, 2003) of recovery-oriented care. Our primary focus, though, will be on what was learned through these efforts that was effective and helpful, hoping in this way to add flesh and bones to what remains a largely skeletal framework for recovery-oriented practice (Davidson *et al.*, 2009).

As we see it, the primary challenge for recovery-oriented practice is how to educate, encourage and support people with serious mental illnesses as they go about trying to figure out how to live a meaningful life with, compensate for and perhaps eventually overcome a serious mental illness. While there remains much for us to figure out in terms of the nature of the illness, its impact on everyday life and what we can do to educate and encourage people, there may also be much to learn from previous efforts to support people in having a life. We will begin to unpack in the following some of those lessons and their implications for ways to transform current practice. The remainder of this chapter provides a brief introduction to and overview of the various areas in which some of these efforts have been made.

1.3 From *traitement moral* to moral treatment

As we mentioned above, some people see the recovery movement as a return to the days of moral treatment. This was roughly a 100-year period between 1790 and 1890 in which people with serious mental illnesses whose families had the financial means could send them to an asylum or 'retreat' for convalescence and recuperation following an episode of mental illness, and during which they were likely to be treated and cared for by a benevolent doctor and staff who would gradually restore them to, or help them to achieve for the first time, a state of mental health, maturity and satisfactory functioning. As also noted above, success or recovery rates for these institutions were estimated to be around 90% for those patients admitted within a year of the onset of their illness, attesting to the effectiveness of this re-educational approach.

In this chapter, we will expand our focus beyond the specific strategies of this period to consider the humanistic elements that led up to the development of '*traitement moral*' by Philippe Pinel and the humanistic aims which this approach was then deployed to achieve. We will begin this section, therefore, with the liberation of mental patients from the chains in which they had been held during the Middle Ages. We will find, perhaps surprisingly, that recognition of the value of hiring people in recovery to provide care to others – what is currently called 'peer support' – can be traced back to this era, when Jean-Baptiste Pussin, the governor of the Bicêtre when Pinel arrived there and himself a former patient of the hospital, was not only the first to remove the inmates' chains but also the first to use the strategy of hiring convalescing patients to provide *traitement moral* to the patients of the asylum.

We will then follow Pussin and Pinel's approach as it crossed the English Channel and then eventually the Atlantic Ocean, being transformed into what has come to be known since as 'moral treatment' proper. We will see that some things were lost from, and others added to, Pinel's original vision in the translation from the French, with mental illness and its care taking on a much more paternalistic and moralistic tone under the influence of the Tukes and their like-minded contemporaries in Victorian England. Where previously there had been treatment for illnesses that were most likely to affect people of extraordinary sensitivity and talent, there came to be an educational and disciplinarian approach to promoting self-control and restraint in people who had come to be seen as 'wayward children'. Although the precise factors that account for the transformation of *traitement moral* into moral treatment are not clear, we suggest that one possible source of explanation is the difficulty involved in managing large institutions, regardless of their stated or explicit aims. It certainly was in part the rapid growth, over-crowding and under-staffing of these moral treatment retreats which led to their rapid demise.

1.4 Reciprocity in community-based care

After discussing the changes moral treatment underwent when adapted by British and American reformers, we will then consider the Herculean efforts of Dorothea Dix to spread the promise of moral treatment to all those afflicted with mental illnesses, despite their social class or their family's ability to pay. Dix was particularly concerned with individuals who had ended up in jails and prisons and who, therefore, were not receiving any of the benefits of the available moral treatments. Within this context, we suggest that the magnitude of the work that remains to be done is indicated, in part, by the fact that there are even more individuals with mental illness in jails and prisons now than there were when Dorothea Dix began her crusade in the 1840s.

Acknowledging her importance to the recovery movement – as representing advocates who wish to secure appropriate and effective care for all those in need – we then turn to question the central belief that Dix held in common with both Pinel and the moral treatment proponents in the United Kingdom and the United States, namely that people with serious mental illnesses needed to be extracted from their everyday and interpersonal context in order to recover. In order to offer an alternative vision of how care can be provided in a person's home environment and community, we take up the thinking and practice of Jane Addams, founder of the settlement house movement in the United States. Perhaps more than anyone else, the work of Addams provides a counterpoint to Dix and her wish to rescue people from their everyday lives. Coming from outside of psychiatry altogether, Addams offered the first model of what a comprehensive and holistic approach can offer in a community, as opposed to institutional, setting. Rather than bringing people to care, Addams and her colleagues brought care to the people they viewed as being in need, offering them the opportunities, encouragement and support needed for them to reclaim their lives out of the ravages of illness, addiction, poverty, discrimination, oppression, immigration and disability. Addams was perhaps the first to point out how it is not enough to establish a trusting relationship with someone who is suffering or in need, but that the way in which care, compassion and resources are offered to that person can also influence the degree to which, or the ways in which, that person will then be able to make use of such gifts.

The work of Addams offers us hints as to ways in which help can be offered to people in need without locking them into a second-class status or engendering their further dependency on help-givers. By reviewing the principles and lessons learned by the settlement house movement, this chapter considers the positive characteristics required of community-based services and supports if they are not to perpetuate segregation and chronicity. 'Care', in this sense, is not something that is given by one person to be passively received by another, but rather involves creating or expanding access to opportunities for people to take advantage of in pursuing their own hopes and dreams and in giving to others. Indeed, within this framework the notion of 'giving back', which is frequently cited by people in recovery as an important foundation for their efforts, is given a central role in re-establishing and expanding the person's sense of self and agency. These key concepts will then be taken up again in Section 1.8, when we turn to the central role of agency in recovery.

1.5 The everyday and interpersonal context of recovery

The work of Addams is complemented nicely by turning next to the work of three leading psychiatrists who specialized in serious mental illnesses and the care of individuals experiencing and recovering from them. A contemporary of Addams, Adolf Meyer, considered by some the father of modern American psychiatry, was the first person from within psychiatry to propose a community-based alternative to moral treatment and mental hospitalization. Swiss born and trained, Meyer brought with him from Switzerland intimate knowledge of European psychiatry at the turn of the century and introduced to the newly emerging discipline in America the ideas of Emil Kraepelin and Sigmund Freud, among others. In contrast to their ideas (i.e. Kraepelin's belief that psychosis was an organic and progressively deteriorating condition and Freud's that it was both organic and a pre-Oedipal developmental fixation), Meyer's own view of serious mental illnesses was perhaps closest to Pinel's. Consistent with what we will read from Pinel's *Treatise on Insanity*, Meyer was perhaps the first American psychiatrist to take seriously the ideas that mental illnesses could be illnesses like any other, that many people can recover from them and that, even when they are ill, most people with serious mental illnesses retained areas of healthy functioning relatively in tact, co-existing with the illness.

Where Meyer differed from Pinel was in terms of the nature of the treatment required by this particular form of illness. Rather than viewing the illness as internal to the person, Meyer – like Addams – believed the illness, or what he termed 'problem in living', to arise at the interface between the person and his or her immediate social environment. In this case, it made little sense to extract the person from his or her situation, as the problem did not reside within the person per se. If the problem were to disappear with the person's removal from his or her life circumstances, it would just as surely re-emerge as soon as the person was returned to these same circumstances once the treatment or cure had been effected. In this way, Meyer viewed the person's everyday life within his or her social world as the primary locus for psychiatric research and intervention. Rather than sending them off for rest, respite and recuperation, Meyer believed that people could deal with and manage their difficulties within the context of their ongoing lives, rather, that is, than waiting for the illness to abate before returning to the community and resuming their lives. He saw that it was through the process of navigating and negotiating everyday life, rather than in escaping from it, that people were able to build on their strengths in constructing satisfying lives. Although contemporaneous with him, Meyer in this way set the stage for the Russian psychologist Lev Vygotsky, with whom we will deal in Section 1.8. Both are credited with providing the conceptual foundation for the fields of occupational science and therapy, as both understood the central role of activity and occupation in human growth and development.

Much of the material about Meyer, his work and his influence will come from the one author of this volume who was trained in the era, and in the places, where this influence was most directly and immediately felt. Following this retrospective reflection, we then have asked John Strauss, the second of the leading psychiatrists discussed in this chapter, to summarize the findings from his own groundbreaking research. Being the senior partner in the trio of authors for this book, John has served as an invaluable mentor, friend and inspiration for the other two of us (LD and JR). The papers that he began to publish with his collaborator and friend William Carpenter in the 1970s on the course and outcome of psychotic disorders marked the beginning of the recovery movement for academic psychiatry. Simultaneous with the origins and development of the consumer/survivor/ex-patient movement in the United States, Strauss and Carpenter's work provided the scientific evidence to corroborate and confirm what people in recovery were saying. This body of rigorous longitudinal research, which John describes briefly in this chapter, has been one of the key sources of inspiration and information for the recovery movement since. It paved the way for the next generation of research on recovery and recovery-oriented practice in which we and others have been engaged, and for which we owe John a debt of gratitude.

As the last component of this chapter, we then turn to the work of Harry Stack Sullivan, who, more than anyone else, pioneered the development of a psychotherapeutic approach to working with individuals with serious mental illnesses. Although typically viewed as falling within the psychoanalytic tradition, Sullivan actually was equally, if not more so, influenced by thinkers such as Meyer and his American contemporaries than by Freud and his other followers. Sullivan's major original contribution was to view interpersonal relationships as the central medium for both the development and the treatment of serious mental illnesses. Like Meyer's 'common sense' approach to psychiatry, this point may now seem to be so obvious as to be taken for granted. Prior to Sullivan, however, people with schizophrenia were viewed as impossible to understand, and therefore impossible to relate to or to engage in meaningful, reciprocal relationships. The interpersonal milieu of psychoanalysis was viewed as inappropriate for people suffering from psychosis, leaving them to fall outside the boundaries of the emerging discipline of clinical psychiatry. Sullivan broke with this position, viewing psychosis as a basically human – rather than primitive or alien – condition and showing how interpersonal relationships, particularly with skilled and caring practitioners, could be therapeutic or healing.

Sullivan's early work took place within the context of a psychiatric hospital and could, in this way, be viewed as a continuation of Pinel's *traitement moral*.

Like Pussin before him, he made a practice of hiring recovering patients to staff his inpatient unit, convinced that their own first-hand experience of psychosis and recovery prepared them especially well for the tasks involved in caring for their acutely ill peers. While Pussin, Pinel and the Tukes all placed a premium on human relationships, they gave little thought to how specifically these relationships could effect changes in the person's mental health. Despite having to invent highly idiosyncratic, off-putting, terms to express his original ideas, Sullivan was able to demonstrate through his practice and his teaching that people could be welcomed back from psychosis through the medium of human relationships. The fact that he experienced a psychotic episode himself both lends credence to his views and makes him an especially appealing and relevant figure during this era of 'peer support' in which increasing numbers of people in recovery are being trained and employed to engage with and promote the recovery of their peers.

1.6 Closing the hospital

Following on the demise of moral treatment, it then required someone, or several influential someones, to realize that recovery was more likely to occur outside of the institution, where everyday life in the community naturally unfolded, than inside of the institution, where everyday life was in the hands of, and determined by, others. We focus on two of the central conceptual figures behind de-institutionalization, one of whom, Erving Goffman, primarily documented and demonstrated the destructive influence and iatrogenic effects of the hospital and the other of whom, Franco Basaglia, understood well these effects and went the farthest in actually closing hospitals and beginning to sketch out how life in the community could be supported and sustained among individuals with the most disabling mental illnesses.

As a classic text, Goffman's indictment in *Asylums* of what he terms the 'total institution' may well be understood at an intellectual level by students of the social sciences. There is much in what Goffman wrote about the asylum and institutionalization, however, which has yet to be fully appreciated at the concrete level of practice within psychiatry. As we are beginning to learn in the recovery movement, there are ways in which the effects of stigma and institutionalization extend beyond the walls of the hospital or even take up residence in the lives of individuals who have never been hospitalized. Goffman's understanding of how the institution can be recreated within the person's own psyche or identity may be useful in contending with what is currently being referred to as 'internalized (or self) stigma', which is being reported to pose as formidable a barrier to recovery as discrimination and the illness itself.

With profound insight into the ways in which the institution not only affected its inmates but also affected the very manifestation of the illness itself, Franco Basaglia might have gone further than anyone else before him in envisioning the possibilities that could be created by closing the asylum altogether. This he did at first in Goritzia, then in Parma and Trieste, initiating what has since been called the Italian mental health reform movement. Basaglia's efforts in Italy differed from the majority of parallel de-institutionalization efforts in the United States and elsewhere by being grounded explicitly in an appreciation of the freedom and autonomy of people with mental illnesses and by developing community-based systems of care founded on the principles of social inclusion and participatory governance. Basaglia not only succeeded in securing funds for robust systems of community-based care (unlike the United States, for example) but also recognized that many of the characteristics of his patients that were thought to be intrinsic to their mental illness per se, the vacant stares, the word salad, the perseverative movements and gestures, appeared to melt away as they left the confines of the asylum. From these observations, he concluded that we would not know what mental illnesses were, or what limitations they would intrinsically place on individuals suffering from them, until both patients and staff were liberated from the culture, attitudes and beliefs of the asylum. With poverty, social isolation, discrimination and prolonged unemployment taking the place of the hospital, we suggest in the following that for the most part we still do not know what limitations are intrinsic to the illness per se, if any.

The more innovative aspects of this legacy are now being used as a basis for policy and programme development in Western Europe, Canada, Australia and New Zealand, and have begun to offer insights into how much less disabling mental illnesses may be when they are uncoupled from these attitudes and beliefs, many of which have survived well beyond the tenure of the institutions which gave them birth.

1.7 The rights and responsibilities of citizenship

Following the work of Basaglia to its natural conclusion, we then come to appreciate that a key aim of recovery-oriented care is to enable people who had been thrust to the margins of society to reclaim their basic citizenship as free and autonomous actors. As Rowe (1999) suggests, rather than recovery being a precondition of citizenship, it is achieved actually *through* citizenship. But what is the ideal of citizenship to which such individuals aspire? What exactly is involved in exercising one's citizenship? Is citizenship merely the absence of discrimination or oppression, or do we have a positive notion of citizenship which may provide more concrete guidance to mental health services? In this chapter, we turn to two perhaps unlikely figures to help us understand what is involved in reclaiming one's rights to citizenship along with the responsibilities associated with it.

While only peripherally interested in issues of mental illness and mental health, who better than the Reverend Dr Martin Luther King, Jnr to turn to for guidance on the civil rights dimension of recovery? King learned many valuable lessons about what is entailed in an oppressed minority population staking claim to and winning the battle for their basic human dignity and rights. As we noted above, the recovery movement is first and foremost a civil rights movement initiated and led by, and for the direct benefit of, individuals with serious mental illnesses. There are more parallels between the battles for civil rights among communities of color, women and lesbian/gay/bisexual/transgendered people and those with serious mental illnesses than one would initially or ordinarily think. This chapter considers some of these parallels and what they can teach us about future challenges faced by the recovery movement.

In addition to promoting human and civil rights, both King and the French philosopher and political thinker Gilles Deleuze cautioned people not to feel obliged to adjust or adapt to the world as it currently is, but instead to contribute actively to creating a world that is more like one thinks it could or should be. King, for his part, refused to adjust 'to lynch mobs, segregation, economic inequalities, "the madness of militarism" and self-defeating physical violence.' 'The salvation of the world', he writes, 'lies in the maladjusted' (King, 1981, p. 23). Deleuze took this sentiment further, challenging the very notion of adjustment as a psychological construct and drawing attention to its inevitable political function within a capitalist economic system.

One of the more enigmatic facts that we appear to know about recovery from serious mental illnesses is that it is easier to recover in non-industrial, non-capitalist countries. One of the more promising theoretical explanations for this disparity is that capitalist economies insist more stringently on people 'fitting in' or adjusting to the requirements of the labor force. King apparently was also beginning to understand this association between oppression and capitalism late in his life, as his attention turned more towards poverty and the Vietnam war as posing even more fundamental challenges to civil rights than racism. We look to the thought of Deleuze for guidance as to how to promote civil rights and citizenship among individuals with serious mental illnesses without falling sway to the seduction of a rigid capitalist notion of 'normalcy'. While this line of thinking is still in its early stages, we consider it important enough to preventing individuals with mental illness from trading in one form of oppression for another that we devote the remainder of this chapter to laying out these ideas in admittedly rough and unfinished form.

1.8 Agency as a basis for transformation

Given the emphasis on agency emerging first from Addams and Meyer through Basaglia to Deleuze, we then take up this important notion more fully in this chapter, turning to the thinking of a largely under-appreciated (in the English-speaking world) but influential Russian psychologist, Lev Vygotsky, and an increasingly relevant Nobel Prize-winning political economist, Amartya Sen. What these two disparate thinkers have in common is their fundamental commitment to agency as a defining characteristic of human nature and their corresponding emphasis on activity, doing and occupation as core aspects of determining a person's quality of life. In contrast to their actual chronological order, we will begin this discussion with Sen's work, as it provides a more accessible point of departure and clear parallels to what we have learned thus far about recovery. With that framework in place, we then turn to the thinking of Vygotsky to help us translate these lessons into their implications for recovery-oriented practice.

Sen was an economist by training. But rather than focus in determining quality of life on what people have, as has been conventional in economics (but only within the last century, as Sen points out), he emphasized 'the *actual living* that people manage to achieve' (Sen, 1999, p. 73). Regardless of one's material wealth, it is the capability to act and 'to take part in the life of the community' that is a fundamental expression of the person's freedom and autonomy, without which he or she cannot function as a fully human being (Sen, 1999, p. 73). At the collective level, Sen showed how the investment of resources in enabling the population of a country to become free and active participants and contributors to the economy in the end generates prosperity and capital, whereas no amount of prosperity or capital in and of itself can ensure or bring about freedom. 'The usefulness of wealth', according to Sen, lies only 'in the things that it allows us to do – the substantive freedoms it helps us to achieve' (Sen, 1999, p. 14). Based on this central commitment to the priority of agency over possession, Sen distils three useful principles for a psychiatry that is attempting to help restore to people their sense of agency and efficacy in the world. These three principles are: (i) for choice to be truly free it must be determined by each unique individual for him- or herself; (ii) free choice necessarily results in variability and diversity, as unique individuals will choose different things from each other; and, finally, (iii) we cannot insist that people wait until certain material, social or political preconditions are in place in order for them to begin to choose, as people are born active agents who are always already making choices in their lives on an everyday basis (Davidson *et al.*, in press). We will see, as we turn to Vygotsky, how these principles have direct applicability in recovery-oriented practice.

For Vygotsky, action preceded rather than followed from thought, as did language. It was through the person's active engagement with the world and with others that he or she learned how and what to think, adopted a shared language and eventually came to reflect on him- or herself and his or her place in the world. None of these things could be acquired, not to mention mastered, first or prior to action and activity, but instead were some of its by-products, as were habits, routines, social norms and a common culture. As a developmental psychologist (among other things), Vygotsky studied how these processes unfolded in children as they learned and grew over time. As we now know, people do not stop learning and growing when they reach adulthood, and these same fundamental processes are at play in adults as well. Vygotsky's insights have since proven to have equal relevance for learning and growth processes in adults, including adults who are learning about and trying to figure out how to manage a serious mental illness while pursuing their life goals and aspirations. We close this chapter with two in-depth examples of how these insights shed light on and help us to understand what appear to be some of the central principles of recovery, principles which may have less to do with the nature of serious mental illnesses and more to do with the nature of human beings.

1.9 Why these figures and not others?

Some reviewers of the proposal for this book were concerned that our choices were too slanted to American developments or did not include important figures or traditions from outside of the United States. Others may consider our choices highly idiosyncratic and question our inclusion of people like Jane Addams, Amartya Sen, Martin Luther King, Jnr or Gilles Deleuze who have had little if anything to do with serious mental illness or recovery. We acknowledge that these are not choices that would likely be made by most other proponents of recovery, but we also think it is important that mental health not remain as insular as it has tended to be in the past. There is much valuable knowledge and guidance that can be gleaned from outside of mental health, particularly as it relates to restoring the rights and citizenship of individuals who just happen to have serious mental illnesses. We mentioned this first in the preceding paragraph in relation to Vygotsky, but it applies equally well to others. As there is much more to individuals with serious mental illnesses than the mental illnesses they happen to have, there also is much more to the knowledge we need to acquire and the care we need to offer than what is specific to mental illness per se – especially, as we noted above, as we still do not know what is specific to mental illness per se and what stems from the social conditions under which people with mental illnesses have had to live for the last three centuries.

On the other hand, there are undoubtedly additional people we could have mentioned. Why, for example, would a book that is at least in part about efforts to humanize psychiatry not include representatives of humanistic psychology, such as Carl Rogers, Viktor Frankl or Abraham Maslow? Rogers was certainly a pioneer in the pursuit of active, reflective listening, Frankl understood the importance of having a sense of meaning and purpose in life and Maslow appreciated the urgency of meeting an individual's basic needs for home, income, food, safety and companionship. Although important, these are aspects of recovery that would appear to require less conceptual justification. Perhaps as a result of its success or influence, the aspects of recovery to which this stream of the humanistic tradition speaks are more easily taken for granted or considered of obvious value than those aspects to which we devote our time and attention in this book.

Very few people will argue, for instance, about whether individuals with serious mental illnesses need to have a safe and dignified place to live, food and a sense of meaning and purpose in life. Most practitioners will agree that taking the time to listen carefully to individuals with serious mental illnesses would be a good thing to do – had they the time to do so. What people will argue about, however, is where people should live and eat (e.g. in a hospital or a home, with or without supervision), whether a sense of meaning and purpose can be supplied or given by others (as opposed to needing to be actively chosen by the person him- or herself) and what value or function listening is ultimately to serve (e.g. to identify the person's own goals for his or her life or to identify leverage and evidence that can be used to persuade him or her to adhere to prescribed treatments). In our opinion, answers to these questions are better found in the work of the thinkers and doers we have selected to focus on in this volume than in the humanistic tradition in psychology.

How about other innovations or other innovators in psychiatry? There currently is much stock being placed, at least in certain parts of the world, on treatment advances such as assertive community treatment, cognitive-behavioral psychother-apy, cognitive remediation or re-training and the development of newer and better psychiatric medications. Why don't we discuss these here? The original theoretical impetus of assertive community treatment of *in vivo* skills training and support has since made possible many of the advances made in psychiatric rehabilitation and can be found at the core of supported employment, supported education, supported housing and supported socialization. *In vivo* skills training, unfortunately, is one of those aspects of assertive community treatment which receives the least attention in the literature and in practice, resulting in many assertive community treatment teams becoming little more than mobile crisis or intensive case management pro-grammes which, as Floersch has aptly described, have narrowed their focus to 'meds, money and manners' (Floersch, 2002). While there are efforts underway to make assertive community treatment more recovery-oriented (Salyers and Tsemberis, 2007), these efforts are limited primarily to decreasing the amount of coercion used and increasing the degree to which care is driven by the person's own goals, failing to constitute significant advances or breakthroughs in practice.

Cognitive-behavioral psychotherapy may constitute a significant breakthrough, especially as it relates to medication-resistant positive symptoms of psychosis. The underlying framework for this approach can already be found, however, in the work of Harry Stack Sullivan and his colleagues. While they did not develop the specific technical interventions involved in cognitive-behavioral psychotherapy in any explicit way, their practice was already an effort to explore the patient's own mental processes and ways of perceiving and understanding the world within the context of a collaborative and respectful relationship. We will, for this reason, take up briefly the topic of cognitive-behavioral psychotherapy in our chapter on Meyer and Sullivan. As a highly technical intervention addressing only a very narrow swath of psychotic symptoms, however, cognitive-behavioral psychotherapy can only be considered one useful tool among many in the recovery-oriented practitioner's toolbox. As there is much more to recovery than the reduction and/or management of the positive symptoms of psychosis, there needs to be much more to the care of individuals with serious mental illnesses than cognitive-behavioral psychotherapy alone.

The same case could be made for psychiatric medications, as they traditionally have only been effective in targeting these same positive symptoms of psychosis. We can certainly hope that new and more effective medications will be developed in the future, both with a broader focus than hallucinations and delusions and with fewer potentially lethal side effects. The modest progress made since the 1950s, however – especially when contrasted to the marketing claims made by pharmaceutical companies and zealous investigators – does not give us much hope for the near term in terms of significant breakthroughs. It is also difficult to imagine making such breakthroughs, other than through accidental discoveries, when we know so little about the nature of the serious mental illnesses we are trying to treat. As we noted above more than once, we still do not know what mental illness will look like once freed from the institution *and* from the layers of poverty, unemployment, isolation, discrimination and social disadvantage layered on top of it in contemporary society. As Strauss suggested in 1994, it will continue to be difficult to make genuine breakthroughs in developing effective medications until we have a more focused and accurate descriptive base of what serious mental illnesses look like in the person's everyday life experience, until, that is, we know what it is we are trying to treat (Strauss, 1994a). We are still a long way from having such a descriptive understanding of these disorders (Flanagan, Davidson and Strauss, 2007).

We are more hopeful that such a process is now underway in the development and testing of approaches to cognitive remediation or cognitive re-training. We know from research that the cognitive impairments that appear to be associated with serious mental illnesses are among their most disabling features (along with negative symptoms). There are many efforts currently underway to better identify, understand and begin to address these impairments, and early results have shown promise. This is a genuinely new area of research that has opened up only within the last decade or so, made possible by revolutionary new insights into the plasticity of the brain and central nervous system. Once thought to be permanent and irreversible, we are now learning that damage to the brain can be lessened, compensated for and at times even reversed through the generation of new neuronal connections. These processes of regeneration can be stimulated both by somatic interventions, including psychiatric medications, and by life experiences, including the kind of mental challenges and exercises involved in cognitive remediation or re-training. We look to this area of research for exciting new developments in ways to address, compensate for and possibly reverse some of the more disabling aspects of serious mental illness, and expect these interventions to play increasingly prominent roles in the recovery-oriented systems of the future. If so, these interventions would figure prominently within the framework we describe in Chapter 7, as part of the activity analysis and rehabilitative approach inspired by Vygotsky. At this time, however, there is not much more we can say about such interventions other than to hope and pray for their eventual success in lessening some of the least visible, but most distressing, elements of the disorder.

Finally, the humanistic(-existential)-inspired work of R.D. Laing in the 1960s and 1970s, and of Loren Mosher and others since, is worthy of comment. These have been efforts to offer humane and supportive alternatives to inpatient care and forced medication for people experiencing acute episodes of psychosis, first in democratically governed therapeutic communities inspired by the communes of the 1960s and then later in crisis respite and residential programmes staffed by tolerant and understanding people who sought to guide people gently back from the abyss to which their emotional distress had unwittingly taken them. We have not included a fuller discussion of this area of work for three reasons.

First, despite their protestations to the contrary, these approaches have tended to romanticize psychosis as a spiritual journey of discovery or self-actualization and have, in principle, denied people access to certain interventions, such as medication, that they might have found useful in lessening their distress out of a conviction that the distress needed to be 'worked through'. In our experience, there is very little that is romantic or spiritual about psychosis per se, which is not to deny that spirituality and faith may play a key role in the recovery process. We view psychosis primarily as a serious and potentially fatal illness (e.g. one out of 10 people with schizophrenia commit suicide) which tragically disrupts a person's life and from which he or she seeks relief. We do not believe in insisting that people 'work through' their psychosis to 'self-actualize', but rather that they are doing their best to 'actualize' themselves already and are trying to recover from or, if that is not yet possible, to find a way to live a decent and meaningful life in the face of this horrendous condition.

Second, the most promising elements of this approach to providing a humane and accepting environment for people suffering from an acute episode of psychosis as an alternative to inpatient care have been developed further by Shery Mede and others (Dumont and Jones, 2002) as a peer-run respite model which eschews the more controversial and, in our opinion, unnecessary aspects of the Laing/Soteria approach. This model for respite care has been highly successful to date and is beginning to be replicated across the country as one of several peer or consumer-run programmes, and in this sense is included in Chapter 3 under this broader rubric that dates, from our historical perspective, back to the groundbreaking work of Sullivan in the 1920s. As we noted above, at that time, Sullivan – like Pussin before him – made a practice of hiring individuals who had recovered from psychosis to staff his inpatient unit as he believed that they would have an increased sensitivity towards, and acceptance of, others who were suffering from the same condition as they had themselves experienced. He also thought that their life experiences offered them valuable knowledge and expertise that they could lend to the patients in their care, foreshadowing the explosion in peer-delivered services we have seen around the world since the early 1990s.

The third and final reason is important not only for justifying our exclusion of Laing and the Soteria House model but also for the consideration of many other approaches and interventions that others may think useful in promoting recovery. This reason is that Laing's communities and the Soteria House model are acute care settings for acute episodes. Although it is of course important that people receive compassionate and competent care when experiencing an acute episode of psychosis or other serious mental illness, and that it is true that how this episode is handled could have longer-term repercussions for that person's life, it is also true that most people with serious mental illnesses only spend 5% of their lives in acute distress (Wexler et al., 2008). This means that they spend 95% of their lives not in acute distress. The vast majority of recovery thus happens in that 95% of the time when they are not in acute episode, thus limiting the utility or effectiveness of interventions that are only oriented towards resolution of acute episodes.

This fundamental limitation of the Laing/Soteria model applies, therefore, to a much broader range of interventions and approaches and reminds us of Goffman's characterization of institutional care as a whole. Goffman likened hospitalizing someone with a serious mental illness to taking a drowning person out of a lake, teaching the person to ride a bicycle and putting the person back into the lake. While it is important that there are safe, dignified and supportive ways to assist people who are experiencing an acute episode of distress and/or psychosis, we should strive to avoid becoming overly ambitious about what can be accomplished within a short period within the context of a long-term condition. On the one hand, crises may represent opportunities for changing long-standing beliefs or behaviors. In this case, capitalizing on the opportunities represented by acute episodes may prove to be beneficial in the long-term. On the other hand, however, we have little reason to believe that acute cure for serious mental illness is any different from acute care for a heart attack, a particularly severe asthma attack or an episode of ketoacidosis for someone with diabetes. In most cases, people need to recuperate from the acute distress, come to terms with its consequences for their lives, try to understand what might have caused it and, if possible, try to prevent it from happening again in the future. It will be in the remaining 95% of the time, which is typically lived outside of institutional settings, that they will have to contend with, manage and live their lives in the face of, despite, or alongside the illness. It is for this reason that most recovery-oriented interventions address people's everyday lives within the everyday community contexts in which those lives are lived.

1.10 Conclusion

We have laid out the beginnings of a framework for identifying, exploring and learning from various aspects of the recovery movement in psychiatry. At this point, it might have become evident to the reader that there will be a few fundamental or overarching tensions that will emerge from and permeate our study of the various thinkers and doers described above. Looking back from Vygotsky and Sen to Sullivan and Meyer, for example, we can see that there may be a tension between a focus on people as free and autonomous agents and a counterbalancing focus on their needs for social relationships, resulting in a dynamic view of what we will describe as 'self in relation'. Similarly, looking backwards from Goffman and Basaglia to Pinel and Dix, we can see that there may be a tension between an emphasis on choice, creativity and self-determination on the one hand and a counterbalancing emphasis on community membership and reciprocity on the other, resulting in a dynamic of what we will describe as 'self in society'. Finally, there is a related tension between Deleuze's attention to the rights of citizenship and Addams' attention to

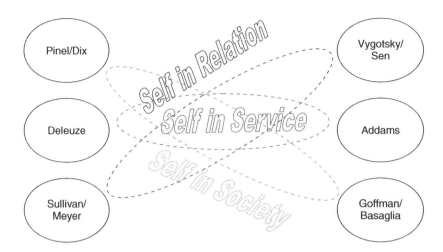

Figure 1.1 A schematic for three fundamental tensions in recovery-oriented practice.

the associated responsibilities, resulting in a dynamic of what we will describe as 'self in service'. These various dynamics are depicted in Figure 1.1. In our concluding chapter, we will envision a dialogue between these various thinkers and doers which will help to explicate these tensions further and begin to establish a coherent conceptual framework for the development and dissemination of recovery-oriented mental health care.

2

From *Traitement Moral* to Moral Treatment

> One cannot ignore a striking analogy in nature's ways when one compares the attacks of intermittent insanity with the violent symptoms of an acute illness. It would in either case be a mistake to measure the gravity of the danger by the extent of trouble and derangement of the vital functions. In both cases a serious condition may forecast recovery, provided one practices prudent management. (Philippe Pinel in his address to the Society for Natural History, Paris, France, 1794; cited in Weiner, 1992, p. 729)

2.1 The birth of psychiatry as a medical speciality

Of the many eloquent and astonishingly contemporary passages that may be found in the writings of Philippe Pinel – a goodly number of which follow below – we chose this particular one with which to begin this chapter because of its paradigm-shifting significance. Understated and modest in its tone, as was Pinel's style, this passage comprising three simple sentences did nothing less than set the stage for the creation of the discipline of psychiatry as a branch of medicine. In addition, it set the stage for the development of 'practices of prudent management', which, as we will see in this chapter, Pinel later came to refer to as '*traitement moral*', a term which later came to be translated into English as 'moral treatment'. In contrast to the meaning this term took on once introduced into England, though, 'it is important to point out', according to medical historian Dora Weiner, 'that "*traitement moral*" meant psychological treatment, in contrast to physical treatment'. 'The term should not be translated into the English "moral" with its connotation of moralizing,' she continues, 'which the French does not convey' (Weiner, 1979, p. 727).

The somewhat unexpected, if not paradoxical, juxtaposition of these two positions captures well the originality and importance of Pinel's contributions. At the same

The Roots of the Recovery Movement in Psychiatry   Larry Davidson, Jaak Rakfeldt, John Strauss
© 2010 John Wiley & Sons, Ltd

time that he was establishing mental illnesses to be illnesses that belonged, like other illnesses, under the purview of medicine, he was arguing that recovery was possible and was to be brought about by primarily psychological, rather than physical, means. The first few sections will deal with the first of these positions, and we will take up the development of moral treatment in the sections which then follow. As Pinel's background and expertise in internal medicine was crucial in shaping his approach to mental illness, and as we still have much to learn from the application of this approach at the present time, we think it worth focusing initially, if briefly, on his establishment of mental illnesses as appropriate phenomena for medicine and for 'the natural history of man'.

Pinel's personal history helps to account somewhat for the uniqueness of his approach and perspective. Born into a family of physicians and surgeons, Pinel returned to the study and practice of medicine after being educated in religion, mathematics and literature. Also interested in botany – an increasingly popular hobby in the Paris of the late eighteenth century – Pinel initially was attracted to studying and classifying diseases in the ways others at the time were studying and classifying plants. His first, and at the time most important, book was *Nosographie Philosophique* published in 1798, in which he put forth his own systematic taxonomy of diseases. His approach to this task involved close observation, the voluminous recording of these observations and then review and analysis of the observations recorded. While sounding somewhat rudimentary today, this practice was only under development at the time, and then only replacing theological and philosophical theorizing in such domains as medicine or botany. It would be yet another century before such an approach would finally be (re-)introduced into psychiatry by the founding fathers of descriptive psychopathology, Kraepelin, Bleuler and Jaspers. Pinel used this approach with much success at the time, with his nosology going through several editions as a popular textbook and his resulting appointment of being physician for life to Napoleon. Also among his original contributions was to create the first inoculation clinic, where he offered the first vaccination in Paris in 1800.

It was the loss of a close friend which turned this accomplished physician's attention to the subject of mental illness and its treatment, a subject which at the time received little medical attention. As he writes in his *Treatise on Insanity* first published in French in 1801, and then quickly translated and published in English in 1806:

> The loss of a friend, who became insane through excessive love of glory, in 1783; and the inaptitude of pharmaceutic preparations to a mind elated, as his was, with a high sense of its independence, enhanced my admiration for the judicious precepts of the ancients, and made me regret that I had it not then in my power to put them into practice. (Pinel, 1806, p. 52)

This loss of a dear friend and his discovery of how little was known or understood about mental illnesses, from antiquity on, led Pinel to devote the remainder of his career to studying and then developing and disseminating treatments for these disorders. In order to do so, he applied the same methods of close observation, written recording of notes and analysis that he had used in internal medicine. As he describes in the *Treatise on Insanity*, once situated within the context of the asylum: 'I viewed the scene that was opened to me with the eye of common sense and unprejudiced observation' (Pinel, 1806, p. 109). Also, given that his interest was piqued by the loss to mental illness of a good friend, he came to this topic without the customary bias of the times, which was to view 'mad' people as either bestial, demonically possessed, witches or of a lesser, perhaps alien, species. He was, in this way alone, already remarkable for his time.

As Weiner describes, this put Pinel in a fortuitous position to set an entirely new standard for how people with mental illnesses were to be viewed and treated by those who cared for them. She writes:

> No physician had yet written case histories as sympathetic and elo-quent as the ones that Pinel read to the Society for Natural History in December 1794. We turn, for example, to the vignette of the clockmaker who believed himself seized by perpetual motion or the white-haired 70-year-old who was convinced that he was a young woman. These would soon be quoted in the whole Western literature of the nascent psychiatric speciality. By speaking of these destitute mentally ill men with understanding and respectful kindness toward each inmate, Pinel initiated a new tone, lowered fear of the insane, and facilitated a more evenhanded, democratic approach to public medicine in large hospitals. (Weiner, 1992, p. 727)

Not only did Pinel paint such pictures in sympathetic terms with kindness and understanding, but he went so far as to suggest that many people with mental illnesses – far from being from an inferior race or species – were in fact suffering from an over-abundance of sensitivity and other highly valued human qualities. Pinel begins his groundbreaking 1794 address to the Society for Natural History with the following words, containing an implicit appeal for respect, if not even admiration, for this population of formerly despised and dispensable people:

> A large gathering of madmen inspires an undefinable thoughtful tenderness when one realizes that their present state derives only from a vivid sensitivity and from psychological qualities that we value highly. I find that truth ever more convincing and confirmed by my daily notes. Here is the father of a family whom unexpected losses have thrown into despair; here is a son exhausted by work and vigils to provide for his parents' subsistence; elsewhere a passionate and sensitive young man, victim of unrequited love; there a tender husband, distracted by suspicions and the justified or false umbrage of jealousy; a young warrior thirsting for glory whose vast and ambitious projects failed, his spirit crushed by the harsh experience. Religious zeal claims its

victims, as does ardent military fervor, which often expresses all the reveries and excesses of manic fanaticism. Man is most often led from the free use of reason to madness by overstepping the limits of his good qualities and of his generous and magnanimous inclinations. (Cited in Weiner, 1992, p. 728)

Pinel then continues at length with a variety of examples and illustrations that cover a range of intellectual and artistic pursuits. One can imagine that his intention was in part to plant the seed of doubt in his distinguished audience that they, too – they, who would surely count themselves among the company of 'very talented persons' – should consider themselves vulnerable to the development of mental illness. Given Pinel's stature and influence at the time as one of the most highly regarded physicians in France, we can appreciate the magnitude of the impact this address was to have for decades to come. We also can think of no more eloquent or impassioned a plea to respect and value people who happen to suffer from mental illnesses issued since. He writes:

> The excessive sensitivity that characterizes very talented persons may become a cause for the loss of their reason: I mention this as a well-meant warning without the intention of discouraging them. Groups as diverse as investigators, artists, orators, poets, geometers, engineers, painters, and sculptors pay an almost annual price to the hospice for the insane. I have on more than one occasion stopped at the cell of a madman speaking about current affairs in the most elaborate terms and with great verve. The exalted imagination of poets also leads sometime to madness, and I am often importuned by a confabulator who urges me to read his productions, while I see only the need to subject him to treatment for madness. Recently I watched one of the most distinguished sculptors of the Pantheon die in the hospice for the insane. One of the most skillful clockmakers in Paris, infatuated with the fantasy of perpetual motion, spent a long time in the hospice but has now been returned to his family. Patriotism is pained to find among the inmates an engineer employed during the siege of the town of Condé who exhausted himself by work and sleep deprivation. There are usually some famous painters, at the moment two skilled artists named after the famous Le Sueur. I also give special care to a man versed in the most profound mathematical meditations who lost his reason because of ever-renewed fears that Vandalism visited upon True Knowledge. How many talents lost to Society and what great efforts are needed to salvage them! (Cited in Weiner, 1992, p. 728)

In publishing this text in English for the first time in recent history in 1992, Weiner offered a similar assessment of its significance:

> Pinel, physician of the Enlightenment and the French Revolution, expresses a genuine empathy with the sufferings of ordinary men – a

distraught father, a jilted lover – and points out that gifted and sensitive
persons are particularly vulnerable to mental anguish. He claims for
them the attention and care that the natural rights of man imply. This
is a classic text because of its permanent human and humane qualities.
(Weiner, 1992, p. 728)

We have quoted these passages at length for two reasons. One, to give the reader
a taste of Pinel's literary gifts and style and, two, because we agree with Weiner that
the insights and lessons offered by Pinel are not limited to the place and time of
their creation. Whether they prove to be 'permanent', it will become clear to the
reader as we proceed with this volume that these revolutionary insights of Pinel's
are at least as equally relevant today as they were 200 years ago. We are still far from
appreciating the scope and magnitude of the talents that are lost to society every day
owing to the ravages of mental illness, and farther still from persuading our society
to expend the efforts needed to salvage them. In this sense, Pinel may be considered
the father of a science of psychiatry which has yet to be fully born.

In addition to observing that mental illnesses afflict ordinary people and perhaps
even more often people of extraordinary sensitivity, Pinel's observational, natural
history approach to mental illness generated two other insights which remain equally
valuable – and unfortunately equally uncommon – today.

The first of these was that recovery is possible in many, if not most, cases. To
expand upon the analogy to physical illnesses with which we began this chapter,
Pinel continued: 'The ways of nature are no less admirable in the termination of
attacks of madness than in the critical resolution of other illnesses and the gradual
recovery of health' (cited in Weiner, 1992, p. 730). He understood this to contradict
the popular beliefs of the day, which held 'madness' to be incurable. It was this
belief of incurability that had justified or at least excused the brutality and neglect
that had become accepted practices in the asylums of the day; the staff of these
institutions had to exert such coercive measures, and could be allowed not to feed,
clothe or care for their charges because these were not, or were no longer, people
like themselves. They were, more likely, brute beasts indifferent to the elements and
to pain or suffering (a view surprisingly still held by some contemporary figures; cf.
Andreasen, 1982). In challenging this view, Pinel asserts that: 'To consider madness
as a usually incurable illness is to assert a vague proposition that is constantly refuted
by the most authentic facts' (cited in Weiner, 1992, p. 730). It was just such facts
that he then went to great pains to document in his *Treatise on Insanity*.

Pinel's second insight into the nature of 'madness' may be equally as important as
his first, as it too remains unappreciated to a large extent to this day. This insight has
two related parts: (i) 'madness' can be episodic and can be precipitated in response
to external, social or environmental events, from unrequited love or the loss of
a parent to changes of the seasons and (ii) 'madness' can affect or compromise
certain functions while leaving others intact, even when the person is in an active
or acute phase. Introducing a distinction that is often thought to have originated
with Kraepelin a century later, Pinel first explains that there are at least two different

forms of 'madness'. He writes: 'Madness may be continuous during a large part of life or show long remissions, increase steadily, without interruption, or occur in regular or irregular attacks. This points to two kinds of madness: one continuous or chronic, the other intermittent' (cited in Weiner, 1992, p. 728). This discovery, or recognition, that at least some forms of 'madness' could be intermittent, with periods of long if not permanent remission, had its own important implications. As Weiner describes:

> As for periodic insanity, it was a new concept with profound implica-
> tions for therapy. If the patient was intermittently insane, then he or
> she was intermittently sane. Knowing this, the therapist could attempt
> to establish confidence and a good relationship with the sane part of
> the person and involve the patient in the therapeutic process. (Weiner,
> 1992, p. 727)

Were this Pinel's only insight into the nature of 'madness', it alone might have revolutionized practice. He went on, however, to suggest that even in the acute phase the reach or extent of the illness was rarely absolute or all-encompassing. Even behind the ravings of the 'lunatic' or beneath the mantle of despair of the 'melancholic', the vestiges of a person remained who could be reached through the ministrations of a caring doctor. He writes:

> The idea of madness should by no means imply a total abolition of the
> mental faculties. On the contrary, the disorder usually attacks only one
> partial faculty such as the perception of ideas, judgment, reasoning,
> imagination, memory, or psychologic sensitivity . . . A total upheaval
> of the rational faculty . . . is quite rare. (Cited in Weiner, 1992, p. 729)

As an example of this principle, he describes how the reasoning of many 'insane' individuals is easily understood and quite correct as long as one accepts the premises upon which their use of reasoning is based. While the premise itself may be faulty, the resulting reasoning may be quite sound, reflecting the preservation and persistence of this important human faculty. He writes:

> Errors of reasoning are much rarer among madmen than is commonly
> thought, for they derive reliable inductions from a particular sequence
> of ideas that preoccupies them. The white-haired 70-year-old still living
> at Bicêtre who believes that he is a young woman is in perfect agreement
> with himself when he obstinately refuses other than feminine clothing,
> adorns himself with care, is flattered by the polite behavior of the staff
> and their talk of his prospects of an approaching marriage, or when his
> modesty seems alarmed at the least indecent gesture. (Cited in Weiner,
> 1992, p. 729)

Such an appreciation of the humanity that remains at the heart of mental illness, and of the fact that mental illness remains an integral part and parcel of the human condition, is rarely found before or after Pinel within the confines of medicine. In fact, one would have to look to Shakespeare to find examples of equal sensitivity elsewhere.

2.2 Philippe Pinel and Jean-Baptise Pussin

So what did Pinel do with this exquisite sensitivity? As we noted above, when he first turned to medicine following his friend's onset of mental illness to see what could be done, he was dissatisfied with what he found, or did not find, there. As he notes in his 'Memoir on Madness': 'It is true that a person who seeks to acquire the right ideas and fixed principles about the psychologic treatment of madness hardly knows where to turn' (cited in Weiner, 1992, p. 730). This should not be taken to suggest, however, that Pinel created moral treatment out of nothing. Owing to the widespread influence of the Enlightenment, similar efforts to find more humane ways of treating asylum inmates were being made across Europe, particularly in Italy, Spain and Great Britain (England and Scotland). But, as Pinel complains, he could learn little from these efforts other than the fact that they were being made and were purported to be highly successful. His frustration over this state of affairs was directed mostly towards England – with whom France happened to be at war at the time – and which he accused of hiding its valuable 'secrets'. As he explains to the Society for Natural History:

> The rights of man are too little respected in Germany to make the study of their ways of handling the insane in public establishments worthwhile. Spain has taken only a few steps toward this great goal, as I showed a few years ago in a periodic publication: the inmates of a public asylum dedicated to their custody are managed with the greatest gentleness and assigned to regular work which has served to cure most of them. But it is mainly England one must envy for the artful wisdom of managing a large group of madmen and effecting the most unexpected cures. Why does that haughty and self-righteous nation spoil such a great gift to humanity by keeping a mysterious silence and guiltily casting a veil over its skills to restore distracted reason? The English proudly display the majestic sight and the internal arrangements of the asylums that Philosophy has dedicated to the unfortunate insane. But they keep the art of managing the insane a deep secret which they apparently want to control and keep from other peoples. I have therefore been restricted this first year to the slim resources of the preliminary studies I had done and to the observations I was making daily. (Cited in Weiner, 1992, p. 730)

The observations of which he speaks were those of day-to-day life within the Asylum at Bicêtre, the Paris hospital where he had just a year earlier been appointed as chief physician. It is at this asylum that Pinel is famously credited with removing the shackles from the 'mad' inmates and restoring their liberty as a path to ultimately restoring their reason, a dramatic scene depicted in oil paintings shortly thereafter and used widely as a symbol of the victorious values of the French Revolution. History, however, is not that simple; but it also is much more interesting.

Note that in the speech quoted above, given one year after he joined the Bicêtre as chief physician, Pinel describes relying on *preliminary studies* and making *observations*. He does not describe providing treatment, making interventions or effecting cures. That is because when he joined the staff of the Bicêtre it was out of interest rather than expertise. He was not made chief physician because he had actually treated people with mental illnesses successfully before, but rather because he wanted the opportunity to observe what was to him a new category of diseases about which little was known and for which there were few effective treatments. In most cases, the only measures that were instituted that were thought to have any therapeutic benefit at all were the popular somatic treatments of the day, including bloodletting and various forms of hydrotherapy (Woods and Carlson, 1961, p. 17). Far more common was the brutality, cruelty and punishment directed towards the inmates by the asylum staff, who were typically untrained and unskilled workers. These staff, who spent the majority of the time with the inmates, had the unenviable job of trying to keep order among the hordes and, when possible, to feed, clothe and occasionally bathe them. While Pinel had heard reports that British asylum superintendents were trying other approaches, these, as he remarked above, were kept secret or at least were not being described in any format to foreigners. He thus begins his *Treatise on Insanity* with the following complaint:

> Few subjects in medicine are so intimately connected with the history and philosophy of the human mind as insanity. There are still fewer, where there are so many errors to rectify, and so many prejudices to remove. Derangement of the understanding is generally considered as an effect of an organic lesion of the brain, consequently as incurable; a supposition that is, in a great number of instances, contrary to anatomical fact. Public asylums for maniacs have been regarded as places of confinement for such of its member as are become dangerous to the peace of society. The managers of those institutions, who are frequently men of little knowledge and less humanity, have been permitted to exercise toward their innocent prisoners a most arbitrary system of cruelty and violence; while experience affords ample and daily proofs of the happier effect of a mild, conciliating treatment, rendered effective by steady and dispassionate firmness. Availing themselves of this consideration, many empirics have erected establishments for the reception of lunatics, and have practiced this very delicate branch of the healing heart with singular reputation. A great number of cures have undoubtedly been effected by those base born children of the profession; but, as might be expected, they have not in any degree contributed to the advancement of science by any valuable writings . . .
> Thus, too generally, has the philosophy of this disease, by which I mean the history of its symptoms, of its progress, of its varieties, and of its

treatment in and out of hospitals, been most strangely neglected.
(Pinel, 1806, pp. 3–5)

How, then, was Pinel to know how to deliver 'mild, conciliating treatment, rendered effective by steady and dispassionate firmness'? Was there, in fact, anything to learn about the care of people considered 'mad'? Or was it simply a matter of removing their chains and treating them with kindness and respect? In this regard, Pinel considered himself to have been extremely fortunate to find at the Bicêtre both a governor and a governess of considerable knowledge, tact and skill. As he writes in the *Treatise on Insanity*:

> I am indebted to a fortunate concurrence of circumstances. Among these may be first enumerated, the eminent qualities, both of body and mind, of the governor of the Asylum de Bicêtre. He possesses the principles of a pure and enlightened philanthropy ... [By observing him] I then discovered, that insanity was curable in many instances, by mildness of treatment and attention to the state of the mind exclusively, and when coercion was indispensable, that it might be very effectually applied without corporal indignity ... My faith in pharmaceutic preparations was gradually lessened, and my skepticism went at length so far, as to induce me never to have recourse to them, until moral remedies had completely failed. (Pinel, 1806, pp. 108–109)

In addition to observing the behaviors of the governor and their effects on the inmates, one of the first things Pinel did when he arrived at the asylum was to ask the governor to give him an account of the population and to describe his approach to care. Specifically, he asked the following series of questions:

1 What is the number of insane patients admitted? Has the Revolution brought changes?

2 What is the incidence of mortality?

3 What therapy succeeds best?

4 Is work useful to patients?

5 Is bleeding helpful?

6 What diet should the insane receive?

7 Does the treatment administered at the Hospice of Humanity aid recovery?

8 What methods work best in dealing with insane patients?
(Cited in Weiner, 1979, p. 1129)

It is in response to these questions that we find the first written account of the removal of the shackles from the inmates at the Bicêtre and the first written description of the principles of what Pinel would come to call '*traitement moral*'. He appears to be both generous and sincere in crediting the approach of this governor, and later also of 'his esteemed wife', accordingly:

> The gentleman, to whom was committed the chief management of the hospital . . . was not deficient either in the knowledge or the execution of the duties of his office. He never lost sight of the principles of a most genuine philanthropy. He paid great attention to the diet of the house, and left no opportunity for murmur or discontent on the part of the most fastidious. He exercised a strict discipline over the conduct of the domestics, and punished, with severity, every instance of ill treatment, and every act of violence, of which they were guilty towards those whom it was merely their duty to serve. He was both esteemed and feared by every maniac; for he was mild, and at the same time inflexibly firm. In a word, he was master of every branch of his art, from its simplest to its most complicated principles. Thus was I introduced to a man, whose friendship was an invaluable acquisition to me. Our acquaintance matured into the closest intimacy. Our duties and inclinations concurred in the same object. Our conversation, which was almost exclusively professional, contributed to our mutual improvement. With those advantages, I devoted a great part of my time in examining for myself the various and numerous affections of the human mind in a state of disease. I regularly took notes of whatever appeared deserving of my attention . . . Such are the materials upon which my principles of moral treatment are founded. (Pinel, 1806, pp. 53–54)

The name of this governor was Jean-Baptiste Pussin, and it was he who actually first removed the shackles from the inmates of the Bicêtre and who, along with his courageous and ingenious wife, taught Pinel the basics of how to engage, manage and facilitate the recovery of 'madmen' and 'lunatics'. It was in response to question eight above that Pussin writes:

> I have tried so hard to improve the condition of these unfortunates that in the month of Prairial of the Year V I managed to eliminate their chains (used until then to contain the furious) and to replace them with straitjackets that permit freedom of movement and the enjoyment of all possible liberty without any added danger. (Cited in Weiner, 1979, p. 1133)

Pussin was to go well beyond the use of straitjackets as well, and to articulate fully several of the key principles of his humane approach, as we will see in the following section.

We dwell on this little-known fact of history not to detract from Pinel's importance or to diminish his contributions, which are considerable. Rather, we dwell on this fact because of the nature of the life experiences that prepared Pussin for this role and an even lesser-known aspect of his approach, that also was adopted by Pinel but mentioned only briefly in his *Treatise on Insanity*. Pussin was a tanner by trade and had no formal training in medicine or any other field that might have prepared him for being governor of an asylum (Weiner, 1979). What did prepare him for this role was that he had himself been an inmate at the Bicêtre in 1771 and had recovered fully. 'As often happened with former patients', explains Weiner, Pussin 'found employment at the hospital, first on the boys' ward and then, in 1784, as superintendent of the ward for incurable mental patients . . . That was where Pinel met Pussin in September 1793' (Weiner, 1979, p. 1128). Pussin had worked his way up through the hospital hierarchy to become governor of the asylum, and as one of his core strategies for managing the hospital and delivering effective care, he continued the tradition of hiring former and recovered inmates as staff. In fact, in response to Pinel's third question ('What therapy succeeds best?'), Pussin writes the following:

> 3. Moderate work and distraction are very favorable to the recovery of these unfortunates. I have often noticed that when I employed a madman who had just recovered his senses either to sweep or to assist a servant, and then to become himself a servant – I have noticed, I say, that his state improved every month, and that somewhat later he was totally cured. There are few instances where this method has not succeeded. Therefore, as much as possible, all servants are chosen from the category of mental patients. They are at any rate better suited to this demanding work because they are usually more gentle, honest, and humane. (Cited in Weiner, 1979, p. 1132)

It was not only Pussin who emphasized the importance of hiring former 'mental patients' as staff, but Pinel as well. In the following summary of the humane and effective treatment he witnessed at the Bicêtre, Pinel highlights this strategy of hiring convalescents to staff the hospital as the 'simple' but central method of the approach:

> In lunatic hospitals, as in despotic governments, it is no doubt possible to maintain, by unlimited confinement and barbarous treatment, the appearance of order and loyalty. The stillness of the grave, and the silence of death, however, are not to be expected in a residence consecrated for the reception of madmen. A degree of liberty, sufficient to maintain order, dictated not by weak but enlightened humanity, and calculated to spread a few charms ever the unhappy existence of maniacs, contributes, in most instances, to diminish the violence of the symptoms, and in some, to remove the complaint altogether. Such was the system which the governor of Bicêtre endeavoured to establish on his entrance upon the duties of his present office. Cruel treatment of every description, and in all departments of the institution, was unequivocally proscribed. No man was allowed to strike a maniac even in his own defence. No concessions however humble, nor complaints nor threats were allowed to interfere with the observance of this

law. The guilty was instantly dismissed from the service. It might be supposed, that to support a system of management so exceedingly rigorous, required no little sagacity and firmness. The method which he adopted for this purpose was simple, and I can vouch my own experience for its success. His servants were generally chosen from among the convalescents, who were allured to this kind of employment by the prospect of a little gain. Averse from active cruelty from the recollection of what they had themselves experienced; disposed to those of humanity and kindness from the value, which for the same reason, they could not fail to attach to them; habituated to obedience, and easy to be drilled into any tactics which the nature of the service might require, such men were peculiarly qualified for the situation. As that kind of life contributed to rescue them from the influence of sedentary habits, to dispel the gloom of solitary sadness, and to exercise their own faculties, its advantages to themselves are equally transparent and important. (Pinel, 1806, pp. 89–91)

Taken together, Pussin and Pinel offer many reasons to hire and value the contributions former patients can make to the functioning of the asylum. In addition to being 'gentle, honest and humane', former patients are less likely to abuse or mistreat the inmates and are more likely to respect them as fellow human beings, having been recently in the same shoes. Work is not only beneficial to the staff, but may be responsible to some degree for their recovery as well. We will return to this point below. In addition, former inmates do not fall prey to the social biases and prejudices against individuals who became afflicted, knowing personally that they have remained people of value and may even grow from the experience. Finally, perhaps owing to feelings of gratitude for the care they received, they were more likely and more willing to follow the instructions of the governor and governess, even in cases involving seemingly trivial issues which others, who had not been through the experience themselves, might not appreciate. We will find a similar strategy of hiring people in recovery and a sense of appreciation for these contributions in a later chapter, when we discuss the work of Harry Stack Sullivan. For the moment, though, we return to the broader topic of Pussin's and Pinel's *traitement moral*.

2.3 *Traitement moral*

Of what, then, did Pussin's and then Pinel's *traitement moral* consist, other than hiring staff from among the population of former or convalescing 'mental patients'? We have both in Pussin's answers to Pinel's questions and in Pinel's own descriptions of the sensitivity, skill and talents demonstrated by Pussin and his wife a wonderful collection of maxims and examples of what was eventually to become *traitement moral*. Since the content and tone of moral treatment as it was later developed and practised in England and the United States was to diverge considerably from these early roots in Paris, we will devote the next two sections to the descriptions and examples offered by Pussin and Pinel. In the sections which follow, we will then examine what became of this approach as it crossed first the English Channel and then the Atlantic Ocean.

We quote first from Pussin's responses to Pinel, as it will become evident as we proceed how much of Pussin's perspective and thinking is reflected in Pinel's writing. Once again, this is not to suggest that Pinel somehow plagiarized these ideas from someone else; Pinel is the first to acknowledge Pussin's generosity and his influence on Pinel's own thinking and practice. The fact that Pussin's central contributions to these historic developments have not been fully acknowledged or appreciated falls entirely on the shoulders of history rather than on any faults or failures of Pinel's. It is possibly due to the needs of an emerging medical speciality to emphasize and give credit to the investigations and innovations of physicians that the genius and discoveries of others who are perhaps less educated or well-trained have to be overlooked. We unfortunately will see this same tendency to ignore or overlook the contributions of non-physicians to the care and understanding of mental illnesses recur in the chapters which follow. For our own purposes, it is important to correct the record and counterbalance this tendency, as we will suggest several times throughout this volume that the first-hand experiences of individuals who have suffered from mental illnesses and recovered have been and remain invaluable in helping us to understand and develop more effective treatments for mental illness – at least as much as, if not in fact more so than, medical science.

We return to Pussin. Pussin considered most of the men in his care to be responsive to humane treatment and to have a good chance of recovery. In some cases, however, he found cure to be more difficult. This was typically true in cases of 'madness if caused by pride or by religion'. Even in these cases, however, he found work to play a constructive and useful role. In response to Pinel's fourth question ('Is work useful to patients?') Pussin thus writes that even in these cases:

> Work also seems to me the only means, if not of cure, at least of relief for those whose madness is caused by pride or by religion, and who have hitherto been considered as almost totally incurable ... I say that, since there is hardly any hope of cure after a number of years, the greatest service one could render these men is to give them work to do. Almost all of them are able to work and would do so gladly, if one could give them a little encouragement. Also their work would help to cover a part of the cost of their upkeep and somewhat lessen their unhappiness. (Cited in Weiner, 1979, p. 1132)

Pussin did not speculate as to the different categories or forms of madness, nor did he suggest why treatment worked for some as opposed to others. His role was rather to offer humane care, employment and sympathetic understanding and to encourage his inmates' efforts to recover. His wife, the governess, is described by Pinel to apply more ingenuity to engaging with some of the more challenging inmates and to experimenting with ways to persuade or cajole them out of their convictions to firmly held false beliefs (which would be considered today delusions). In retrospect, one could suggest that she was naively exploring various cognitive-behavioral interventions. It was left up to Pinel, though, to theorize about the possible psychological mechanisms underlying both symptoms and effective approaches to their management. In the particularly stubborn cases of 'insanity' due to pride or religion, which he found equally difficult to treat, he speculated that these particular forms of 'madness' offered their victims a too lofty and gratifying sense of purpose and identity to trade in for the lowly status of 'mental patient'. In a sensitive, respectful manner still lacking from most mental health settings today, he describes, for example, the case of a man who believed he was Louis XIV:

> The madman who believes he is Louis XIV and who often hands me Dispatches for the Governments of his provinces is so enchanted with his exalted power that his imagination holds on to it: he would make too great a sacrifice in stepping down from his imaginary throne. (Cited in Weiner, 1992, p. 729)

It is in his response to Pinel's eighth question ('What methods work best in dealing with insane patients?') that Pussin describes most fully his overall approach. His first emphasis is to deplore the treatment that was being received by most inmates in most asylums at the time, and to point out how such treatment only aggravates rather than ameliorates their 'madness'. Notable in the following passage is Pussin's recognition that inmates retained their memory and use of reasoning and his sympathetic tone in regard to the 'hapless heads of family' in his care, a tone which we may recall from Pinel's address to the Society for Natural History. He writes:

> Until now, and in most hospices, furious madmen have always been considered and treated like wild beasts. How long will such an insane and barbarous treatment be followed? How many hapless heads of family have been its victims! When it is so easy to find means of repression without harming people, as I shall tell shortly. Without any doubt, mistreatment angers the insane rather than calming them. Beatings may well tame them for the moment, but they will assuredly not forget. The memory of mistreatment leads the inmates to watch for the moment of vengeance as soon as the opportunity arises and when one expects it the least. What is more, while they are consumed by this thirst for vengeance, anything one might undertake for their cure is, if not harmful, at least absolutely useless. But, as I have already stated, one can use means of repression without mistreatment and even with appropriate tact. One can thereby avoid irritating them and thus induce them, in their lucid moments, to regard you as their benefactor and not as their enemy. (Cited in Weiner, 1979, p. 1133)

Current debates about the use of coercive measures in psychiatry would do well to consider Pussin's insights into the fact that even 'madmen' do not forget how they are treated, how their resentment and thirst for vengeance can render any potentially effective interventions useless and how beneficial it can be to both parties for practitioners to focus first on earning trust and demonstrating to their potential patients how they can be of use to them. Many of these lessons had to be re-learned beginning in the 1980s, when mental health and other social service staff were given the responsibility of conducting outreach to and connecting people to care who had become homeless (Cohen and Tsemberis, 1991; Interagency Council on the Homeless, 1991; Cohen and Marcos, 1992; Vaccaro *et al.*, 1992).

Pussin then goes on to describe his own approach and the steps he had to take to change the culture of the Bicêtre. Both the extent to which he had to go to achieve this degree of change (e.g. dismissing all the staff) and the consequences of doing so are impressive; superintendents of the remaining state hospitals currently operating in the United States would do well to consider these lessons. Writes Pussin:

> When, thirteen years ago, I was made supervisor of the insane at Bicêtre, I saw only men full of hatred and vengeance against all the administrative personnel around them. I almost fell victim to it myself when a priest, Citizen A, a strong and powerful man, grabbed me by the hair from behind and hit me several times on the head with the back of his breviary – so hard that I lost consciousness on the spot and, without the attendants who plucked me from his hands, I would unquestionably have perished.
>
> I held to the principle that in no case would I permit the insane to be beaten and I had formally declared my intentions in this respect. The attendants tried to rebel against me, saying that they were not safe and objecting that, if I myself was not spared, they were all the more exposed, etc. But, despite their clamors, I persisted in my resolve and, to reach my goal, I was forced to dismiss almost all of them in turn when they disobeyed. It is thus not without trouble that I realized my purpose, but I finally managed to achieve that the servants never beat any of the insane, even when victimized by their violence. I know that those who care for the insane run great risks, but I am also certain that the danger is less when gentleness rather than severity prevails.
>
> I have had as many as three hundred madmen under my supervision and many of them have always been violent and very dangerous, especially during the hot season. To control them I have never used anything but repressive measures without mistreatment, and I have never permitted that they be beaten in any way. And yet I have always managed not only to impress them but even to gain their confidence to such a point that they are the first to protect me. They even help maintain order and calm in their own midst and these regulations are so well observed that most of the time one does not seem surrounded by madmen. Strangers have often told me of their surprise. It is true that very active supervision is required to achieve this. (Cited in Weiner, 1992, p. 1133)

In the following, final, passage from Pussin the attentive reader will notice again his description of the inmates as 'unfortunates', his suggestion that everyone is vulnerable to mental illness and his suggestion to Pinel that this 'class of men' (i.e. 'madmen') is 'most worthy of attention' given that their 'sensitivity is the cause of their illness' – all themes that again are reflected in Pinel's address to the Society for Natural History. Writes Pussin:

> This class of men which has until now been virtually abandoned is nevertheless most worthy of attention since their sensitivity is the cause of their illness. If one seeks upright men, it is among these that a large number can be found. And, in any case, who can flatter himself to have spent his life without any misfortune and without fear of a similar fate? What government can provide protection against it?
>
> My experience has shown, and shows daily, that to further the cure of these unfortunates one must treat them with as much kindness as possible, dominate them without mistreatment, gain their confidence, fight the cause of their illness, and make them envision a happier future. I have always fought this illness by psychological means and thus known the happiness of some favorable results. Yet I am far from denying the usefulness of physical treatments. On the contrary, I believe them to be very advantageous, even urgent, when they are adequately supervised. Work, among other things, seems to me almost necessary, not only because it provides for exercise but also because it offers distraction. Work, in fact, belongs to the category of psychological remedies on which I especially insist. (Cited in Weiner, 1992, p. 1133)

2.4 Pinel's psychological interventions

In his *Treatise on Insanity*, published a few years after Pussin's letter, Pinel would agree with all of Pussin's recommendations and then go on to introduce, via explanations and case examples, a few of his own. While he drew most heavily from his observations of Pussin and his wife, Pinel also incorporated his knowledge of other reports from abroad and, as we showed above, began to develop theories as to the curative effects of these new psychological treatments. In terms of work, for example, he agreed wholeheartedly with Pussin's insistence on employing inmates in productive activities and derived further confirmation for the central importance of work from reports from northern Scotland. He writes:

> We are informed by Dr. Gregory, that a farmer, in the North of Scotland, a man of Herculean stature, acquired great fame in that district of the British empire, by his success in the cure of insanity. The great secret of his practice consisted in giving full employment to the remaining faculties of the lunatic. With that view, he compelled all his patients to work on his farm. He varied their occupations, divided

their labour, and assigned to each, the post which he was best qualified to fill. (Pinel, 1806, p. 64)

It is worth noting that this farmer did not simply force his patients to work the farm, as would become standard practice in many state hospitals a few generations later. Rather, assigning to each person the post 'he was best qualified to fill' required getting to know each person as a unique individual with 'remaining faculties' and finding work that matched each person's interests and skills. Pinel developed this approach still further, and described how it might unfold over a longer period, providing a kind of bridge from active mental illness through convalescence to full recovery. Writes Pinel:

> Convalescent maniacs, when, amidst the languors of an inactive life, a stimulus is offered to their natural propensity to motion and exercise, are active, diligent, and methodical . . . The first ray of returning talent ought to be seized with great avidity by the governor, and tenderly fostered, with a view of favouring and accelerating the development of mental faculties . . . The return of convalescents to their primitive tastes, pursuits, and habits, has always been by me considered as a happy omen of their final complete re-establishment. To discover those promising inclinations, a physician can never be too vigilant; nor to encourage them, too studious of the means of indulgence. (Pinel, 1806, pp. 193, 196, 217)

Based on his, and others', experiences with this approach, Pinel draws the following conclusion:

> It is no longer a problem to be solved, but the result of the most constant and unanimous experience, that in all public asylums as well as in prisons and hospitals, the surest, and, perhaps, the only method of securing health, good order, and good manners, is to carry into decided and habitual execution the natural law of bodily labour, so contributive and essential to human happiness. This truth is especially applicable to lunatic asylums: and I am convinced that no useful and durable establishments of that kind can be founded excepting on the basis of interesting and laborious employment. (Pinel, 1806, p. 216)

Being vigilant in discovering a person's 'promising inclinations' and then systematically exploring ways for the person to pursue those inclinations and re-establish his or her habits as central aspects of convalescence and recovery are themes to which we will return in Chapter 7 when we suggest directions for future rehabilitative practice. This represents only one strand, albeit an important one, of what we think a future psychiatry – one which finally lives up to Pinel's ideals – will look like.

In addition to 'accelerating the development of mental faculties', Pinel suggests that there are at least two other significant benefits to engaging inmates in 'interesting and laborious employment'. The first of these is to restore hope, offer meaningful alternatives to empty time spent dwelling on one's problems and encourage people to 'look forward to better days'. The second is that the person is able to secure some disposable income, no matter how trivial, which also picks up his or her spirit or countenance. These two related elements of *traitement moral* are identified as key therapeutic factors in the following case described at length by Pinel:

> A young man, already depressed by misfortune, lost his father, and in a few months after a mother, whom he tenderly loved. The consequence was, that he sunk into a profound melancholy; and his sleep and appetite forsook him. To these symptoms succeeded a most violent paroxysm of insanity. At a lunatic hospital, whither he was conveyed, he was treated in the usual way, by copious and repeated blood-letting, water and shower baths, low diet, and a rigorous system of coercion. Little or no change appeared in the state of the symptoms. The same routine was repeated, and even tried a third time without success, or rather with an exasperation of the symptoms.
>
> He was at length transferred to the Asylum de Bicêtre, and with him the character of a dangerous maniac. The governor, far from placing implicit confidence in the accuracy of this report, allowed him to remain at liberty in his own apartment, in order more effectually to study his character and the nature of his derangement. The sombrous taciturnity of this young man, his great depression, his pensive air, together with some broken sentences which were heard to escape him on the subject of his misfortunes, afforded some insight into the nature of his insanity. The treatment most suitable to his case was evidently to console him, to sympathize with his misfortunes, and, after having gradually obtained his esteem and confidence, to dwell upon such circumstances as were calculated to cheer his prospects and to encourage his hopes.
>
> These means having been tried with some success, a circumstance happened which appeared at once to give countenance and efficiency to the consolatory conversations of the governor. His guardian, with a view to make his life more comfortable, now thought proper to make small remittances for his use, which he promised to repeat monthly. The first payment dispelled, in great measure, his melancholy, and encouraged him to look forward to better days. At length, he gradually recovered his strength. The signs of general health appeared in his countenance. His bodily functions were performed with regularity, and reason resumed her empire over his mind. His esteem for the governor was unbounded. This patient, who had been so egregiously ill treated in another hospital, and consequently delivered to that of Bicêtre as a furious and dangerous maniac, is now become not only very manageable, but, from his affectionate disposition and sensibility, a very interesting young man'. (Pinel, 1806, pp. 101–102)

So convinced was Pinel of the therapeutic benefits of *traitement moral* that he insisted that people afflicted with 'madness' be placed in an asylum based on these principles not only for the safety and convenience of the community but also for the person's own welfare as well. That is, he insisted that 'madness' could not be cured through other means and that people had to be extracted from their usual everyday lives and family in order to receive therapeutic care. He not only tried to make the most of the asylum experience he had taken on but also concluded from that experience that the life situation from which the patient had come had had at least a hand in causing the illness to begin with and would continue to exert a deleterious effect as long as the person remained there. He asserts:

> It is found by experience, that maniacs are seldom or never cured as long as they are kept at home, subject to the influence of family intercourse ... Insanity is much more certainly and effectually cured in places adapted for their reception and treatment, than at home amidst the various influences of family interests. (Pinel, 1806, pp. 212–214)

On this score, Pinel does not speculate further. While he argues that psychological, rather than physical, treatments are effective, and that mental illness often occurs in response to social or environmental events, he does not offer detailed theories that would account for either the aetiology or the cure of mental illness. What he has done, nonetheless, is to leave a legacy in which mental illnesses are understood to be illnesses that affect ordinary and extraordinary human beings and that are, for the most part, curable given the appropriate care and resources. The care and resources required involve removing the person from his or her present social environment, offering safe and dignified respite from these circumstances, engaging the person's mental faculties and offering the person hope that life can improve along with perhaps glimpses into what such a better life might be like. Most of these treatments are psychological and social in nature, but have very real and enduring effects on the person and the illness. What remains to be determined is the mechanism through which these salutary effects are derived.

Before turning to theories offered to account for such effects, we close this section with a final passage from Pinel which summarizes his perspective. At its most simple, he characterizes *traitement moral* as based on the decision 'to govern by wisdom rather than to subdue by terror' (Pinel, 1806, p. 207). This distinction he elaborates more fully as follows:

> In all cases of excessive excitement of the passions, a method of treatment, simple enough in its application, but highly calculated to render the disease incurable, has been adopted from time immemorial: – that of abandoning the patient to his melancholy fate, as an untameable being, to be immured in solitary durance, loaded with chains, or otherwise treated with extreme severity, until the natural close of a life so wretched shall rescue him from his misery, and convey him from the cells of the madhouse to the chambers of the grave. But this treatment convenient indeed to a governor, more remarkable for his indolence

and ignorance than for his prudence or humanity, deserves, at the present day, to be held up to public execration, and classed with the other prejudices which have degraded the character and pretensions of the human species.

To allow every maniac all the latitude of personal liberty consistent with safety; to proportion the degree of coercion to the demands upon it from his extravagance of behaviour; to use mildness of manners or firmness as occasion may require, – the bland arts of conciliation, or the tone of irresistible authority pronouncing an irreversible mandate, and to proscribe, most absolutely, all violence and ill treatment on the part of the domestics, are laws of fundamental importance, and essential to the prudent and successful management of all lunatic institutions ... Experience has uniformly attested the superiority of this method of managing the insane. (Pinel, 1806, pp. 82–83, 218)

2.5 The Retreat at York

There is much analogy between the judicious treatment of children, and that of insane persons. (Tuke, 1813, p. 150)

The motives, the influences, and, as a general rule, the means necessary for the good government of children, are equally applicable, and equally efficient for the insane. (Pliny Earle, Superintendent of Bloomingdale Hospital, 1845, cited in Bockoven, 1956, p. 300)

We consider it an understatement to suggest that moral treatment underwent a profound transformation when it crossed the Channel and then the Atlantic Ocean. The quotes above from Samuel Tuke of the York Retreat and Pliny Earle, one of the leading American psychiatrists of the second half of the nineteenth century, give some glimpse into the nature of this transformation. While developed at almost the same time, and while crediting Pinel and his work at the Bicêtre with the first articulation of what they came to call moral treatment, the British developed an approach to managing their 'retreats' which differed significantly from that of Pussin and Pinel. How much of this difference was due to the differences between the two countries in terms of their culture, religion, politics and morality, how much was due to Pinel's medical training and perspective and how much was due to other influences is not clear. As the reader will see in this section, however, the result, even prior to being exported to the United States, was based on different assumptions, implemented through different means and most likely produced different effects.

The discontinuity between the two is to such an extent that we suggest that 'traitement moral' should no longer be equated with 'moral treatment'. Weiner's caution that the French term did not contain the moralistic connotations of the English translation gave us an initial clue. Recognizing these differences, Borthwick and her colleagues at the Retreat suggest that Tuke borrowed Pinel's terminology, not because their approaches were so similar, but rather as a way 'to justify, explain and publicize the methods at The Retreat' (Borthwick *et al.*, 2001, p. 429). Reference to Pinel was to give the work of the Retreat credibility. In this section, we will describe in some depth the degrees to which Pinel's original vision informed the work of the Retreat and to which the Retreat charted an alternative path in the century following publication of the *Treatise on Insanity*.

We recall that Pinel first turned to 'madness' and its cure when he lost a good friend to mental illness. In this respect, the work of the Tukes in England began in a similar fashion, only in this case it was the loss of a member of their Quaker community. Samuel Tuke, the grandson of William Tuke – the man who was credited with founding the York Retreat as the first moral treatment asylum in England – gives the following account in his 1813 *Description of the Retreat, An Institution near York for Insane Persons of the Society of Friends*:

> The origin of the Institution which forms the subject of the following pages, has much the appearance of accident. In the year 1791, a female, of the Society of Friends, was placed at an establishment for insane persons, in the vicinity of the City of York; and her family, residing at a considerable distance, requested some of their acquaintance in the City to visit her. The visits of these friends was refused, on the ground of the patient not being in a suitable state to be seen by strangers: and, in a few weeks after her admission, death put a period to her sufferings.
>
> The circumstance was affecting, and naturally excited reflections on the situation of insane persons, and on the probable improvements which might be adopted in establishments of this nature. In particular, it was conceived that peculiar advantage would be derived to the Society of Friends, by having an Institution of this kind under their own care, in which a milder and more appropriate system of treatment, than that usually practiced, might be adopted; and where, during lucid intervals, or the state of convalescence, the patient might enjoy the society of those who were of similar habits and opinions. It was thought, very justly, that the indiscriminate mixture, which must occur in large public establishments, of persons of opposite religious sentiments and practices; of the profligate and the virtuous, the profane and the serious; was calculated to check the progress of returning reason, and to fix, still deeper, the melancholic and misanthropic train of ideas, which, in some descriptions of insanity, impresses the mind. It was believed also, that the general treatment of insane persons was, too frequently, calculated to depress and degrade, rather than to awaken the slumbering reason, or correct its wild hallucinations. (Tuke, 1813, pp. 22–23)

Several aspects of this passage are worthy of note and already indicate divergences in tone and perspective from those of Pinel. The Quakers in general, and the Tukes in particular, were in agreement with Pinel that the usual 'treatment' and care that was being provided to the 'insane' at the time was harsh and cruel and more likely exacerbated rather than cured the illness. They were in agreement also that better, more humane methods could be developed and implemented that would have a better chance of promoting recovery. But in contrast to Pinel's sympathy for those who we should consider 'unfortunate', and who may suffer from an over-abundance of sensitivity and other highly valued human attributes, it is difficult not to be taken aback by the moralistic tone that permeates this passage (e.g. 'the profligate and the virtuous, the profane and the serious'). Tuke's suggestions that the 'indiscriminate mixture ... of persons of opposite religious sentiments and opinions' likewise exacerbates the person's condition and slows the return of reason, while enjoying the company 'of those who were of similar habits and opinions' was thought to speed recovery are also to be questioned. The discrimination and marginalization that the Quakers had experienced in the prior century may help somewhat to account for this desire to keep people of different religious faiths apart. But it quickly becomes apparent as one reads Tuke's *Description* that these are not isolated comments but also suggest a religious and moralistic understanding of the nature of 'insanity' itself.

Note, for example, that Tuke speaks of awakening 'slumbering reason' and 'correcting' its hallucinations. For the Tukes and their followers, 'madness' was to be equated with the loss of reason and recovery with its rediscovery or restoration. In continuing his justification for why the Society of Friends chose to build its own retreat, Samuel Tuke explains:

> There also has been occasion to observe the great loss, which individuals of our Society have sustained, by being put under the care of those, who are not only strangers to our principles; but by whom they are frequently mixed with other patients, who may indulge themselves in ill language, and other exceptionable practices. This often seems to leave an unprofitable effect upon the patients' minds, after they are restored to the use of their reason, alienating from those religious attachments which they had before experienced; and sometimes even corrupting them with vicious habits, to which they had been strangers. (Tuke, 1813, p. 50)

The mission of the Retreat appears to be to restore people 'to the use of their reason'. Contrast this statement to Pinel's treatment of the 'white-haired 70-year-old' man who thought he was an attractive young woman and who was 'in perfect agreement' with himself (i.e. being perfectly rational) by being willing only to wear women's clothing. For Pinel, the faculty of reason was only one faculty among many, and he was convinced that 'errors of reasoning are much rarer among madmen than is commonly thought'. The Tukes, however, speak of the 'perversion' of reason and the need for it to be 'corrected'. While they agreed with Pinel that only one faculty may be impaired at a time, the impairment in that faculty, regardless of its nature, was to be understood as its loss or perversion of reason. Tuke writes:

> Insane persons generally possess a degree of control over their wayward propensities. Their intellectual, active, and moral powers, are usually rather perverted than obliterated; and it happens, not unfrequently, that one faculty only is affected. The disorder is sometimes still

more partial, and can only be detected by erroneous views, on one particular subject. On all others, the mind appears to retain its wonted correctness ... The same *partial* perversion, is found to obtain in this disease with regard to the affections. (Tuke, 1813, pp. 133–134; italics in the original)

We appear no longer to be dealing with illnesses of the mental faculties analogous to physical illnesses, illnesses to which we are all susceptible, illnesses which affect only some faculties and leave others intact, and illnesses to which those of us who are the most sensitive, artistic or creative may be the most susceptible. Rather, we are dealing with perversions of reason, 'erroneous views' and 'wayward propensities', which it is our obligation to correct. Even though both Pinel and William Tuke credit John Locke with providing inspiration for their ideas, it appears that at least Pinel's concept of 'insanity' as an illness, and the preservation of reason even during bouts of 'insanity', was not shared by Tuke. This had profound implications for the nature of the treatments and care provided to address these different forms of 'madness'.

How did the Tukes envision 'correcting' the 'erroneous views' and 'perverted reason' of their charges? Given the fact that 'insanity' was no longer considered an illness by the Tukes, it is not surprising that the Retreat eschewed all somatic treatments, with the exception of warm baths. While Tuke devotes one chapter of his *Description* to medical treatments, he begins this chapter with the following preface:

> The experience of the Retreat, if it should contribute in some degree to the improvement, will not add much to the honour of extent of medical science. I regret that it will be the business of the present chapter, to relate the pharmaceutic means which have failed, rather than to record those which have succeeded. (Tuke, 1813, p. 110)

Medicine, Tuke concludes, 'as yet, possesses very inadequate means to relieve the most grievous of human diseases' (Tuke, 1813, p. 111). This passage suggests that the Tukes initially might have considered 'insanity' a disease, and indeed the first years of the Retreat saw experiments with various medications and other somatic therapies. After a few years, however, they came to recognize that the most medicine had to offer was temporary relief from some of the symptoms of the disease, but that it could not effect a cure or recovery. It was left to 'management' and moral treatment to pick up where the somatic therapies failed. In this respect, Samuel Tuke felt that they were in complete agreement with the approach of Pinel, as he writes:

> In the present imperfect state of our knowledge, of the very interesting branch of the healing art, which relates to the cure of insanity; and unable as we generally are to ascertain its true seat in the complicated labyrinths of our frame, the judicious physician is frequently obliged

to apply his means, chiefly to the alleviation and suppression of symptoms.

Experience, however, has happily shown, in the Institution whose practices we are attempting to describe, that much may be done towards the cure and alleviation of insanity, by judicious modes of management, and by moral treatment. The superintendent . . . fully unites with the intelligent Dr. Pinel, in his comparative estimate of moral and medical means. (Tuke, 1813, p. 132)

2.6 Moral treatment or moral management?

To this point, we appear to have agreement as to what does not work well in addressing mental illness and as to the important role of moral treatment. But it is interesting, and not an accident, that Tuke mentions 'management' first and moral treatment only secondarily. This otherwise trivial point underscores the difference in how the British came to view the role of moral treatment in contrast to how it was understood by the French. For the French, in part because of Pinel's background and status as a physician, *traitement moral* was primarily a form of treatment, a non-physical form of treatment, but a form of treatment nonetheless. For the Tukes and their followers, we suggest that moral treatment was viewed as, and came almost entirely to be, a form of management. Although Tuke's early *Description*, which is clearly influenced by Pinel, retains the language of disease and disorder, there is little else in this book, or in the many descriptions of moral treatment which followed, that addresses mental illnesses as illnesses or that frames moral treatment as a treatment.

This shift becomes evident as soon as one looks to how Tuke conceptualized and then described moral treatment, to which he devotes the second section of his *Description*. This section he divides into the following three components of which moral treatment is thought to consist. They are:

1 By what means the power of the patient to control the disorder, is strengthened and assisted.

2 What modes of coercion are employed, when restraint is absolutely necessary.

3 By what means the general comfort of the insane is promoted
(Tuke, 1813, p. 138)

The majority of description and discussion is devoted to the first component, as this is the central focus of moral treatment: to help the patient to develop better self-control. While again it is here framed in terms of controlling the disorder, this concept comes to encompass anything that may challenge or undermine the patient's possession and use of reason. Therefore controlling the disorder is also referred to as 'self-control' or 'self-restraint', just as moral treatment is referred to also as 'moral management'. In fact, the title of the section of the text where he addresses the first component above is entitled: 'Of the means of assisting the patient to control himself' (Tuke, 1813, p. 139). The following passage offers additional examples of this shift in language, along with the suggestion that religion, in particular, may be useful in combating the 'disorder' and restoring reason. Writes Tuke:

> Hitherto we have chiefly considered those modes of inducing the patient to control his disordered propensities, which arrive from an application to the general powers of the mind; but considerable advantage may certainly be derived, in this part of moral management, from an acquaintance with the previous habits, manners, and prejudices of the individual. Nor must we forget to call to our aid, in endeavouring to promote self-restraint, the mild but powerful influence of our holy religion. Where these have been strongly imbued in early life, they become little less than principles of our nature; and their restraining power is frequently felt, even under the delirious excitement of insanity. To encourage the influences of religious principles over the mind of the insane, is considered of great consequence, as a means of cure. For this purpose, as well as for others still more important, it is certainly right to promote in the patient, an attention to his accustomed modes of paying homage to his Maker. (Tuke, 1813, pp. 160–161)

In addition to the influence of religion, Tuke identifies two principles for the management of the Retreat and its inhabitants to which one can appeal in inducing the patient to regain control of his or her disordered propensities, promote self-restraint and reawaken reason. The first of these is fear. 'The principle of fear, which is rarely decreased by insanity', writes Tuke, 'is considered as of greatest importance in the management of the patients' (Tuke, 1813, p. 141). Given that the second and third components mentioned above involve using restraint only when necessary and promoting the general comfort of the patient, we should not conclude from Tuke's willingness to use fear that he argued for perpetuating the cruelty and brutality found in other asylums at the time. He did not. His approach, that is the approach of his grandfather, was based on humane and kind treatment, and did emphasize both offering as comfortable and warm a home-like environment as possible and avoiding the use of restraint except as a last resort. Based in part on Pinel's experience and in part on their own religious principles, the Quakers suggested that these measures could be taken to ensure proper management of the Retreat because 'the insane' were not, as a population, considered or expected to be violent. Inmates of other asylums might behave violently, but that was only because they themselves had been treated violently by the staff. We can recall here Pussin's observation that it is 'the memory of [their] mistreatment [that] leads the inmates to watch for the moment of vengeance'.

Aware of the popular perception of 'the insane' as dangerous, and of other asylums' pre-occupations with decreasing risk, Tuke suggested that these concerns were misplaced. He writes:

> Many errors in the construction, as well as in the management of asylums for the insane, appear to arise from excessive attention

to *safety*. People, in general, have the most erroneous notions of the constantly outrageous behaviour, or malicious dispositions, of deranged persons; and it has, in too many instances, been found convenient to encourage these false sentiments, to apologize for the treatment of the unhappy sufferers, or admit the vicious neglect of their attendants.

In the construction of such places, cure and comfort ought to be as much considered, as security; and, I have no hesitation in declaring, that a system which, by limiting the power of the attendant, obliges him not to neglect his duty, and makes it his interest to obtain the good opinion of those under his care, provides more effectually for the safety of the keeper, as well as of the patient, than all the apparatus of chains, darkness, and anodynes. (Tuke, 1813, pp. 106–107; italics in the original)

In other words, it is better to treat 'deranged persons' kindly and solicitously, and to earn their trust and admiration, than to try to beat, punish or torture them into submission. In this spirit, Tuke quotes from Haslam, the esteemed superintendent of the Bethlehem Hospital, who remarked that: 'I can truly declare, that by gentleness of manner, and kindness of treatment, I have seldom failed to obtain the confidence, and conciliate the esteem, of insane persons; and have succeeded by these means in procuring from them respect and obedience' (Tuke, 1813, pp. 134–135). He then goes on to assert that the superintendents of the Retreat 'give precisely the same evidence', concluding accordingly:

I firmly believe, that a large majority of the instances, in which the malevolent dispositions are peculiarly apparent, and are considered as characterizing the disorder, may readily be traced to secondary causes; arising from the peculiar circumstances of the patient, or from the mode of management. (Tuke, 1813, p. 135)

If patients treated in the Retreat are not in general prone to violence owing to their disorder, and if the mode of management utilized by the staff of the Retreat does not generate a secondary kind of disorder manifesting as violence, why, then, is fear to be the first principle of treatment? What function, other than containing the behavior of 'deranged persons', then, was to be served by promoting fear? The Tukes' use of fear was meant more to inculcate in the patients the proper or correct way to behave, to ensure their 'obedience', than to contain their dangerous behavior. Avoidance of the use of restraint should thus not be taken to suggest that coercion was not to be used at the Retreat. Rather, coercion becomes, in fact, the primary tool of management. It is just that it is a more sophisticated and humane form of coercion in which the superintendent and staff attempt to shape the person's behavior, instilling ever greater degrees of self-control and self-restraint, until the person has been restored to his or her rightful ('correct') use of reason. As Tuke succinctly expresses this overarching foundation for moral management, the patients 'quickly perceive, or if not, they are informed on the first occasion, that their treatment depends, in great measure, upon their conduct' (Tuke, 1813, p. 141).

The first principle of fear (the proverbial 'stick') thus is complemented quite naturally by a second principle, which is that of providing incentives (the 'carrots') for good or desired behavior. The more Tuke writes of this second principle, the more evident it becomes that the main mission of the Retreat had shifted from providing treatments for an illness to a person who has unfortunately fallen ill to correcting the problematic behavior of a morally deficient person who lacks the appropriate degree of self-control. The following passage conveys this shift well:

> In an early part of this chapter, it is stated, that the patients are considered capable of rational and honourable inducement; and though we allowed *fear* a considerable place in the production of that restraint, which the patient generally exerts on his entrance into a new situation; yet the *desire of esteem* is considered, at The Retreat, as operating, in general, still more powerfully. This principle in the human mind, which doubtless influences, in a great degree, though often secretly, our general manners; and which operates with peculiar force on our introduction into a new circle of acquaintance, is found to have great influence, even over the conduct of the insane. Though it has obviously not been sufficiently powerful, to enable them entirely to resist the strong irregular tendencies of their disease; yet when properly cultivated, it leads many to struggle to conceal and overcome their morbid propensities; and, at least, materially assists them in confining their deviations, within such bounds, as do not make them obnoxious to the family. (Tuke, 1813, p. 157; italics in the original)

The patients at the Retreat were to be taught to overcome or at least conceal their perverted propensities so that they would no longer be considered 'obnoxious' to their families. At that point, we might imagine, they could be returned to their families and considered 'recovered' from their disorders.

If this approach is beginning to sound parental, as well as moralistic, to the reader, then he or she is on the right track. The Tukes, and even more so the superintendents of other retreats who followed them, spoke increasingly of the role of superintendent as that of a benevolent but firm parent and the role of the patient as that of the wayward child needing correction and the instillation of discipline. It is for this reason that we opened the previous section with the two quotations from Tuke and Pliny Earle. While Tuke considered there to be 'much analogy between the judicious treatment of children, and that of insane persons', the analogous nature of this relationship disappears to be replaced by one of equivalence for Earle, who argues that 'the means necessary for the good government of children, are equally applicable, and equally efficient for the insane' (Pliny Earle, Superintendent of Bloomingdale Hospital, 1845, cited in Bockoven, 1956, p. 300). So blatant was this application of a paternalistic model to the moral management of the Retreat that it was not at all lost on the patients themselves. Without the least sense of irony or appreciation for how this may be considered objectionable to patients, Tuke observes that: 'Hence it has been frequently remarked by the patients at The Retreat, that a stranger who has visited them, seemed to imagine they were children' (Tuke, 1813, p. 159).

2.7 From treatment to education

> Institutions for the care and cure of those affected by mental disorders will be made to resemble those for education, rather than hospitals for the sick ... and when we call to mind that the greater part of those committed to such establishments are not actually sick, and do not require medical treatment, but are suffering from deranged intellect, feelings and passions, it is evident that a judicious course of mental and moral discipline is most essential for their comfort and restoration. (Amiriah Brigham, 1847; cited in Bockoven, 1956, pp. 301–302)

The same people whom Pinel described as 'very talented persons' whose mental illness 'derives only from a vivid sensitivity and from psychological qualities that we value highly' have now been transformed into misbehaved children whose 'perverse propensities' are found to be 'obnoxious' to their families. As we noted above, such a transformation in how 'madness' and 'mad' people are viewed leads to substantially different approaches in terms of how they are managed and, to the degree that any therapeutic mission lingers, treated. Before describing these different approaches, it is worth noting that the Tukes did retain or confirm some of Pussin's and Pinel's strategies for recovery, even though at times they understood these strategies and their mechanisms of influence in very different terms. The two strategies they retained were those of identifying and building on the patient's individual strengths and the value of engaging in work whenever and to whatever degree was considered possible at the time.

Let us take the example of work first. For Pussin and Pinel, many functions were served by engaging their patients in employment. Some of these benefited the hospital, such as the labor involved in taking care of the facility and its grounds, in preparing and serving meals and so on. But all of the work was to be consistent with a patient's personal interests and talents, was to appeal to the patient's sensibility and, most importantly, was to benefit the patient and his or her recovery. The therapeutic mechanism was not fully described, but was characterized first as eliciting, building on and exercising those faculties of the patient that were involved in the activity. If these were faculties that had remained relatively intact, then only good could come from their deployment as a way of expanding the healthy arenas and activities in the person's life. If the faculty were one that had been impaired, then engaging that faculty by eliciting the person's interest in a meaningful or pleasurable activity would begin to repair and enhance its use. For Pussin, meaningful work was considered the primary route to cure, and for Pinel effective hospitals could only be 'founded on the basis of interesting and laborious employment'.

How was this same activity viewed by the Tukes? Samuel Tuke agreed with Pinel that work provided the most effective route to cure, but he explains the primary function of work as follows: 'Of all the modes by which the patients may be induced to restrain themselves, regular employment is perhaps the most generally efficacious' (Tuke, 1813, p. 156). Employment is most highly valued as a way to promote self-restraint. Why is this? Because, as Tuke continues: 'As indolence has a natural tendency to weaken the mind, and to induce ennui and discontent, every kind of rational and innocent employment is encouraged' (Tuke, 1813, pp. 180–181). Rather than building up the person's faculties and strengths from the inside, so to speak, based on his or her interests, employment is a way to rescue the person from his or her indolence, a state which we must assume preceded his or her entrance into the asylum and might even have caused it. It was therefore important that this perverse propensity also be corrected, along with all the others that were part and parcel of the disorder, for reason to be rightfully reinstated. The other function that might be served by employment was to distract the person from his or her morbid thoughts and to prevent his or her 'indulgence of gloomy sensations'. Writes Tuke:

> In describing the particular benefits of this undertaking, it seems proper to mention that of occasionally using the patients to such employment, as may be suitable and proper for them, in order to relieve the languor of idleness, and prevent the indulgence of gloomy sensations. (Tuke, 1813, p. 51)

While the Tukes appeared to consider themselves the experts in which types of work would be considered 'suitable and proper' for whom, they did attempt to identify and build on a person's unique interests and strengths as well. The point of doing so, however, was not to enhance these strengths for their own sake but rather to allow them 'to display their knowledge to the greatest advantage'. This is consistent with the second major principle of moral treatment being the 'desire of esteem', as noted above. That is, patients were encouraged to display their knowledge or provide useful service to the Retreat in order to gain the esteem of others, most importantly of the superintendent and attendants. Writes Tuke:

> It is probably from encouraging the action of this principle, that so much advantage has been found in this Institution, from treating the patient as much in the manner of a rational being, as the state of his mind will possibly allow. The superintendent is particularly attentive to this point, in his conversation with the patients. He introduces such topics as he knows will most interest them; and which, at the same time, allows them to display their knowledge to the greatest advantage. If the patient is an agriculturist, he asks him questions relative to his art; and frequently consults him upon any occasion in which his knowledge may be useful. I have heard of one of the worst patients in the house who, previously to his indisposition, had been a considerable

grazier, give very sensible directions for the treatment of a diseased
cow. (Tuke, 1813, pp. 158–159)

Using those remaining faculties that have not been perverted by the disorder
is considered of the greatest importance not because the faculties themselves can
be useful in compensating for or overcoming the disorder but because the esteem
the patient derives from others who observe his or her useful behavior will lead
the patient to want to continue to behave in ways that will continue to generate
their esteem. In other words, getting a taste for how good it feels to be valued and
esteemed by others, to feel oneself to be 'of some consequence', intensifies the desire
for more of the same. As a result, the person eventually will act more in accordance
with good manners and etiquette so as not to lose the esteem he or she has now
gained. Instilling a taste for the approval of others and helping the patient to secure
at least a modicum of esteem that he or she will not want to lose not only facilitates
the proper management and smooth functioning of the Retreat but also constitutes
a 'cure' of the disorder. Writes Tuke:

> These considerations are undoubtedly very material, as they regard
> the comfort of insane persons; but they are of far greater importance,
> as they relate to the cure of the disorder. The patient feeling himself
> of some consequence, is induced to support it by the exertion of his
> reason, and by restraining those dispositions, which, if indulged, would
> lessen the respectful treatment he receives; or lower his character in
> the eyes of his companions and attendants. (Tuke, 1813, p. 159)

Here end the parallels between the modes of management of the Retreat and those
of the Bicêtre. The remaining strategies employed by the Tukes have as their aim the
cultivation of the religious, intellectual and moral capacities of the person so as to
encourage and assist him or her in regaining self-control or exercising self-restraint
in the face of the lower, less desirable, human qualities. We have already noted the
importance accorded to religion in the life of the Retreat, a component we might
not find surprising given that it was established by the Society of Friends. It was not
only that attendance at weekly religious services was promoted as an expected part
of everyday life, though, but also that adherence to Quaker values and principles in
one's behavior was promoted directly by the superintendent and staff. While 'many
patients attend the religious meetings of the Society', notes Tuke, 'most of them are
assembled, on a first day afternoon, at which time the superintendent reads to them
several chapters in the Bible' (Tuke, 1813, p. 161).

The proper sentiments and conduct were also encouraged by careful selection
and approval of which reading materials the patients were allowed. These choices
appeared to depend as much on the particular values of Quaker society as on the
person's disorder, as we read below from Tuke's *Description*:

> There certainly requires considerable care in the selection of books for
> the use of the insane. The works of the imagination are generally, for

obvious reasons, to be avoided; and such as are in any degree connected with the peculiar notions of the patient, are decidedly objectionable. The various branches of the mathematics and natural science, furnish the most useful class of subjects on which to employ the minds of the insane; and they should, as much as possible, be induced to pursue one subject steadily. (Tuke, 1813, p. 183)

Similar care was taken related to the issue of whether patients would be allowed writing utensils and paper, as writing about certain topics appeared to be considered as ill-advised as reading about them. This was especially true in the case of patients who had false beliefs, for whom the opportunity to write would only allow them to elaborate on these notions and become even more convinced of them. 'The means of writing', explains Tuke, are 'sometimes obliged to be withheld from the patient, as it would only produce continual essays on his peculiar notions; and serve to fix his errors more completely in his mind' (Tuke, 1813, p. 182).

Given the purported salutary effect of mathematics and natural science on the mind of 'the insane', it is perhaps not so surprising that the Retreat model of moral management shifted so completely to that of an educational model that superintendents began to give lectures on these topics as well. Pliny Earle, the superintendent cited at the opening of Section 2.5, equating the management of 'the insane' to the management of children – and one of the most influential psychiatrists in the United States in the later part of the nineteenth century – provided the following description in his account of his approach to moral treatment:

> Soon after the writer of this article first directed his attention to the treatment of the insane, he became convinced that lectures upon scientific and miscellaneous subjects might be made an object of interest, as well as of utility, in the moral treatment of patients in public institutions. Accordingly, being at that time connected with the Frankford Asylum, near Philadelphia, he induced the managers of that institution to purchase an air pump and other philosophical apparatus, and with the aid of these he gave a series of experimental lectures before the patients ... the 38 lectures included:

Topic	# of lectures
Natural Philosophy	4
Chemistry	6
Animal Physiology	9
Astronomy	10
Physical, Intellectual, and Moral Beauty	2
Recitations of Poetry	1
History and Description of Malta	2
Greece as it was in 1838	2
Characteristics of the Americans and Europeans	2

(Cited in Bockoven, 1956, p. 300)

It is hard to imagine what a lecture on 'Animal Physiology' or 'The History and Description of Malta' was to do to help a suffering person regain control of his or her mind, so we are left to assume that these were topics of some interest to the superintendent personally, which he was moved to share with his patients. Regardless of their efficacy, or lack thereof, Earle had become so convinced of the importance of these lectures as a cornerstone of moral treatment that he concludes:

> As a simple method of exerting disciplinary restraint, simultaneously, over a large number of patients . . . we believe that there is no other plan, hitherto adopted in the system of moral treatment, which will prove more generally and extensively useful than that of judicious and well managed lectures. (Cited in Bockoven, 1956, p. 301)

Apparently not thinking much of the intellectual capacity of his patients, Earle, who now speaks of 'a school for the insane', is clear to remind the reader that the purpose of such lectures is not to impart knowledge but rather to exert 'moral control'. We will return to the issue of his need to exert this control 'over large numbers' in the next section. For now, it suffices to demonstrate the degree to which the Retreat model had now been transformed by the time it reached the United States. Writes Earle:

> It is not to be expected that great advancement in valuable knowledge can ever be attained in a school for the insane. The only subject generally within reach, and the only one the acquisition of which needs be expected – and this indeed is much – is the exercise of a moral control over large numbers at once; subduing excitement, rousing the inactive, and giving a new current to their thoughts. (Cited in Bockoven, 1956, p. 301)

2.8 Re-shaping character

It is perhaps the most important strategy introduced by Tuke – it certainly has been the most influential and longest-lasting strategy – that we have reserved for last. All of the strategies described above were deployed within the context of the culture of the Retreat. Establishing and maintaining this culture was perhaps the most central element of the superintendent's role. It was through this culture that the work of reshaping the person's character from that of a wayward child to that of a rational, civilized and well-socialized adult was to unfold. Attendance at religious services, readings from the Bible, engagement in productive labor and listening to lectures were only some of the activities which sustained this culture. Equally, if not more, important were the ways in which this culture operated implicitly and outside of the person's conscious or reflective awareness.

For the reader to appreciate the degree to which this same culture continues to operate implicitly and outside of awareness to the present day and throughout the mental health system, all that he or she need do is to visit an extended stay unit at one of the remaining state hospitals, or a group home or other congregate site housing programme for individuals with serious and persistent mental illness, in the United States. Odds are that this ward or programme will employ some version of a 'level system' in which people with mental illnesses are expected to conform their behavior to the expectations of the programme in order to progress in their treatment and enjoy the privileges and rewards which come from achieving higher and higher 'levels' within the system. As one participant in a recent qualitative study said: 'You come in as a five and the goal is to leave as a one.' In other wards or programmes you might come in as a one with the goal of leaving as a five. Regardless of the direction of the numbers attached to the levels, you are expected to gain increasing levels of self-control and control over your disorder in order to regain some of the rights and benefits you typically enjoyed prior to admission into the programme. This includes such privileges as being able to leave a locked unit, being able to spend unstructured time with peers, being able to use a knife and fork, being able to participate in community activities without supervision, being able to watch television or being allowed access to your own possessions (e.g. a radio, a computer).

This type of level system, which remains unquestioned as providing the foundation for many mental health programmes to this day, appears to have been an original contribution of the Tukes and the Retreat at York. We mentioned earlier how Samuel Tuke chastised asylum superintendents for overemphasizing safety at the expense of patient comfort. This should not be taken to suggest, however, that the Tukes were unconcerned with safety. They were, in fact, very concerned with the risks posed by potentially dangerous patients, it is just that they thought they had developed a more effective and more humane approach to preventing and managing aggression should it occur. These approaches were relevant to the lowest level of a somewhat elaborate system that had several different levels of behavioral expectations and consequences through which they hoped their patients would advance in a relatively linear fashion. Although they did not describe the system as a whole as such, they did describe the various levels patients could attain in their progress towards discharge and, as a result, created the first level system in the history of psychiatry.

At the Retreat, these levels typically differed in terms of where the patients took their meals, with whom they were allowed to eat and the degree to which they were allowed out of their rooms and outside the asylum altogether. Decisions as to which privileges the person could enjoy when appear to have been made based on two primary factors: the person's social class or access to resources and the person's control over his or her behavior. Patients could pay a higher daily rate to enjoy more privileges, and also 'there are apartments in which patients, with a servant, may be accommodated, without mixing with the others' (Tuke, 1813, p. 49). This was important not only for the patient's comfort but also for the speed and completeness of the cure. Rather than risking 'the promiscuous exposure to such company as is mostly found in public Institutions of this kind' and being dragged down to their crass level (Tuke, 1813, p. 37), a person of sufficient means could be isolated from the commoners and take his or her cure in private. This opportunity also continues to the present day in private institutions for the wealthy.

Aside from wealth and social standing, decisions were made based on patients' behavior and, more specifically, their willingness and ability to follow the rules of communal life. At the bottom of the hierarchy are the potentially dangerous or disorganized patients who could not be trusted and who required almost constant supervision. Of these patients, Tuke describes their care as being provided in public spaces and under staff supervision and control:

> The patients, who take their meals in the galleries or dayrooms, are not allowed the use of knives or forks. Their meat is divided into small pieces by the attendant, and they eat it with a spoon. It also is the business of the attendant to take the patient's clothes out of the lodging-room, and examine the pockets every night. (Tuke, 1813, pp. 173–174)

Seclusion rooms could also be used for these patients, described as 'an opportunity of temporary confinement, by way of punishment, for any very offensive acts', but, according to Tuke, were only used very rarely (Tuke, 1813, p. 98).

As patients improve, or should their social standing require it, they are able to move up the ladder of privilege, one primary indicator of this being where they take their meals. This opportunity is not only considered as a reward for appropriate behavior but also to have a curative function itself, creating a kind of upward spiral of functioning. If you behave well enough, you can dine with the superintendent and his family and other people of prestige and high standing and, as a result of this experience, you will want to improve your behavior even more so as to keep and enhance the esteem of these companions. Writes Tuke:

> Patients of the higher class, in regard to property, and who can be intrusted to leave the gallery, take their meals with the superintendent and the female patients of the same class, in the dining-room, of the centre building. The convalescents of the lower class, many of whom have been, previously to their disorder, in respectable situations, are frequently admitted to take their meals in this room; as the change is found essentially to promote their recovery. (Tuke, 1813, p. 99)

Once patients proved themselves capable of carrying on civilized dinner-table discourse with the superintendent, his family and other convalescing patients, then exposure to the outside world could be considered. At first, this could be provided by having selected (i.e. upstanding) people from the community come in to visit with the convalescing patients. For women, in particular – since most of the staff were male – this required bringing in respectable young ladies from the neighboring town to take tea with female patients. Patients who reached this level of returning reason could also begin to be treated like 'normal' adults, resuming more and more the lifestyle they had prior to admission and that they would presumably have again once discharged. Writes Tuke:

> It is, however, very certain, that as soon as reason begins to return, the conversation of judicious, indifferent persons, greatly increases the comfort; and is considered almost essential to the recovery of many patients. On this account, the convalescents of every class, are frequently introduced into the society of the rational parts of the family. They are also permitted to sit up till the usual time for the family to retire to rest, and are allowed as much liberty as their state of mind will admit. (Tuke, 1813, p. 179)

The final level then involves going outside of the asylum for visits to attend religious services, to visit family and friends and to begin to re-establish a life following treatment. Patients who handled these visits well, and did not suffer a relapse or setback in their illness, could then be considered for discharge and considered cured.

As a final point of divergence with Pinel and *traitement moral*, it is interesting to see what strategy Tuke suggests to ensure the smooth and effective functioning of the culture we have just described. We recall that for Pussin, and then for Pinel, the 'simple method' used to ensure that patients received humane and compassionate care was to hire back as staff people who were convalescing or recovering from their own disorder. This strategy does not appear to be an option for the Tukes, as their model requires authority and expertise to lie in the managers of the asylum, not in the patients themselves. While perhaps a seventh-grader could attempt to teach mathematics to fifth graders, it is better to have an experienced teacher with expertise in mathematics, so too with the asylum. It is best to have rational, principled and ideally moral people staffing the asylum, people equally influenced by the religious values of the Quakers, and who can embody and role model these values for the patients. As Tuke is frank enough to admit, such people can be very difficult to come by. He writes that it is:

> exceedingly difficult to ensure the proper treatment of deranged persons. To consider them at the same time both as brothers, and as mere automats; to applaud all they do right; and pity, without censuring, whatever they do wrong, requires such a habit of philosophical reflection, and Christian charity, as is certainly difficult to attain. (Tuke, 1813, pp. 175–176)

As the history of moral treatment following the Retreat clearly demonstrates, it is difficult, indeed, to set such expectations for the staff of any hospital to achieve on a consistent basis.

2.9 The demise of moral treatment

We hope that with the picture we have painted of moral treatment thus far, the reader will be disabused of the notions that we reached the pinnacle of psychiatry during this period and that all of our answers for the future lie in resurrecting this past. The past is seldom as unambiguous and pretty as we prefer to remember it. This is certainly true of moral treatment. At the time, though – in the first half of the nineteenth century – the idea and practice of moral treatment caught on like wildfire and spread rapidly. The Retreat itself went through three expansion projects in its first five years, going from a bed capacity of 25 to 35 and eventually to 45. Similar developments were occurring in Connecticut, Philadelphia, Boston, New York and many other major cities in the United States, leading to the construction of 17 additional hospitals by the late 1940s (Bockoven, 1956, p. 173). It was this rapid expansion of asylums and asylum beds that accounted, in part, for the demise of this model, as the patient population quickly outgrew the existing expertise and personnel. While the founders argued that retreats should not exceed 200 patients, so that the superintendent could come to know each person individually, their census quickly exceeded this limit. As Samuel Tuke recognized as early as 1813, after the three expansions mentioned above: 'The necessity for such an establishment has, on every account, been found much greater than was at first imagined' (Tuke, 1813, p. 70).

At their peak, during this thirty-year period between 1813 and 1843, retreats were reporting success or recovery rates of between 70 and 90% for people admitted within the first year of the onset of their disorder and between 45 and 65% of the total population being recovered upon discharge (Bockoven, 1956). There has been some debate about the veracity of these numbers, as some sceptics have suggested that people were counted as recovered if they left the hospital well but then relapsed or were re-admitted later. A careful and rigorous study conducted by Bockoven in the 1950s, however, suggests that these numbers were most likely accurate, at least for the general population. We now know that these same numbers have been found by over 30 studies conducted in over 30 countries in the 30 years between 1969 and 1999, studies which have consistently demonstrated a recovery rate for individuals with serious mental illnesses between 45 and 65%. Because these studies, and the body of work they represent, remain relatively unknown in the field, we collected some of these papers in a two-volume set that we published in 2005–2006 (cf. Davidson, Harding and Spaniol, (2005, 2006)). As these studies do not control for treatment effects, but find similar recovery rates across cultures, countries and health care systems, one is left to conclude that between 45 and 65% of people with serious mental illnesses will recover over time with or without treatment, including moral treatment.

At the time, however, the recovery rates seen in and published by the moral treatment asylums in the United States and elsewhere fuelled optimism about the possibility of recovery from serious mental illness and enthusiasm about the efficacy of moral treatment. As we will see in the next chapter, the rapid and uncontrolled growth of mental hospitals exploded exponentially after the success of Dorothea Dix's crusade to build a hospital in every state of the country. But even as Dix was beginning her advocacy work in the 1840s, increasing numbers of people were being referred to these asylums. These people did not necessarily match the profile of the typical patient of the Retreat or the other private asylums, being primarily property owners and people of culture and means. Rather, the influx beginning in the 1840s included the poor, immigrants and people who were not welcomed elsewhere in society, and for whom placement in a mental hospital provided an expedient solution to their disposition. This change in population was not missed by the early fathers of moral treatment, and, as early as 1854, an annual report from a Massachusetts mental hospital included 'the lament ... that the state hospital was fast becoming a hospital for Irish immigrants rather than for the intelligent Yeomanry of Massachusetts' (cited in Bockoven, 1956, p. 179).

2.10 Summary of lessons learned

From this review of the evolution of moral treatment, we suggest the following lessons:

- Many people recover from serious mental illnesses, either with or without treatment.

- Even when acutely ill, many people with serious mental illnesses retain certain of their mental faculties intact, with domains of health and competence co-existing with domains of dysfunction and impairment.

- Some individuals recovering from serious mental illnesses may be particularly well suited to taking care of others suffering from these conditions, as they will have more empathy and compassion for their struggles and will likely treat them with more dignity, respect and kindness.

- When provided the opportunity, most people with serious mental illnesses remain capable of working without any particular accommodations or supports.

- Engaging in work that the person finds interesting and/or enjoyable appears to promote recovery, perhaps more than any other single factor.

- Individuals with serious mental illnesses are rarely violent or aggressive towards others, unless they have experienced violence or aggression at the hands of others.

Lessons to avoid repeating:

- Level systems, which continue to be in use today, are based on paternalistic and moralistic approaches which view mental illnesses as being due to developmental and moral failures on the part of patients and their families.

- When institutions are created for the purpose of extracting problematic people from their families and their communities, the number of beds will always be insufficient for the number of people to be admitted.

3
Reciprocity in Community-based Care

3.1 The advocacy of Dorothea Dix

It was at the height of the enthusiasm for moral treatment and prior to the wholesale 'dumping' of the elderly, the poor and immigrants into mental hospitals that Dorothea Dix entered the scene. Her intercession at this time in history is instructive for us on several scores, even as an example of the unintended adverse consequences of humane and progressive social policies. Given her own life experience, her single-minded dedication to the cause of securing appropriate care and treatment for individuals with mental illnesses and her impassioned advocacy on their behalf, it would be ungenerous not to include Dix in a book on the conceptual roots of the recovery movement. She represented at the time, and continues to represent, an important and compassionate point of view that must be addressed in current debates about mental health policy. Even if we do not wish to return to the days of large, custodial mental hospitals, we are still faced with the challenge of what to do with and for individuals who do not think they need, or who do not willingly seek or accept, care on their own. A little background about Dix's life and her work provides a useful context for such a discussion (Tiffany, 1890; Marshall, 1937; Browne, 1969; Greenstone, 1979; Gollaher, 1995; Brown, 1998).

Dorothea Dix was born the year after the publication of Pinel's *Treatise on Insanity*. By all accounts, her childhood was not a happy one, running away from her parents' home in Maine when she was only 12 years old to live with her paternal grandmother and then with an aunt in Massachusetts. Showing an impressive degree of determination, leadership and energy that would last for most of her life, she opened two schools by the age of 20. Also showing a keen sense of duty and a commitment to social justice, she ran a private school during the day but then also opened her school in the evening for poor children, whom she taught for free. By the time she was 22, she had written the first of a number of children's books as well,

The Roots of the Recovery Movement in Psychiatry   Larry Davidson, Jaak Rakfeldt, John Strauss
© 2010 John Wiley & Sons, Ltd

a highly popular book for parents entitled *Conversations on Common Things*. She pursued this career in education with steadfast devotion until 1836, at which point, at the age of 34, she developed serious health problems and left for England for an extended period of rest and recuperation at the family home of a friend. Accounts of the nature of these problems vary considerably, from a severe upper respiratory infection to unexplained bleeding and fatigue to an ambiguous nervous ailment. A number of more recent studies suggest that this was actually the first of two bouts of a serious mental illness, most likely of bipolar disorder, accounting both for her periods of sustained and concentrated energy and singular productivity and her extended periods of withdrawal and lethargy.

Dix's experiences during the period between 1836 and 1841 appear to be crucial to the remainder of her career and to her legacy, particularly as revealed through her correspondence. Apparently, she found the warm and generous family in England with whom she stayed to offer her a level of love, acceptance and support that she had not experienced in her own family. Dix found this to be a surprisingly pleasant and curative experience. At the same time, her stern grandmother chastised her for being ill and for taking the time off from work to convalesce, insisting that she was shirking her duties and being irresponsible and even indolent, faults of major significance at the time – as well as being associated with mental illness – as we have seen in the previous chapter. She remained with this family for over a year, describing it as perhaps the best year in her life and feeling that what she had received from this loving family had filled a void left by her own neglected and perhaps even abusive childhood. Shortly thereafter, Dix's grandmother died and she remained out of work, living off of family savings and the royalties from her books.

Her now famous experience in the East Cambridge Jail happened in 1841, when she was approached by a seminary student who did not feel comfortable teaching a Sunday school class to female inmates. The student thought that the women would do better with a female teacher, and his mother had recommended he ask the well-known female educator Miss Dix for advice. Rather than recommending available female teachers in the area, Dix volunteered to take on the responsibility herself, agreeing to return to teaching for this worthy cause. What she found at the East Cambridge Jail, however, was not at all what she had anticipated. She found women who were suffering from serious mental illnesses housed with female inmates who had committed violent crimes. All of them were housed in filthy and unheated cells, were poorly clothed and shivering from cold in the New England winter. When she enquired how the jailers could treat the women with mental illness in such a deplorable way, the jailers assured her that the mentally ill could not feel the cold and that, furthermore, they would not be safe around a heater, should they provide one. As mentally ill people were unpredictable and dangerous, they might very well set fire to the jail.

Dix's almost immediate reaction to the squalid conditions she found there was to launch a state-wide, then national and eventually international movement to rescue individuals with mental illnesses from languishing in jails, prisons and almshouses and to secure for them the same quality care and treatment that at the time was only being afforded to the wealthy. Just as she was committed to seeing that poor children could have the same quality education in the evening that she had offered to children of means during the day, she was committed to seeing that adults with serious mental illnesses who were poor could have the same kind of humane and effective treatment that was available at that time to those of means in the retreats described in Chapter 2. Given her experience in England, we also could imagine that she wanted the women she met at the jail to have the same opportunity she had recently had during her own convalescence.

As a result, she undertook at first an extensive investigation of all of the poor houses, alms houses and jails in the state of Massachusetts, visiting each personally and taking copious notes. She studied the works of Pinel, the Tukes and other leaders of the moral treatment era, and talked at length with physicians about the various mental illnesses and their care. She found people with mental illnesses living in over-crowded and deplorable conditions across the state, including people being chained to walls (as they had in the Bicêtre prior to Pussin), sitting in their own excrement, malnourished and shivering in the cold. She forged alliances with other advocates for people with mental illnesses and by 1843 had prepared eloquent and impassioned testimony for the Massachusetts legislature documenting her observations of these conditions and making a plea for reform. Mindful of the limited and largely subservient role accorded to women at the time, she asked an esteemed colleague who was a male physician and member of the legislature to deliver the testimony. After some debate and further investigation that confirmed her observations, the Massachusetts legislature allocated funds for a state mental hospital at Worcester; emboldened, Dix marched on.

She took the same approach to reform in other states, preparing testimony for well-known and respected male figures in New York in 1844 and in New Jersey and Pennsylvania in 1845, each time visiting, observing and documenting conditions in the jails and almshouses herself. She continued this work indefatigably and with much success, and by 1847 she had visited 18 state penitentiaries, 300 county jails and over 500 almshouses, resulting in the construction or renovation and expansion of mental hospitals in 20 states, Nova Scotia and Newfoundland. At this point she turned her attention to the federal level and began drafting and lobbying for an ambitious plan to set aside 12 225 000 acres of land as a public endowment, with the income to be used to secure adequate accommodations, treatment and support for people who were either deaf and mute (2 225 000 acres) or suffering with a mental illness (10 000 000 acres). She finally secured passage of this plan by both the Senate and the House of Representatives in 1854, after six years of strenuous lobbying and behind-the-scenes efforts. By this point, however, it was too late for Millard Fillmore, the president she had been lobbying and preparing for receipt of this bill, to sign it. Much to her disappointment, the new president, Franklin Pierce, vetoed the bill, arguing that caring for people with mental illnesses and other disabilities was the responsibility of the states, not the federal government.

This setback, which we can imagine could have been devastating, precipitated another episode of illness, and Dix returned to Europe for rest and recuperation.

She did not rest long this time, however, and, finding conditions in Europe equally distressing among the poor, began her lobbying for reform with earnest once more. Between 1854 and 1856, she travelled to 14 countries, spreading the seed for the creation of mental hospitals everywhere she went. Her travels included an audience with the Pope in Rome (who compared her to Saint Theresa) and meetings with representatives of other countries she could not visit herself, such as Japan, where she was instrumental in the creation of two hospitals. She returned to the United States in 1856 after this worldwide tour, but soon thereafter got caught up in the American Civil War along with the rest of the country. A week after the attack on Fort Sumter inaugurating the war, Dix volunteered her services to the Union Army. By then a well-known and admired advocate, she was appointed Superintendent of Female Nurses and was responsible for overseeing the work of over 3000 nurses during the war – which she did for no pay. She brought to this work the same persistence, resourcefulness and tirelessness with which she had lobbied for mental health reform, and left the army nursing corps in a much better shape than she had inherited. She was apparently better suited to working alone than to supervising others, however, as she not-so-affectionately came to be known as 'Dragon Dix' by her army colleagues and subordinates.

By the time the war ended, Dix was in her sixties and largely withdrew from public life. By this time, 22 of the 33 states had public mental hospitals and the wake of the Civil War was not an opportune time to push for additional costly social reforms. In addition, Dix became discouraged over what had already become of the hospitals she had been instrumental in creating a mere 20 years earlier. She died at the age of 85 in 1887, having spent her last two decades refusing to talk about her work or career, but is still considered by some the foremost and most visible crusader for humanitarian causes of the nineteenth century.

3.2 The legacy of Dorothea Dix

Informed by both her personal experience of her own family and by her reading of Pinel, Tuke and others, Dix firmly believed that people with mental illnesses needed to be taken out of their family contexts and provided kind and compassionate care by professionals in home-like settings. In addition, she reportedly was very reluctant to seek care for herself early in the course of her own episodes of illness, doggedly pursuing her agenda of helping others at her own mental and physical expense until her physician insisted that she take time off work for a rest. Even after finally agreeing to seek respite in the face of exhaustion, Dix still had to deal with her own conflicts over receiving care from others, most likely embodied in and exacerbated by her stern grandmother's disapproval and chastisement.

She finally found confirmation for her eventual decision to allow herself to be cared for by the warm and accepting family she discovered in England when she turned to the writings of Pinel, Tuke and others. As we saw above, Pinel had insisted that 'maniacs are seldom or never cured as long as they are kept at home, subject to the influence of family intercourse' and that 'Insanity is much more certainly and effectually cured in places adapted for their reception and treatment, than at home amidst the various influences of family interests' (Pinel, 1806, pp. 212, 214). On this score, Tuke had been in full agreement and had even gone one step further, encouraging friends and family to seek removal of the person early in the course of the disorder so as to enhance his or her prospects for a quick recovery. The Tukes placed such a premium on early removal and treatment that they offered to admit appropriate patients for free for an initial period of treatment if they could not afford the usual fees. Writes Tuke:

> As experience demonstrates, that the recovery of insane patients, frequently depends on their being removed from their connexions, and put under proper care and treatment, in the early stages of the disorder, it is earnestly recommended to their friends, to remove them at an early period after the disorder appears to be fixed. (Tuke, 1813, p. 88)

Although the Tukes did not themselves appear to speculate as to why removal from the family and home was necessary for recovery, other proponents of moral treatment did, and they invariably agreed with Pinel's sentiment that people needed to be protected from family interests and intercourse. While for Pinel this might have been required to create a protected space in which he could identify and treat the problematic aspects of the illness – for example engaging delusional patients in rational investigations of their beliefs or reviving the interest and passion of someone who had succumbed to melancholy – for the proponents of moral treatment, removal from the family was increasingly viewed and justified based on the assumption that it was the family who had caused the disorder in the first place. Given that mental illnesses were largely viewed as the results of failures to develop adequate self-control and restraint over one's lesser desires and propensities, it is understandable how the culpability for these failures could be laid at the feet of the patients' families. We can imagine that Dix might have derived some comfort from this shift in responsibility, being able to stop blaming herself for her difficulties and placing the fault instead on the moral failings of the parents from whom she had run away at the age of 12. From the sequence of events we have now described, we can see how Dix had attempted to secure for poor people the same kind of care from which she had herself benefited so fully, offering them safe havens from their families and home-like environments in which they could recuperate and recover themselves even if they did not know enough, or have the financial means, to seek out such settings for themselves.

In terms of the further evolution of moral treatment, Bockoven suggests that the later adherents of moral treatment became increasingly 'impressed with the importance of child rearing to mental health'. As one example, he cites a Dr Butler, who 'categorically stated that he had traced the cause of insanity to the malign influences of childhood in a large proportion of over 3000 patients he had personally studied' (Bockoven, 1956, p. 175). It would not be too long before this approach would be picked up and codified by Freud, issuing in an entirely new way of studying, understanding and treating mental illnesses.

3.3 Jane Addams' community alternative

We will return to the childhood roots of mental illness, Freud and the psychoanalytic approach when we take up the work of Harry Stack Sullivan in the next chapter. Before turning back to American psychiatry, though, we think it worth a sizable detour to explore an alternative to the approach pioneered by Pinel, the Tukes and Dix. In other words, is there any way to support a person in recovering from a serious mental illness *without* removing the person from his or her family influences, home and other 'connexions'? Can assistance be offered to the person, and the illness and its sequelae addressed, outside of an asylum, retreat or hospital setting? While Jane Addams did not specialize in mental illness or mental health per se, the settlement house movement and its model of community-based services and supports which she and a few of her good friends launched in Chicago in the late nineteenth century provides just such an alternative. We think it important, therefore, to describe this model and Addams' thinking about its essential elements and principles prior to taking up the more focused psychiatric thinking of Sullivan and his predecessor, Adolf Meyer. In the end, we will suggest that this model provides perhaps the most appealing and effective framework for the delivery of community-based care developed to date. As such, it will offer a foundation for the efforts that we will later describe as inspired by Sullivan, Basaglia and Vygotsky.

By all accounts, Jane Addams grew up in very different circumstances from those experienced by Dorothea Dix. Nonetheless, she was Dix's successor in terms of assuming the role of being the foremost female reformer, advocate and humanitarian of her age. Again by all accounts, Addams was a remarkable and indefatigable woman whose efforts spanned a wide range of social issues, beginning with urban poverty and ending with global peace. In addition to initiating the settlement house movement in the United States, she founded or co-founded numerous organizations, entities and collaboratives across the country, including the American Civil Liberties Union and the NAACP (National Association for the Advancement of Colored People). A staunch advocate for social justice and peace, she also became a leading figure internationally, finally being awarded the Nobel Peace Prize in 1931 for her long-standing and highly productive efforts to protect and promote human rights around the globe. Our focus in the following, however, will largely be restricted to the settlement house movement and the model it offers for the provision of services and supports in community-based settings for people facing various challenges.

Even though she lost her mother at the age of two, Addams described an almost idyllic childhood in the Illinois countryside, growing up the eighth of nine children in a warm and loving family. She idolized her father, who owned a local grain mill and was a banker, a senator, a founder of the Republican Party and a long-standing supporter of Abraham Lincoln. Her first of two autobiographical accounts of the development of Hull-House, the first Settlement House founded in the United States by Addams and her colleagues in an inner-city neighborhood in Chicago in 1889, is replete with stories of her father and his social and political influence on her life and thought. As the following story – and the fact that she dedicated her first book about Hull-House to him – attest, she clearly credited her father with being her major influence and inspiration. Here she recounts her father's response to her putting on a new cloak for the first time with the intent of wearing it to Sunday School:

> Although I constantly confided my sins and perplexities to my father, there are only a few occasions on which I remember having received direct advice or admonition ... I can remember an admonition on one occasion, however, when, as a little girl of eight years, arrayed in a new cloak, gorgeous beyond anything I had ever worn before, I stood before my father for his approval. I was much chagrined by his remark that it was a very pretty cloak – in fact so much prettier than any cloak the other little girls in the Sunday School had, that he would advise me to wear my old cloak, which would keep me quite as warm, with the added advantage of not making the other little girls feel badly. I complied with the request but I fear without inner consent, and I certainly was quite without the joy of self-sacrifice as I walked soberly through the village street by the side of my counselor.
>
> My mind was busy, however, with the old question eternally suggested by the inequalities of the human lot. Only as we neared the church door did I venture to ask what could be done about it, receiving the reply that it might never be righted so far as clothes went, but that people might be equal in things that mattered much more than clothes, the affairs of education and religion, for instance, which we attended to when we went to school and church, and that it was very stupid to wear the sort of clothes that made it harder to have equality even there. (Addams, 1910, pp. 13–14)

One surmises from Addams' other accounts of her father that the scorn expressed at the end of this passage was her own self-criticism rather than an admonition by him directly. The reader is struck, in fact, by how much of a social conscience she had developed at a very young age, due in part no doubt to her father's influence, but also enhanced in part by the degree to which she had already chosen by this time to begin to assume responsibility for redressing 'the inequalities of the human lot'. The following story, with which she begins her account of the development of Hull-House, not only illustrates the sense of personal responsibility for addressing social ills and inequities she had accepted prior to the age of seven years old, but also foreshadows the experience she was to have in London two decades later that was to result in her creation of Hull-House in the centre of one of Chicago's poorest communities. She writes:

> I recall an incident which must have occurred before I was seven years old, for the mill in which my father transacted his business that day

> was closed in 1867. The mill stood in the neighboring town adjacent
> to its poorest quarter. Before then I had always seen the little city of
> ten thousand people with the admiring eyes of a country child, and it
> had never occurred to me that all its streets were not as bewilderingly
> attractive as the one which contained the glittering toyshop and the
> confectioner. On that day I had my first sight of the poverty which
> implies squalor, and felt the curious distinction between the ruddy
> poverty of the country and that which even a small city presents in
> its shabbiest streets. I remember launching at my father the pertinent
> inquiry why people lived in such horrid little houses so close together,
> and that after receiving his explanation I declared with much firmness
> when I grew up I should, of course, have a large house, but it would
> not be built among the other large houses, but right in the midst of
> horrid little houses like those. (Addams, 1910, pp. 4–5)

In essence, this is what Hull-House was to become over 20 years later, except for that in addition to living in a large house in the midst of poverty, by that point Addams was to have given much thought and some beginning attempts to figure out what a person could do in such circumstances to improve the lot of those around her. Her conviction in the necessity of doing so, and her initial ideas about what to do once 'settled' in such an environment, she traces to the life's work of Lincoln and to a series of three events in her early adulthood. As she describes: 'It required eight years – from the time I left Rockford in the summer of 1881 until Hull-House was opened in the autumn of 1889 – to formulate my convictions even in the least satisfactory manner, much less to reduce them to a plan for action' (Addams, 1910, p. 64).

3.4 A series of unfortunate, but influential, events

The first of these events occurred in East London in 1881, at the beginning of a European tour suggested by the prominent physician Weir Mitchell, who Addams described as giving her a 'prescription of spending the next two years in Europe' (Addams, 1910, p. 65). This prescription had been given to address a state of 'nervous exhaustion' and 'deep depression' she had experienced after a prolonged convalescence from the development of a 'spinal difficulty' due to a condition with which she had been born (Pott's disease) and that was to result in recurring health problems throughout her life (Addams, 1910, p. 65). As a result of this spinal difficulty, she had had to withdraw from the Woman's Medical College of Philadelphia and spend six months 'bound to a bed' in her sister's house. She described finding the combination of medical school, for which she felt poorly suited, and her protracted medical problems to precipitate this depression, and was, at the time, happy to follow Dr Weir's 'prescription' as offering a possible antidote.

Upon her arrival in England, however, her experience of this prescribed respite could not have been more different from Dix's experience of the warm and loving family with whom she had stayed while recuperating from her own episode of illness a half a century earlier. Upon arriving in East London, Addams encountered the following scene, the description of which we quote at length, as we did with Pinel, in order both to convey her characteristic writing style and to highlight for the reader how she was moved by, made sense of and responded to the horrors she witnessed. She writes:

> One of the most poignant of these experiences, which occurred during the first few months after our landing upon the other side of the Atlantic, was on a Saturday night, when I received an ineradicable impression of the wretchedness of East London, and also saw for the first time the over-crowded quarters of a great city at midnight. A small party of tourists were taken to the East End by a city missionary to witness the Saturday night sale of decaying vegetables and fruit, which, owing to the Sunday laws in London, could not be sold until Monday, and, as they were beyond safe keeping, were disposed of at auction as late as possible on Saturday night. On Mile End Road, from the top of an omnibus which paused at the end of a dingy street lighted by only occasional flares of gas, we saw two huge masses of ill-clad people clamoring around two hucksters' carts. They were bidding their farthings and ha'pennies for a vegetable held up by the auctioneer, which he at last scornfully flung, with a gibe for its cheapness, to the successful bidder. In the momentary pause only one man detached himself from the groups. He had bidden in a cabbage, and when it struck his hand, he instantly sat down on the curb, tore it with his teeth, and hastily devoured it, unwashed and uncooked as it was. He and his fellows were types of the 'submerged tenth,' as our missionary guide told us, with some little satisfaction in the then new phrase, and he further added that so many of them could scarcely be seen in one spot save at this Saturday night auction, the desire for cheap food being apparently the one thing which could move them simultaneously. They were huddled into ill-fitting, cast-off clothing, the ragged finery which one sees only in East London. Their pale faces were dominated by that most unlovely of human expressions, the cunning and shrewdness of the bargain-hunter who starves if he cannot make a successful trade, and yet the final impression was not of ragged, tawdry clothing nor of pinched and sallow faces, but of myriads of hands, empty, pathetic, nerveless and workworn, showing white in the uncertain light of the street, and clutching forward for food which was already unfit to eat.
>
> Perhaps nothing is so fraught with significance as the human hand, this oldest tool with which man has dug his way from savagery, and with which he is constantly groping forward. I have never since been able to see a number of hands held upward, even when they are moving rhythmically in a calisthenic exercise, or when they belong to a class of chubby children who wave them in eager response to a teacher's query, without a certain revival of this memory, a clutching at the heart reminiscent of the despair and resentment which seized me then.
>
> For the following weeks I went about London almost furtively, afraid to look down narrow streets and alleys lest they disclose again this hideous human need and suffering. I carried with me for days at

a time that curious surprise we experience when we first come back into the streets after days given over to sorrow and death; we are bewildered that the world should be going on as usual and unable to determine which is real, the inner pang or the outward seeming. In time all huge London came to seem unreal save the poverty in its East End. (Addams, 1910, pp. 66–69)

This experience, and others like it, took Addams back to her first experience of poverty which she had shared with her father on their country stroll and planted the seed in her that her destiny lay in joining with such people and helping to improve their lot. 'Before I returned to America', she explains, 'I had discovered that there were other genuine reasons for living among the poor than that of practicing medicine upon them' (Addams, 1910, pp. 65–66). As a result, she abandoned her medical career but remained unsure of exactly how she should proceed in channelling her outrage and her empathy.

She described the next few years as difficult and full of listless wandering as she tried to figure out what she, personally, could do in the face of such inequities. After consulting both classical and contemporary literature to see how others had approached such circumstances – as she knew that they were more or less 'eternal' – she became increasingly dissatisfied with the efforts of her predecessors. Her reading led only to 'a sense of futility, of misdirected energy, the belief that the pursuit of cultivation would not in the end bring either solace or relief' (Addams, 1910, p. 70). 'No comfort came to me then from any source', she writes, as the scene of the East London auction continued to haunt her (Addams, 1910, p. 69). Eventually, she came to the conclusion that she, as well as her socially conscious literary forefathers, had fallen into what she came to call 'the snare of preparation': thinking that in order to respond adequately to such horrors one first needed to be prepared, that is educated, informed and cultivated (Addams, 1910, p. 65). In reality, however, all they were doing was trying to numb themselves to the awful realities they had encountered, becoming indifferent to them rather than engaging with and trying to change them. She had come to the conclusion, as she described above, that it was in fact the scene in the East London slum that was the real rather than the 'outward seeming' of civil society. All we were doing, Addams concludes, was 'lumbering our minds with literature that only served to cloud the really vital situation spread before our eyes' (Addams, 1910, p. 70). These first experiences thus left her, in her own words, 'clinging only to the desire to live in a really living world and refusing to be content with a shadowy intellectual or aesthetic reflection of it' (Addams, 1910, p. 64).

It remained for another event several years later, also in England, to begin to give her ambiguous and ambitious ideas about what to do with this reality some shape. Having heard of the newly emerging 'settlement' movement there, she spent two days at Oxford University with the director of Toynbee Hall, the home of the first such programme in the United Kingdom that had been founded just three years earlier. Based on what Addams came to regard as a semi-romanticized vision of poverty and manual labor, the purpose of Toynbee Hall was to attract, recruit and deploy Oxford students – who at that time were invariably men of means – to live and work, on a temporary basis, in the poor neighborhoods of British cities. In addition to contributing their efforts to the greater good, the Oxford students would benefit from such time-limited experiences by being exposed to and 'rubbing elbows' with common people, people who they otherwise might never view as people in their own right (as opposed, e.g., to being servants). While Addams praised these efforts for what they were, and came to adopt the same term of 'settlement' for the movement she subsequently founded in the United States upon her return, she found Toynbee Hall and its derivatives to represent a uniquely British model which offended her American sensibilities. The model fell short, in particular, by its failure to capture the full measure of democracy, especially that version of democracy with which Addams associated her (and her father's) hero, Abraham Lincoln. She writes:

> I was naturally much interested in the beginnings of the movement whose slogan was 'Back to the People', and which could doubtless claim the Settlement as one of its manifestations. Nevertheless the processes by which so simple a conclusion as residence among the poor in East London was reached, seemed to me very involved and roundabout. However inevitable these processes might be for class-conscious Englishmen, they could not but seem artificial to a western American who had been born in a rural community where the early pioneer life had made social distinctions impossible. Always on the alert lest American Settlements should become mere echoes and imitations of the English movement, I found myself assenting to what was shown me only with that part of my consciousness which had been formed by reading of English social movements, while at the same time the rustic American looked on in detached comment.
>
> Why should an American be lost in admiration of a group of Oxford students because they went out to mend a disused road, inspired thereto by Ruskin's teaching for the bettering of the common life, when all the country roads in America were mended each spring by self-respecting citizens, who were thus carrying out the simple method devised by a democratic government for providing highways. (Addams, 1910, pp. 38–39)

Simply stated, there is nothing so noble about choosing to live among the poor and to lend one's assistance to their plight when this should be, in fact, the duty of every citizen in a fully democratic society. Contributing one's effort to the cause, and to the greater good, is not a learning experience for the wealthy – for which they should be praised – but a moral obligation for everyone. Addams tried to argue this case with an Oxford professor who had recently written a book on Lincoln, but found her words to fall on deaf ears. Placing the argument within this framework, however, did help her to clear her own head and to begin to give some direction to her development of a uniquely American model. As she writes:

> The memory of Lincoln, the mention of his name, came like a
> refreshing breeze from off the prairie, blowing aside all the scholarly
> implications in which I had become so reluctantly involved, and as
> the philosopher spoke of the great American 'who was content merely
> to dig the channels through which the moral life of his countrymen
> might flow', I was gradually able to make a natural connection between
> this intellectual penetration at Oxford and the moral perception which
> is always necessary for the discovery of new methods by which to
> minister to human needs. In the unceasing ebb and flow of justice
> and oppression we must all dig channels as best we may, that at the
> propitious moment somewhat of the swelling tide may be conducted
> to the barren places of life.
>
> Gradually a healing sense of well-being enveloped me and a quick
> remorse for my blindness, as I realized ... that vision and wisdom
> as well as high motives must lie behind every effective stroke in the
> continuous labor for human equality. (Addams, 1910, pp. 40–41)

In the end, upon leaving England once more, Addams had decided that 'both
the English and American settlements could unite in confessing [to be] perpetually
disturbed over the apparent inequalities of mankind' (Addams, 1910, p. 41). They
would have to differ, however, in how they went about understanding and correcting
those inequalities.

Her final impetus for returning to America and setting about the work of starting
the first American-model Settlement House came from perhaps a surprising, and
certainly unanticipated, source. Following on her visit to Toynbee Hall, she had
been thinking about offering women who had been in her own earlier shoes – that
is women of means who were becoming educated and cultivated through American
colleges – a similar opportunity (though markedly different experience) to those
offered the male students at Oxford. She writes:

> I gradually became convinced that it would be a good thing to rent a
> house in a part of the city where many primitive and actual needs are
> found, in which young women who had been given over too exclusively
> to study might restore a balance of activity along traditional lines and
> learn of life from life itself; where they might try out some of the things
> they had been taught and put truth to 'the ultimate test of the conduct it
> dictates or inspires'. I do not remember to have mentioned this plan to
> anyone until we reached Madrid in April, 1888. (Addams, 1910, p. 85)

It was then in Madrid that the unexpected happened. We have already seen
Addams' gift in recalling and describing moving moments from her past. In this case,
the moment that moved her and that she then recalled and described for the benefit
of the reader was her first, and we assume only, experience of a bullfight. She writes:

> We had been to see a bullfight rendered in the most magnificent
> Spanish style, where greatly to my surprise and horror, I found that

I had seen, with comparative indifference, five bulls and many more horses killed. The sense that this was the last survival of all the glories of the amphitheater, the illusion that the riders on the caparisoned horses might have been knights of a tournament, or the matadore a slightly armed gladiator facing his martyrdom, and all the rest of the obscure yet vivid associations of an historic survival, had carried me beyond the endurance of any of the rest of the party. I finally met them in the foyer, stern and pale with disapproval of my brutal endurance, and but partially recovered from the faintness and disgust which the spectacle itself had produced upon them. I had no defense to offer to their reproaches save that I had not thought much about the bloodshed; but in the evening the natural and inevitable reaction came, and in deep chagrin I felt myself tried and condemned, not only by this disgusting experience but by the entire moral situation which it revealed. It was suddenly made quite clear to me that I was lulling my conscience by a dreamer's scheme, that a mere paper reform had become a defense for continued idleness, and that I was making it a *raison d'être* for going on indefinitely with study and travel. It is easy to become the dupe of a deferred purpose, of the promise the future can never keep, and I had fallen into the meanest type of self-deception in making myself believe that all this was in preparation for great things to come. Nothing less than the moral reaction following the experience at a bullfight had been able to reveal to me that so far from following in the wake of a chariot of philanthropic fire, I had been tied to the tail of the veriest ox-cart of self-seeking.

I had made up my mind that next day, whatever happened, I would begin to carry out the plan. (Addams, 1910, pp. 85–87)

It was, apparently, one thing to identify and diagnose the 'snare of preparation', something Addams had already done a few years before. It was quite another thing to finally liberate one's self from it, which, in her case, it apparently took the experience of a bullfight to effect. Her own internal dialogues about the relative merits of education, culture and inaction, or of the British class system versus American democracy, she came to recognize as being themselves merely more instances of the same type of inaction. Studying the British settlement movement in order to better prepare for the work she would eventually do in America was, after all, just another form of studying – no different in principle from reading the classic texts of philosophy. The only way to truly escape from this internal merry-go-round of idleness and condemnation would be to act. The only way to truly appease her conscience was to act. And so she did.

3.5 The founding of the first American 'settlement'

Hull-House was founded upon Addams' return from Europe in the autumn of 1889. Along with a close and like-minded friend, Ellen Gates Starr, Addams had searched out a suitable (i.e. large) house in one of Chicago's poorest, predominantly immigrant, neighborhoods and moved in. Unlike the Oxford students at Toynbee Hall, however, she lived there until her death 46 years later. Initially, she secured, renovated and operated Hull-House (named after the first owner of the home, Charles Hull, one of Chicago's 'pioneering citizens' (Addams, 1910, p. 93)) using the $50 000 she had inherited from her father's estate. Following her initial personal investment, Addams became a highly productive fund-raiser.

It is both interesting and important to note that, above and beyond these initial steps of 'settling' down in an impoverished neighborhood, Addams still had no clear plans about what exactly she or Miss Starr were to do to be of assistance to their neighbors. This might have been the result of several factors, including her dissatisfaction with Toynbee Hall and others' previous efforts to address poverty, either in reality or in literary and theoretical works, as well as her own limited, direct experience of poverty herself. While clearly moved and deeply concerned about what she had witnessed earlier (first when seven years old and then later in East London), these experiences remained at a safe distance from the actual circumstances and lives of the people most immediately affected. Having decided now to give up that cushion of safety in order to become engaged in the reality of poverty, the primary thing Addams lacked when moving into Hull-House was experience. Her primary asset, though, might have been her genuine sense of humility in acknowledging how little she did know and in accepting what was at that time – and apparently and unfortunately continues to this day to be – a radical notion: that she could learn primarily from the affected people themselves.

There are many examples of people who knew equally little but were moved to conceal their ignorance behind grand and ambitious theories of what 'must' be the case and what therefore 'must' be done. We have generations of social policy based on little more than this kind of hubris. Addams stands out as one of the rare people who were willing to acknowledge their ignorance and yet remain committed to action despite it. This left her in what most others would consider a highly vulnerable position, especially given the attitudes of the day towards 'the poor' and towards immigrants of various nationalities, all sharing in common the perceived status of being uncultivated, unprincipled, inferior and, as Addams had herself seen in the East London alley, reduced to the appearance of being sub-human. In the face of these kinds of stereotypes, Addams was happy to note that: 'In our enthusiasm over "settling", the first night we forgot not only to lock but to close a side door opening on Polk Street, and we were much pleased in the morning to find that we possessed a fine illustration of the honesty and kindliness of our new neighbors' (Addams, 1910, pp. 95–96).

But what were Misses Addams and Starr to do now, once they had indeed 'settled'? Their first task was to make Hull-House a warm and welcoming home, not only for themselves but also for any neighbors who might choose to stop by. They therefore decorated it as a home, not in order to stand apart from their neighbors and surely not to make their neighbors feel bad or inferior (recall the lesson Addams had learned relative to her new cloak), but more matter-of-factly, consistent with how they would choose to decorate a home wherever it might be located. In other words, they neither dressed up their house to announce their social standing and to separate themselves from their neighbors, nor did they dress down their house out of some self-conscious sense of charity or pity. They outfitted their house as they would ordinarily do, as would be comfortable for them, both to be transparent about who they were (i.e. not pretending to be poor) and to make it clear that they would both be neighbors and accept their neighbors as guests on these same terms (i.e. not saving their prized possessions for 'safer' quarters). As we have learned since, physical environments do make a difference in how people perceive the assumptions and expectations of their hosts, and consequently how they behave. Regardless of whether Addams thought about this explicitly or made such decisions more intuitively, the message appeared to get through. As she writes:

> The fine old house responded kindly to repairs, its wide hall and open fireplace always insuring it a gracious aspect ... We furnished the house as we would have furnished it were it in another part of the city, with the photographs and other impedimenta we had collected in Europe, and with a few bits of family mahogany. While all the new furniture which was bought was enduring in quality, we were careful to keep it in character with the fine old residence. Probably no young matron ever placed her own things in her own house with more pleasure than that with which we first furnished Hull-House. We believed that the Settlement may logically bring to its aid all those adjuncts which the cultivated man regards as good and suggestive of the best of the life of the past. (Addams, 1910, p. 93–94)

In those days, Addams notes, 'the house stood between an undertaking establishment and a saloon' (Addams, 1910, p. 93). The establishment of such a well-furnished and welcoming home in the midst of such a neighborhood was lost neither on the residents of the neighborhood nor on the local press and politicians. For their part, the press and some politicians were sceptical and even derided the lofty purpose of Hull-House, with one 'Chicago wit' describing Hull-House and its immediate neighbors (i.e. the undertaker and the saloon) as the 'Knight, Death and the Devil' (Addams, 1910, p. 94). Addams' true neighbors, however, the residents of the community, were not so inclined. As she astutely perceived on her first morning upon waking up to unlocked and still open doors and her possessions and home intact, the residents, from the first, accepted the establishment and welcomed the newcomers. If they questioned their motives at all, this was never made explicit. Rather, it appeared that their matter-of-fact attitude and genuine interest in the life of the community was enough to earn them acceptance. As she concludes: 'Any mock heroics which might be implied by comparing the Settlement to a knight quickly dropped away under the genuine kindness and hearty welcome extended to us by the families living up and down the street' (Addams, 1910, p. 94).

Before turning to describe what Addams and her colleagues learned about the plight of 'the poor' and how to be of some help to them over the 40-plus years of her experiences at Hull-House, we think it important to justify these claims that the house was accepted on its own terms by the residents, as well as by the city at large, as it is crucial to our choice of Addams and her body of work as it relates to recovery-oriented practice. How this is so will be the focus of the following sections. That this was so, however, we can demonstrate by the rapid expansion of Hull-House and its use by increasing numbers of people during Addams' lifetime. The spring after Hull-House opened, for example, their landlord decided to allow them to lease the property for free. Shortly thereafter, the landlord increased her gift to Hull-House to include the entire city block on which the house stood, so that the undertaker, the saloon and various other buildings could be torn down or renovated for the purpose of accommodating the expanding Hull-House programmes, which we will describe shortly.

As we noted, Addams and Starr moved into Hull-House in the autumn of 1889. By 1891, they had added an art gallery, by 1893 a coffee house and a gymnasium, by 1898 a club house for their various social programmes and by 1899 a theatre. By 1907, 18 years later, when this initial construction and expansion period was finally complete, there was a total of 13 buildings on the property, with approximately 70 people living there full-time. The number of full-time residents paled, however, in comparison to the number of people availing themselves of the diverse range of programmes that had developed by this time. By the time Addams had written her book *Twenty Years at Hull-House* in 1910, there were 1500 boys who were members of the Hull-House boys club and the House and its programmes saw approximately 2000 guests or participants per week. This kind of rapid expansion certainly exceeded Addams' initial expectations and ambitions, but was presaged by her first experience with the first programme she developed at Hull-House in its initial days.

The first community need that she perceived once 'settled' into the house was the need for day care for young mothers and for structured educational opportunities for preschool-age children. Consequently, she hired a kindergarten teacher and opened a kindergarten at the original Hull-House building. Within three weeks of opening, the kindergarten had enrolled 24 children and so had reached its maximum size for the one teacher who had been retained. By that point, however, it had also accumulated a waiting list of 70 additional children. Predating the *Field of Dreams* movie by a century, Hull-House was perhaps one of the earliest American experiences of the power of the premise that 'if you build it, they will come'. In Addams' early experience at Hull-House, though, she and her colleagues had a difficult time building fast enough to accommodate the increasing numbers of people who came.

3.6 Forty years at Hull-House

For what, precisely, did they come? At first, it was not clear to anyone, including Addams herself, what exactly Hull-House could do for its neighbors. Her only sentiment at the beginning was that she somehow belonged there, amongst 'the poor', and that, once situated, she would figure out what to do next. She wrote that her 'early contention' was 'that the mere foothold of a house, easily accessible, ample in space, hospitable and tolerant in spirit, situated in the midst of the large foreign colonies which so easily isolate themselves in American cities, would be in itself a serviceable thing for Chicago' (Addams, 1910, p. 90). Sure enough, this proved to be true fairly quickly, with the neighbors' 'hearty welcome' being followed soon after with their expression of some of their most pressing needs. Writes Addams: 'From the first it seemed understood that we were ready to perform the humblest neighborhood services. We were asked to wash the new-born babies, and to prepare the dead for burial, to nurse the sick, and to "mind the children"' (Addams, 1910, p. 110). It was the need to 'mind the children' that led early on to the creation of the kindergarten and its lengthy waiting list mentioned above.

It would be a grave error to infer from these initial examples, though, that Addams and her colleagues were simply dishing out charity to the needy. It was crucial for Addams, and proved to be crucial to the success of Hull-House, and is crucial to our inclusion of Addams and Hull-House in this volume, that these 'services' were not considered or offered as charity. She was decidedly not taking pity on those less fortunate than herself, nor was she using them to create a learning experience for the well-off who needed to be exposed to real life, as she had seen at Oxford. Rather, she writes: 'Hull-House was soberly opened on the theory that the dependence of classes on each other is reciprocal; and that as the social relation is essentially a reciprocal relation, it gives a form of expression that has peculiar value' (Addams, 1910, p. 91).

To understand the operation of Hull-House, one must first understand Addams' personal perspective on democracy, particularly that American brand of democracy that she associated so closely with Abraham Lincoln and her own father. As she writes: 'In our early effort at Hull-House to hand on to our neighbors whatever of help we had found for ourselves, we made much of Lincoln' (Addams, 1910, p. 37). They made much of Lincoln not only, or not primarily, in theory but also, as this passage suggests, in practice as well. In practice, Addams saw no distinction between herself, her friends and their needs on the one hand and her neighbors and their needs on the other. Whatever had been of help to her could equally be of help to her neighbors. This, in itself, may not seem radical, but when phrased in the reverse, based on the reciprocity she emphasized in the above, the more interesting and useful implications of this view for practice begin to emerge. Phrased in the reverse order, the principle becomes: what is found to be helpful for her neighbors is the same thing that Addams would find helpful herself, were she in their situation. The major implications of this principle are first, when someone appears to be in need, ask the person what it is that she or he may find helpful or useful; most often that person will know just as well, if not better, than someone else what it is that he or she could use under the present circumstances. Second, when the person does not know or cannot identify what would be useful, put yourself in his or her situation and identify what you would yourself find useful under those circumstances; chances are, what you would find useful in that situation will often be found to be useful by the other person as well.

Before the reader dismisses these implications as obvious, consider how rarely such principles had been invoked to this point in the care of individuals with serious mental illnesses. The assumption that the presence of mental illness had somehow made the person *other* (i.e. other than who he or she used to be, other than me, other than human) had made it unlikely, if not impossible, that people with mental illnesses would be treated in this way. The same was true during Addams' time of people who were poor, unemployed, physically disabled or immigrants – they too were being oppressed and discriminated against and viewed as fundamentally *other*. As Addams had witnessed, and participated in, during her visits to London, debates were raging at the time about how such individuals should best be managed, punished or helped within the context of a civilized society. What she saw as largely missing from these debates was the notion that these individuals were no different from any other individuals in any kind of fundamental or basic way, and that these individuals therefore didn't really require anything different from what anyone else would value under the same circumstances. It was primarily the circumstance, the life situation, the material conditions, that were foreign, dehumanizing, unacceptable and in need of urgent intervention – not the people themselves. The people were no different, no less human and no more or less in need of the same things as others; the major difference was rather in their access to opportunities and resources. These were things that could be made available to them in relatively immediate and direct ways. This was what Hull-House had to offer.

The other thing Hull-House had to offer, and the way in which Addams protected Hull-House from deteriorating into a charitable institution founded on misplaced pity, was Addams' conviction in the importance of reciprocity, not just in principle in terms of how people should understand and address each others' unmet needs but also in practice in terms of how people, all people, share responsibility for each other through action. She credited Lincoln with the origins of this value, and suggested that he knew that 'if this tremendous experiment [of American democracy] was to come to fruition, it must be brought about by the people themselves; that there was no other capital fund upon which to draw' (Addams, 1910, p. 35). She relates the following story as one of the significant times in her life when this value was driven home to her by her father's actions:

> I remember an incident occurring when I was about fifteen years old, in which the conviction was driven into my mind that the people themselves were the great resource of the country. My father had made a little address of reminiscence at a meeting of 'the old settlers of Stephenson County', which was held every summer in the grove beside the mill, relating his experiences in inducing the farmers of the county to subscribe for stock in the Northwestern Railroad, which was the first to penetrate the county and make a connection with the Great Lakes at Chicago. Many of the Pennsylvania German farmers doubted the value of 'the whole new-fangled business', and had no use for any railroad, much less for one in which they were asked to risk their hard-earned savings. My father told of his despair in one farmers'

community dominated by such prejudice which did not in the least give way under his argument, but finally melted under the enthusiasm of a high-spirited German matron who took a share to be paid for 'out of butter and egg money'. As he related his admiration of her, an old woman's piping voice in the audience called out: 'I'm here to-day, Mr. Addams, and I'd do it again if you asked me'. The old woman, bent and broken by her seventy years of toilsome life, was brought to the platform and I was much impressed by my father's grave presentation of her as 'one of the public-spirited pioneers to whose heroic fortitude we are indebted for the development of this country'. (Addams, 1910, pp. 35–36)

How did this view of democracy in action influence the operation of Hull-House? In many subtle and not so subtle ways. In the first place, Hull-House was founded on the American ideal that everyone is equal in worth and should have equal access to opportunities. The fact that this has not been true historically is not to be justified or excused on moral, ethical or religious grounds (e.g. as in poor people deserve their lot based on sin or sloth) but is to be viewed as an injustice that needs to be corrected in the present. Following her experience of the bullfight in Madrid, for Addams this was no longer a theoretical issue to be studied or debated but was now instead an impetus for action. Recognizing this fact, one had no choice but to question the status quo and act in ways that would correct the existing inequities. She describes her emerging and maturing perspective:

> There was also growing within me an almost passionate devotion to the ideals of democracy, and when in all history had these ideals been so thrillingly expressed as when the faith of the fisherman and the slave had been boldly opposed to the accepted moral belief that the well-being of a privileged few might justly be built upon the ignorance and sacrifice of the many? (Addams, 1910, p. 79)

Her calling in life, and one of the core purposes of Hull-House, would thus be to offer education to those who had not benefited from the opportunity to pursue it in the past and to lessen the social sacrifice that had to be borne by 'the many'. These two purposes were already evident in the way in which Addams described their initial experience of opening the kindergarten for neighborhood children. Her most pressing concerns were not with improving literacy or with freeing up young mothers to become employed and secure an independent income. Her concerns were rather with offering children who otherwise would not have such opportunities the same chances for taking initiative, exercising their imagination and developing friendships that other, more fortunate, children would have had as a matter of course. She writes:

> That first kindergarten was a constant source of education to us . . . The value of these groups consisted almost entirely in arousing a

> higher imagination and in giving the children the opportunity which
> they could not have in the crowded schools, for initiative and for
> independent social relationships. (Addams, 1910, pp. 103, 105)

Note that Addams speaks first of learning from the children and from the kindergarten experience. Within a fully democratic society, everyone can learn and everyone, including even very young children, has things to teach. Human relationships, at least following infancy and prior to dementia, are not uni-directional or asymmetrical in nature; they are, and should be recognized as, reciprocal. To attempt to relate to another person in a non-reciprocal fashion is to distort the human quality of the relationship and to treat the other person as an object. Martin Buber would come a half-century later to define these differences in relating as 'I–thou' and 'I–it' relationships, and both he and Emmanuel Levinas would derive from this basic reciprocity in human relationships the foundations for ethical practice and behavior. With respect to the current volume, we will see this point and distinction take on renewed significance in the work of Franco Basaglia, who was influenced by the existentialist philosophy of Jean-Paul Sartre. For Addams, however, this basic conviction in the reciprocal nature of human relationships was a core aspect of American and Lincolnian democracy.

In addition to encouraging Addams and her colleagues to learn from the children they were teaching, this principle of reciprocity encouraged Addams to focus in particular on what the children were doing, how they were making use of the opportunities offered to them. This brings us to a second implication of democracy in action at Hull-House. The emphasis in Hull-House programming is not on what the few staff do, on what the services are that are being offered or even on what the people being served need. The emphasis is on what the people *do* with the opportunities and resources afforded to them. Once again, they are not objects to be acted on by caring or compassionate others, but they are themselves active agents in their own lives. They need to be engaged as such. This is illustrated in the following story of a woman who might very well have been placed in a nursing home today, had she the resources, or about whom many case conferences would focus on what was to be done *about* her in terms of structure and supervision. At Hull-House, the most immediate focus was on what she was *doing* that was concerning and on what else she could be *doing* instead. Writes Addams:

> In spite of these flourishing clubs for children early established at
> Hull-House, and the fact that our first organized undertaking was a
> kindergarten, we were very insistent that the Settlement should not be
> primarily for the children, and that it was absurd to suppose that grown
> people would not respond to opportunities for education and social
> life. Our enthusiastic kindergartner herself demonstrated this with an
> old woman of ninety who, because she was left alone all day while her
> daughter cooked in a restaurant, had formed such a persistent habit of
> picking the plaster off the walls that one landlord after another refused
> to have her for a tenant. It required but a few weeks' time to teach

her to make large paper chains, and gradually she was content to do it all day long, and in the end took quite as much pleasure in adorning the walls as she had formally taken in demolishing them. Fortunately the landlord had never heard the aesthetic principle that exposure of basic construction is more desirable than gaudy decoration. In course of time it was discovered that the old woman could speak Gaelic, and when one or two grave professors came to see her, the neighborhood was filled with pride that such a wonder lived in their midst. To mitigate life for a woman of ninety was an unfailing refutation of the statement that the Settlement was designed for the young.

The older settlers as well as their children throughout the years have given genuine help to our various enterprises for neighborhood improvement, and from their own memories of earlier hardships have made many shrewd suggestions for alleviating the difficulties of that first sharp struggle with untoward conditions. (Addams, 1910, pp. 107–109)

It is true, of course, that this focus does not offer a panacea for human misery, that there are not always such happy endings. Addams offers the following examples from her first days at Hull-House to show that she is far from Pollyanna-like in her attitude towards the human race:

Occasionally these neighborly offices unexpectedly uncovered ugly human traits. For six weeks after an operation we kept in one of our three bedrooms a forlorn little baby who, because he was born with a cleft palate, was most unwelcome even to his mother, and we were horrified when he died of neglect a week after he was returned to his home; a little Italian bride of fifteen sought shelter with us one November evening to escape her husband who had beaten her every night for a week when he returned home from work, because she had lost her wedding ring; two of us officiated quite alone at the birth of an illegitimate child because the doctor was late in arriving, and none of the honest Irish matrons would 'touch the likes of her' . . . (Addams, 1910, p. 111)

Such experiences, while tragic and likely to engender feelings of despair, hopelessness and even perhaps impotence in the face of certain realities of human existence, did not dissuade Addams or her colleagues from their fundamental convictions that people are more alike than different and that the best way to help people who are struggling is to offer them the opportunities and resources needed for them to set things right. Importantly, she notes that 'in spite of some untoward experiences, we were constantly impressed with the uniform kindness and courtesy we received'. She continues:

Perhaps these first days laid the simple human foundations which are certainly essential for continuous living among the poor; first, genuine preference for residence in an industrial quarter to any other part of the city, because it is interesting and makes the human appeal; and second, the conviction, in the words of Canon Barnett, that the things that make men alike are finer and better than the things that keep them apart, and that these basic likenesses, if they are properly accentuated, easily transcend the less essential differences of race, language, creed, and tradition. (Addams, 1910, pp. 111–112)

Hull-House remains to this day a testament to the fact that diverse peoples can join around common concerns and missions and overcome these kinds of differences. Situated in a predominantly immigrant neighborhood, Hull-House hosted guests from numerous ethnicities and nationalities, and served as a hub for the American dialogue about race relations unfolding at the time (recall that Addams was a co-founder of the NAACP). In the following paragraph, she tries to illustrate the approach of the Settlement House to these issues, including the ways in which the sum of efforts from both the staff and the neighborhood residents leads to a whole that is much greater than the sum of its parts. With the contributions of all parties to the common good, things become possible that otherwise would have remained impossible. This is the hope and the work of Hull-House, which included, as mentioned in the passage below, a prominent role for spirituality. Writes Addams:

In a thousand voices singing the Hallelujah Chorus in Handel's 'Messiah', it is possible to distinguish the leading voices, but the differences of training and cultivation between them and the voices in the chorus, are lost in the unity of purpose and in the fact that they are all human voices lifted by a high motive. This is a weak illustration of what a Settlement attempts to do. It aims, in a measure, to develop whatever of social life its neighborhood may afford, to focus and give form to that life, to bring to bear upon it the results of cultivation and training; but it receives in exchange for the music of isolated voices the volume and strength of the chorus ... The subjective necessity which led to the opening of Hull-House combined the three trends: first, the desire to interpret democracy in social terms; secondly, the impulse beating at the very source of our lives, urging us to aid in the race progress; and, thirdly, the Christian movement toward humanitarianism. (Addams, 1910, pp. 124–125)

3.7 Distilling the active ingredients

So what can we learn from Addams' 40-plus years at Hull-House that can be useful to us in our attempts to understand and implement recovery-oriented practice in mental health? In order to answer this question in the following sections, it will be important first to distil the active ingredients in Addams' innovative approach to the social problems she and her colleagues addressed. We have already noted the strong foundation laid in the principles of American democracy and Addams' particular interpretation of these principles through the eyes and work of Abraham Lincoln. For Addams, one of the obvious assumptions of this view is that human beings need more than food and shelter in order to live truly human lives, to exist and flourish rather than simply survive. These additional needs include the need for freedom to exercise one's agency and pursue one's own view of happiness; the need for pleasure, enjoyment and a sense of personal meaning and purpose in life; the need for social relationships and to have a sense of belonging to a community and the need for the shared rituals and rhythms of collective life. Each of these needs is as basic to a person's psychological, social and spiritual survival as bread and water would be to his or her physical survival. As a result, each of these domains is equally relevant to the work of the Settlement House. Writes Addams: 'If it is natural to feed the hungry and care for the sick, it is certainly natural to give pleasure to the young, comfort to the aged and to minister to the deep-seated craving for social intercourse that all men feel' (Addams, 1910, p. 116).

For our purposes – as well it appears as for her own – Addams placed special emphasis on the first two of these needs for freedom, agency and the pursuit of pleasure, enjoyment and a sense of meaning and purpose. That is, she viewed people as primarily active agents in their own lives, constantly setting and seeking new aspirations, goals and relationships. Perhaps owing in part to her own dissatisfaction with the contemplative or purely literary life – that 'snare of preparation' in which she felt she had become trapped early in her adult life – she even came to view action as the only sure path to truth. The mind, the imagination and even the senses could be lulled into a false complacency or an illusory sense of what is real. It is only through embodied action in the world that one can find out for sure what is true. She writes of a growing conviction to which she attributes religious significance 'that action is the only medium man has for receiving and appropriating truth; that the doctrine must be known through the will' (Addams, 1910, p. 123). From this conviction comes her consistent focus not only on her own action or that of the other staff at Hull-House but also on the actions of the people she hoped to assist. They also could only access the truth through the medium of action; they also could only improve their own lot in life through their own actions. While their actions could be aided, encouraged and supported by others, the primary focus remained on those actions that they themselves needed to make in order to move ahead in their own lives. Addams saw her role as primarily increasing the person's access to the opportunities to undertake those actions and providing material and social and emotional support for them to do so, when needed.

Within such a perspective, the primary evil or hardship the Settlement House had to address was not poverty, discrimination, abuse or trauma per se but rather the 'want of a proper outlet' for the person to exercise his or her 'active faculties'. She writes: 'It is true that there is nothing after disease, indigence and a sense of guilt, so fatal to health and to life itself as the want of a proper outlet for active faculties' (Addams, 1910, p. 118). With whatever particular situation Addams was faced, her attention therefore was drawn purposefully and pointedly to what the person in question could do, or could not do, for him- or herself. When the actions required were possible, assistance might take the simple form of advice, education, encouragement or material assistance with such things as transportation, child care or money for new clothes. When the actions required were not possible because of some barrier or obstacle lying in the way or because of a lack of opportunities owing to social, cultural or political forces, then those barriers or obstacles would have to be removed or the social, cultural or political forces would have to be addressed and altered to be made more consistent with American/Lincolnian democratic principles. It was in her pursuit of this last avenue of recourse that Addams founded, co-founded or led numerous political, social and cultural causes and movements, all of which shared the common purpose of ensuring equal rights for all citizens, including the right to be free from exploitation and abuse. For example, in addition to fighting against child labor and the exploitation of women, Addams was a strong supporter of organized labor, the protection of civil liberties and the advancement of people of color. To illustrate how Addams and the Settlement House approached such issues, we will offer a few examples that unfolded at each of the various levels of the immediate people involved, the city as a whole and the nation at large.

Before turning to these examples, though, it is important for us to highlight that one of the most important characteristics of the Settlement House, according to Addams, was its flexibility and its willingness to 'experiment' (Addams, 1910, p. 126). This was important for a number of reasons, but at the outset we can suggest that it was especially important early on in the history of Hull-House because Addams and her colleagues admittedly did not know what to do. We saw this when they first moved into the house in 1889, solely on the conviction that such a welcoming establishment would be 'a serviceable thing for Chicago'. This same sense of open-ended eagerness tempered with humility continued throughout the early days of Hull-House, and perhaps persisted there until Addams' death. She certainly retained the sense that in the affairs of the human heart and soul precious little could be understood, not to mention predicted, beforehand. She offers the following example from early in the history of Hull-House to demonstrate how, even in cases where the outcome is at best unclear and at worst a failure, experimenting alongside of people in need is sure to offer an education in the nature of human beings – even if that is not appreciated at the time. The experience that Addams describes in the following passage has surely been had by thousands of social workers since, and the answers, according to some, remain just as elusive today as they were a century ago. She writes:

> Many experiences in those early years, although vivid, seemed to contain no illumination; nevertheless they doubtless permanently affected our judgments concerning what is called crime and vice. I recall a series of striking episodes on the day when I took the wife and child, as well as the old godfather, of an Italian convict to visit him in the State Penitentiary. When we approached the prison, the sight of its heavy stone walls and armed sentries threw the godfather into a paroxysm of rage; he cast his hat upon the ground and stamped upon it, tore his hair, and loudly fulminated in weird Italian oaths, until

one of the guards, seeing his strange actions, came to inquire if 'the gentleman was having a fit'. When we finally saw the convict, his wife, to my extreme distress, talked of nothing but his striped clothing, until the poor man wept with chagrin.

Upon our return journey to Chicago, the little son aged eight presented me with two oranges, so affectionately and gayly that I was filled with reflections upon the advantage of each generation making a fresh start, when the train boy, finding the stolen fruit in my lap, violently threatened to arrest the child. But stranger than any episode was the fact itself that neither the convict, his wife, nor his godfather for a moment considered him a criminal. He had merely gotten excited over cards and had stabbed his adversary with a knife. 'Why should a man who took his luck badly be kept forever from the sun?' was their reiterated inquiry. (Addams, 1910, pp. 144–145)

3.8 Interventions with individuals

We are not told what outcome Addams had hoped to achieve by accompanying this family to visit their loved one in the penitentiary, nor does she share any more about the sense she made of the trip upon her return. We begin with this experience, however, to ensure the reader that we appreciate that things do not always go well in the world of social services, and that Addams understood that her approach was not guaranteed to succeed, however that would be determined. This leads to another of the reasons why it is important for settlement houses to experiment: in the world of human affairs, it is often impossible to know ahead of time what the outcome will be of any action or series of actions. There are simply too many forces at play and too much that is unknown, even in perhaps what appears to be the simplest of instances.

In the following instance, though, Addams' strategy did pay off more handsomely. In this case, she was moved not by what actions a group of people needed to undertake in the future but rather by the significance of the actions this group had performed in the past and the fact that this significance had been lost to present and future generations. In other words, these were people who had already done what they needed to do; it is just that the passage of time and the crossing from one culture to another had prevented their immigrant children from appreciating these actions and the significant contributions these actions had made to their lives. Addams writes:

> An overmastering desire to reveal the humbler immigrant parents to their own children lay at the base of what has come to be called the Hull-House Labor Museum. This was first suggested to my mind one early spring day when I saw an old Italian woman, her distaff against her homesick face, patiently spinning a thread by the simple stick spindle so reminiscent of all southern Europe. I was walking down Polk Street, perturbed in spirit, because it seemed so difficult to come into genuine relations with the Italian women and because they

themselves so often lost their hold upon their Americanized children. It seemed to me that Hull-House ought to be able to devise some educational enterprise which should build a bridge between European and American experiences in such wise as to give them both more meaning and a sense of relation. I meditated that perhaps the power to see life as a whole is more needed in the immigrant quarter of a large city than anywhere else, and that the lack of this power is the most fruitful source of misunderstanding between European immigrants and their children, as it is between them and their American neighbors; and why should that chasm between fathers and sons, yawning at the feet of each generation, be made so unnecessarily cruel and impassable to these bewildered immigrants? Suddenly I looked up and saw the old woman with her distaff, sitting in the sun on the steps of a tenement house. She might have served as a model for one of Michelangelo's Fates, but her face brightened as I passed and, holding up her spindle for me to see, she called out that when she had spun a little more yarn, she would knit a pair of stockings for her goddaughter. The occupation of the old woman gave me the clue that was needed. Could we not interest the young people working in the neighborhood factories in these older forms of industry, so that, through their own parents and grandparents, they would find a dramatic representation of the inherited resources of their daily occupation. If these young people could actually see that the complicated machinery of the factory had been evolved from simple tools, they might at least make a beginning toward that education which Dr. Dewey defines as 'a continuing reconstruction of experience'. They might also lay a foundation for reverence of the past which Goethe declares to be the basis of all sound progress. (Addams, 1910, pp. 235–237)

The Dr Dewey to whom Addams refers was John Dewey, an extremely influential American philosopher and educator, only one of the many such people with whom she was close friends and colleagues. In this case, through conversations with Dewey and others, she hatched the plan of a Hull-House Labor Museum as offering a possible bridge between the generations. She continues:

My exciting walk on Polk Street was followed by many talks with Dr. Dewey and with one of the teachers in his school who was a resident at Hull-House. Within a month a room was fitted up to which we might invite those of our neighbors who were possessed of old crafts and who were eager to use them.

We found in the immediate neighborhood at least four varieties of these most primitive methods of spinning and three distinct variations of the same spindle in connection with wheels. It was possible to put these seven into historic sequence and order and to connect the whole with the present method of factory spinning. The same thing was done for weaving, and on every Saturday evening a little exhibit was made of these various forms of labor in the textile industry. Within one room a Syrian woman, a Greek, an Italian, a Russian, and an Irishwoman enabled even the most casual observer to see that there is no break in orderly evolution if we look at history from the industrial standpoint; that industry develops similarly and peacefully year by year among the workers of each nation, heedless of differences in language, religion, and political experiences. (Addams, 1910, p. 237)

The aim of the museum was not purely educational, of course, as Addams viewed it primarily as a means of communication between generations. Having been silenced by their travels to a foreign country with a foreign language, and by their increasing age set against the background of an urban industrial culture that only valued the new, older immigrants were able to reclaim their experience and their voices through this medium. By putting them back in touch with what they had done and from whence they had come, these immigrants were able to regain their status as experts, as makers and as contributors to the common good and to the historical progression of humanity. As Addams writes: 'far beyond its direct educational value, we prize [the museum] because it so often puts the immigrants into the position of teachers, and we imagine that it affords them a pleasant change from the tutelage in which all Americans, including their own children, are so apt to hold them' (Addams, 1910, pp. 240–241). From novice to expert, from student to teacher, 'from having been stupidly entertained, they themselves did the entertaining. Because of a direct appeal to former experiences, the immigrant visitors were able for the moment to instruct their American hostesses in an old and honored craft, as was indeed becoming to their age and experience' (Addams, 1910, p. 241).

The museum, in this way, served at least two major functions. First, it put the older generation of immigrants back in touch with their earlier actions and experiences and thus restored to them their sense of dignity and self-worth in the midst of a foreign, if not also hostile, environment. Second, it transferred this sense of value from each individual to the larger social sphere, also restoring to these immigrants their deserved social standing within their families, and within the broader community. The story of Angelina and her mother illustrate these processes well.

I recall a certain Italian girl who came every Saturday evening to a cooking class in the same building in which her mother spun in the Labor Museum exhibit; and yet Angelina always left her mother at the front door while she herself went around to a side door because she did not wish to be too closely identified in the eyes of the rest of the cooking class with an Italian woman who wore a kerchief over her head, uncouth boots, and short petticoats. One evening, however, Angelina saw her mother surrounded by a group of visitors from the School of Education who much admired the spinning, and she concluded from their conversation that her mother was 'the best stick-spindle spinner in America'. When she inquired from me as to the truth of this deduction, I took occasion to describe the Italian village in which her mother had lived, something of her free life, and how, because of the opportunity she and the other women of the village had to drop their spindles over the edge of a precipice, they had developed a skill in spinning beyond that of the neighboring towns. I dilated somewhat on the freedom and beauty of that life – how hard it must be to exchange it all for a two-room tenement, and to give up a beautiful homespun kerchief for an ugly department store hat. I intimated it was most unfair to judge her by these things alone, and that while she must depend on her daughter to learn the new ways, she also had a right to expect her daughter to know something of the old ways.

That which I could not convey to the child, but upon which my own mind persistently dwelt, was that her mother's whole life had been spent in a secluded spot under the rule of traditional and narrowly localized observances, until her very religion clung to local sanctities – to the shrine before which she had always prayed, to the pavement and walls of the low vaulted church – and then suddenly she was torn from it all and literally put out to sea, straight away from the solid habits of her religious and domestic life, and she now walked timidly but with poignant sensibility upon a new and strange shore.

It was easy to see that the thought of her mother with any other background than that of the tenement was new to Angelina, and at least two things resulted; she allowed her mother to pull out of the big box under the bed the beautiful homespun garments which had been previously hidden away as uncouth; and she openly came into the Labor Museum by the same door as did her mother, proud at least of the mastery of the craft which had been so much admired. (Addams, 1910, pp. 243–245)

3.9 Interventions with collectives

Addams, like Meyer and Sullivan who followed, viewed social structures and conditions as much more relevant, and contributive, to mental illnesses and other social problems than their predecessors. While Pinel and Tuke might have viewed the family context and perhaps even the immediate social environment as contributing to, if not actually causing, the person's difficulties, Addams and her contemporaries broadened this scope considerably to include community and societal level forces. The interventions emanating out of Hull-House were thus not limited to individuals and families. If social and political forces were at play in making people sick, both physically and mentally; in driving them into prolonged unemployment and poverty; in severing ties between generations and so on, then social and political forces also could be and needed to be addressed and changed for the betterment of all. An illustrative example of this philosophy in practice is provided at the level of the city of Chicago by the problem of public sanitation. The approach Addams and Hull-House took to this issue was to provide a model for effective advocacy on numerous other issues that emerged further down the road.

As Addams notes, this was one of the first community issues to come to their attention when she and Starr moved into the neighborhood. She begins her chapter

in *Twenty-Years at Hull-House* on 'Public Activities and Investigations' with the
following scene:

> One of the striking features of our neighborhood twenty years ago,
> and one to which we never became reconciled, was the presence
> of huge wooden garbage boxes fastened to the street pavement in
> which the undisturbed refuse accumulated day by day. The system of
> garbage collecting was inadequate throughout the city but it became
> the greatest menace in a ward such as ours, where the normal amount
> of waste was much increased by the decayed fruit and vegetables
> discarded by the Italian and Greek fruit peddlers, and by the residuum
> left over from the piles of filthy rags which were fished out of the city
> dumps and brought to the homes of the rag pickers for further sorting
> and washing.
>
> The children of our neighborhood twenty years ago played their
> games in and around these huge garbage boxes. They were the first
> objects that the toddling child learned to climb; their bulk afforded a
> barricade and their contents provided missiles in all the battles of the
> older boys; and finally they became the seats upon which absorbed
> lovers held enchanted converse. We are obliged to remember that
> all children eat everything which they find and that odors have a
> curious and intimate power of entwining themselves into our tenderest
> memories, before even the residents of Hull-House can understand
> their own early enthusiasm for the removal of these boxes and the
> establishment of a better system of refuse collection. (Addams, 1910,
> pp. 281–283)

What was to be done? Being a firm pragmatist, Addams understood that it
would be difficult to gain the attention and support of politicians who lived a safe
and reassuring distance from these alleyways, people who, unlike her, were not
'constantly surrounded' by the stench of the decomposing refuse. She also guessed
perhaps that her complaints would be dismissed by self-serving or indifferent city
bureaucrats who would be more likely to blame the problem on the neighborhood
residents and their 'filthy' ways than on any shortcomings of the city's public works
operation. Therefore, the initial efforts to clean up this situation had to be local and
home-grown. Addams continues:

> During our first three years on Halsted Street, we had established a
> small incinerator at Hull-House and we had many times reported
> the untoward conditions of the ward to the city hall. We had also
> arranged many talks for the immigrants, pointing out that although a
> woman may sweep her own doorway in her native village and allow the
> refuse to innocently decay in the open air and sunshine, in a crowded
> city quarter, if the garbage is not properly collected and destroyed, a
> tenement-house mother may see her children sicken and die, and that
> the immigrants must therefore not only keep their own houses clean,

> but must also help the authorities to keep the city clean. (Addams,
> 1910, p. 283)

As one might have surmised, however, such local efforts were inadequate to the
scope and magnitude of the problem at hand. After addressing those contributions
to the garbage problem over which she and her neighbors had some control, and
upon the impending visit of her own 'delicate' nephew, Addams realized that she
would have to take her efforts up a notch to a higher authority. She writes:

> Possibly our efforts slightly modified the worst conditions, but they
> still remained intolerable, and the fourth summer the situation became
> for me absolutely desperate when I realized in a moment of panic that
> my delicate little nephew for whom I was guardian, could not be with
> me at Hull-House at all unless the sickening odors were reduced. I
> may well be ashamed that other delicate children who were torn from
> their families, not into boarding school but into eternity, had not long
> before driven me to effective action. Under the direction of the first
> man who came as a resident to Hull-House we began a systematic
> investigation of the city system of garbage collection, both as to its
> efficiency in other wards and its possible connection with the death
> rate in the various wards of the city. (Addams, 1910, pp. 283–284)

As Addams had turned to John Dewey for advice and suggestions for the Labor
Museum, at this point she began to elicit the involvement of other players in
addressing the garbage problem. A male resident of Hull-House at the time had
the expertise to initiate an investigation of the problem on the broader scale of the
city as a whole, and other residents and neighbors were solicited to join the effort.
This became, in fact, one of the first initiatives of the Women's Club which had first
formed around the creation of the Hull-House kindergarten. The members of this
club came together, writes Addams:

> in quite a new way that summer when we discussed with them the high
> death rate so persistent in our ward. After several club meetings devoted
> to the subject, despite the fact that the death rate rose highest in the
> congested foreign colonies and not in the streets in which most of the
> Irish American club women lived, twelve of their number undertook in
> connection with the residents, to carefully investigate the conditions of
> the alleys. During August and September the substantiated reports of
> violations of the law sent in from Hull-House to the health department
> were one thousand and thirty-seven. For the club woman who had
> finished a long day's work of washing or ironing followed by the
> cooking of a hot supper, it would have been much easier to sit on her
> doorstep during a summer evening than to go up and down ill-kept
> alleys and get into trouble with her neighbors over the condition
> of their garbage boxes. It required both civic enterprise and moral
> conviction to be willing to do this three evenings a week during the

hottest and most uncomfortable months of the year. Nevertheless, a certain number of women persisted, as did the residents, and three city inspectors in succession were transferred from the ward because of unsatisfactory services. Still the death rate remained high and the condition seemed little improved throughout the next winter. In sheer desperation, the following spring when the city contracts were awarded for the removal of garbage, with the backing of two well-known business men, I put in a bid for the garbage removal of the nineteenth ward. My paper was thrown out on a technicality but the incident induced the mayor to appoint me the garbage inspector of the ward. (Addams, 1910, pp. 284–285)

Addams acknowledges that eyebrows were raised, both outside and even inside of Hull-House, to see such a woman's 'abrupt departure into the ways of men' (Addams, 1910, p. 287). For her part, however, she was unapologetic, persistent and, as we can see in the mayor's eventual response, persuasive. She was careful to argue the point from an accepted 'woman's perspective', that is from the perspective of home, health and nursing the sick. In an elegant line of reasoning that is unfortunately still debated among the health professions to this day, Addams argued that it was a logical extension of the role of the nurse to eradicate the diseases from which she and other women would then otherwise have to nurse people back to health once infected. She writes: 'It took a great deal of explanation to convey the idea even remotely that if it were a womanly task to go about in tenement houses in order to nurse the sick, it might be quite as womanly to go through the same district in order to prevent the breeding of so-called "filth diseases"' (Addams, 1910, p. 287).

In practice, though, it was not nearly so easy to remain within the narrowly defined roles of women that held sway at the end of the nineteenth century. By becoming ward garbage inspector, Addams not only entered into competition with men for the 'political plum' of the paid position but also put herself into a position of having to observe, scrutinize and enforce appropriate work being done by men on a daily basis. She describes her unpleasant role as follows:

The salary was a thousand dollars a year, and the loss of that political 'plum' made a great stir among the politicians. The position was no sinecure whether regarded from the point of view of getting up at six in the morning to see that the men were early at work; or of following the loaded wagons, uneasily dropping their contents at intervals, to their dreary destination at the dump; or of insisting that the contractor must increase the number of his wagons from nine to thirteen and from thirteen to seventeen, although he assured me that he lost money on every one and that the former inspector had let him off with seven; or of taking careless landlords into court because they would not provide the proper garbage receptacles; or of arresting the tenant who tried to make the garbage wagons carry away the contents of his stable. (Addams, 1910, pp. 285–286)

In addition to this inspector role, Addams and Hull-House residents and neighbors undertook many other activities to clean up the streets and, eventually, to clean up the city bureaucracy that accounted for the filth piling up to begin with. These efforts included starting an additional six incinerators, initiating recycling and holding city officials and businessmen accountable for their own actions or lack thereof. In this regard, Addams provides two examples:

> We made desperate attempts to have the dead animals removed by the contractor who was paid most liberally by the city for that purpose but who, we slowly discovered, always made the police ambulances do the work, delivering the carcasses upon freight cars for shipment to a soap factory in Indiana where they were sold for a good price although the contractor himself was the largest stockholder in the concern. Perhaps our greatest achievement was the discovery of a pavement eighteen inches under the surface in a narrow street, although after it was found we triumphantly discovered a record of its existence in the city archives. The Italians living on the street were much interested but displayed little astonishment, perhaps because they were accustomed to see buried cities exhumed. This pavement became the *casus belli* between myself and the street commissioner when I insisted that its restoration belonged to him, after I had removed the first eight inches of garbage. The matter was finally settled by the mayor himself, who permitted me to drive him to the entrance of the street in what the children called my 'garbage phaeton' and who took my side of the controversy. (Addams, 1910, pp. 286–287)

As a result of the various investigations carried out by Hull-House residents, including studies of the transmission of infectious diseases through faulty plumbing, 11 of the 24 people employed by the Chicago Sanitary Bureau were fired and extensive graft was revealed to be taking place at City Hall and in the plumbers' union, the public exposure of which cost Hull-House some rather large donors and a few influential friends.

A final example of how Addams and Hull-House became engaged in collective issues and intervened at ever higher levels of communities and governments is provided by the labor movement and her role within it. As with everything else, Addams' relationships with the trade and labor unions did not simply travel in one direction. She did, for the most part, support labor in its efforts to secure safe, dignified and reasonable work environments and hours, a decent wage, good benefits and so on. She also was well-respected enough by business leaders and the government to act often as a mediator of disputes or as an ambassador of goodwill between warring parties. But her expectations for the unions were the same as her expectations for the residents and neighbors of Hull-House. They were not just to be the fortunate recipients of her actions on their behalf but also expected to see the ultimate aim of their efforts to be a greater good as well. They were expected to support and share the mission of Hull-House as well as to benefit from its support, and to understand the broader vision of a collective good. As Addams concludes, she and the labor unions were involved in 'a general social movement concerning all members of society and not merely a class struggle' (Addams, 1910, p. 213).

According to Addams: 'This special value of the trades-unions first became clear to the residents of Hull-House in connection with the sweating system' (Addams, 1910, p. 208). In addressing and trying to eliminate the sweatshops, it would not be enough to liberate the workers from such exploitive conditions and to close the shops. As we have now learned many times over, closing one shop often encourages other shops to be opened elsewhere, while pulling individuals out of sweatshops without helping to secure them better employment leaves them destitute. Had they not been destitute to begin with, they might likely not have been entrapped by the sweatshop in the first place. Just addressing the sweatshop therefore does not address the root cause of the problem, a root that extends out beyond the individual sweatshop and individual worker and owner to the community at large. From her numerous efforts in advocating for fair labor laws, for a rehabilitative rather than punitive juvenile justice system, for civil liberties for all, for the advancement of immigrants and minority communities and finally for global peace, she came increasingly to the conviction that:

> without the advance and improvement of the whole, no man can hope
> for any lasting improvement in his own moral or material individual
> condition; and that the subjective necessity for Social Settlements is
> therefore identical with that necessity, which urges us on toward social
> and individual salvation. (Addams, 1910, p. 128)

3.10 Applications to mental health

> The Settlement then, is an experimental effort to aid in the solution
> of the social and industrial problems which are engendered by the
> modern conditions of life in a great city ... The only thing to be
> dreaded in the Settlement is that it lose its flexibility, its power of quick
> adaptation, its readiness to change its methods as its environment
> may demand. It must be open to conviction and must have a deep
> and abiding sense of tolerance. It must be hospitable and ready for
> experiment. It should demand from its residents a scientific patience in
> the accumulation of facts and the steady holding of their sympathies as
> one of the best instruments for that accumulation. It must be grounded
> in a philosophy whose foundation is on the solidarity of the human
> race, a philosophy which will not waver when the race happens to be
> represented by a drunken woman or an idiot boy. Its residents must
> be emptied of all conceit of opinion and all self-assertion, and ready
> to arouse and interpret the public opinion of their neighborhood.
> They must be content to live quietly side by side with their neighbors,
> until they grow into a sense of relationship and mutual interests. Their
> neighbors are held apart by differences of race and language which the
> residents can more easily overcome. They are bound to see the needs
> of their neighborhood as a whole, to furnish data for legislation, and to

use their influence to secure it. In short, residents are pledged to devote themselves to the duties of good citizenship and to the arousing of the social energies which too largely lie dormant in every neighborhood given over to industrialism. (Addams, 1910, pp. 126–127)

But what does any of this have to do with mental health? Have we gone so far afield in pursuing this community-based alternative that we have lost sight of our interest in recovery altogether? We think not. In this section, we will briefly point out the relevant applications of Addams' thought and work for developing a recovery-oriented approach to practice.

The first important implication of her work, and the major reason why she was selected for inclusion in this volume, is that people need not be extracted from their immediate social and physical environment in order to receive assistance. Even if social and environmental factors contribute to the onset and exacerbation of mental illness, this does not necessarily mean that people need to be removed from these factors in order to receive care or enter into and pursue recovery. One could in fact argue the reverse, as Addams did, suggesting that these conditions are best and most effectively treated in the environments where they occur. Removing the person from the environment and relationships which cause difficulty, but with which the person has grown familiar, creates a whole new set of challenges and difficulties that stem from the need to adjust to and function within the new environment. Even if these challenges and difficulties are successfully addressed, even, that is, if the person adapts extremely well to the new situation and no longer appears to experience the old difficulties, there is no reason to believe that these same difficulties will not re-arise as soon as the person returns to the original situation. We will learn more about these processes in Chapter 5, where we discuss the work of Goffman, but for now it can suffice to suggest that learning how to be a good patient within the safe and structured environment of a retreat or hospital appears to show very little benefit for the person once he or she returns to the community (where good patient behaviors are no longer rewarded).

Unless one is willing to make the case that people should never return to the community, but live for the remainder of their lives in this foreign and artificial setting, it is difficult to see how to get beyond the problem that learning theorists characterize as the failure of behavior to generalize from one setting to another. It is especially difficult to justify removing people from their usual life circumstances in order to treat and cure them when Addams and her colleagues, and scores of like-minded people since, have shown how effective it can be to assist people in managing their own difficulties within the life circumstances in which they find themselves. This is the second major implication of Addams' work for the recovery movement: that people need to be assisted in managing their own difficulties and lives to the greatest extent possible, rather than to have those difficulties, and their lives as a whole, taken over by others. Mental illness may be something I can treat, to varying degrees of effectiveness, but it remains something with which you have to live on an everyday basis. What you are likely to find helpful in learning how to deal with the illness are the same kinds of things I would likely find helpful were I in your same life situation, so to figure out how best to help you the most useful thing I can do to start is to ask you what kind of assistance you think you could use in dealing with your current situation. This is not always a question that people know how to, or can, answer, but it provides a very important and useful point of departure for the development of a helping relationship, a much different point of departure, to be sure, than much of the mental health care provided over the previous century. This care has been primarily expert/practitioner-driven, a model of care in which the practitioner knows what is best, is the authority and tells the person what he or she needs to do.

The idea that people with mental illnesses can still identify their own needs and know what is best for them remains a radical notion in much of the current mental health system in the United States.

In addition to asking people with mental illnesses how they might be best helped in their current situation, Addams' work suggests that the person him- or herself plays the central, active role in addressing this situation and moving forward in his or her life. It is both this person's responsibility and his or her right to do so. For Addams, this was primarily so because of her interpretation of 'American democracy' and her conviction in the essential importance of action as offering the most immediate and reliable access to truth. These two concepts came together in her emphasis on reciprocity in human relationships, an emphasis that permeated throughout all of the work of Hull-House. People, regardless of their needs and their perceived limitations, remain active agents in their own lives and it is necessary for social services to be respectful of and to preserve the person's own sense of agency.

We highlight this first in the case of helpers addressing the person's own needs and difficulties, as this is the first concern in providing recovery-oriented care (as it was at Hull-House). It is important to note, however, that this also remains the case in terms of viewing this person as an active agent as a helper as well as a person in need of help. From the perspective of Addams' Lincolnian democracy, a person is never in only one of these categories but is always in both. Even the most disabled person, or the person whose capacities may be severely limited, remains a citizen of the society and therefore retains both the responsibility and the right to contribute to the larger good, to take care of others at the same time as graciously accepting the care offered by others.

As an aside, Addams' work also suggests that the graciousness with which care is accepted is often reflective of the degree to which the person receiving care has the opportunity to give care as well. She cites Huxley as declaring 'that the sense of uselessness is the severest shock which the human system can sustain, and that if persistently sustained, it results in atrophy of function' (Addams, 1910, p. 120). Therefore, one of the most crucial things that need to be addressed among a population being served, and one of the most significant sources of their ongoing difficulties, is the sense of uselessness which might have emerged from out of their tragic life circumstances. Not to do so, not to assist in the restoration of their sense of usefulness to others as well as to themselves, will undermine the effectiveness of any other efforts that might be made on their behalf – perhaps to a lesser degree than the vengeance aroused in the inmates of the Bicêtre prior to Pussin outlawing violent treatment, but undermining nonetheless.

Addams did not address any of these issues specifically in relation to mental illness. In this case, though, she did point out how our society discourages and devalues the contributions of young people, having a similar effect on their ongoing participation as we suggest can be found among people who have experienced persistent mental illnesses. She writes:

> There is a heritage of noble obligation which young people accept and long to perpetuate. The desire for action, the wish to right wrong and alleviate suffering haunts them daily. Society smiles at it indulgently instead of making it of value to itself. The wrong to them begins even farther back, when we restrain the first childish desires for 'doing good', and tell them that they must wait until they are older and better fitted. We intimate that social obligation begins at a fixed date, forgetting that it begins at birth itself. We treat them as children who, with strong-growing limbs, are allowed to use their legs but not their arms, or whose legs are daily carefully exercised that after a while their arms may be put to high use. We do this in spite of the protest of the best educators, Locke and Pestalozzi. We are fortunate in the meantime if their unused members do not weaken and disappear. They do sometimes. (Addams, 1910, pp. 118–119)

To insist on the contributions of all parties does not suggest that this is an easy or straightforward affair in all cases. Some of the more ingenious interventions of Pussin's wife, and some of the more creative projects undertaken by Addams and her colleagues (such as the Labor Museum described above), involved finding ways for people to participate despite their challenges and limitations. We will return to this important issue of enhancing access to existing opportunities, and creating new opportunities when they don't exist, in several of the chapters that follow. It is one of the several recurring motifs of this volume, and, to return to where this chapter began, it is one of the essential elements of recovery-oriented practice that is best developed, and most effectively offered, in community-based as opposed to institutional settings.

A final application of Addams' work to mental health is related to her ability to trace problems to their root causes and her willingness and skill in addressing those causes, regardless of the level (e.g. individual, family, city, national, international) at which these causes function. Several of the figures in this book, from Meyer and Sullivan to King and Deleuze, became increasingly convinced over the course of their careers in the substantive social, cultural and political contributions to mental health and mental illness. As a result, they increasingly shifted their focus from the care, treatment or empowerment of individuals to preventive and proactive interventions at the collective level, whether that be the community or national or international in scope. In their own unique ways, they came to agree with Addams' conclusion that 'without the advance and improvement of the whole, no man can hope for any lasting improvement in his own moral or material individual condition'.

While recovery-oriented practice conceptualized within the context of existing health care systems might appear to be limited to individual or family-level interventions – those, for example, for which practitioners can be reimbursed by insurance or Medicaid – we suggest that this represents an overly narrow view of the range of things required to promote recovery. We included the example of garbage collection within the City of Chicago to illustrate this dilemma. It is not always possible to address the root causes of a person's difficulties, and to assist the person in recovering from and overcoming these difficulties, using solely individual or family-level interventions. There certainly are times when it is possible within mental health, such as the combination of medication and psychotherapy in the treatment of a single episode of depression. The care of people with severe and persistent mental illnesses, however, frequently requires a combination of interventions across a number of levels. We will return to this issue in our next to last chapter when we take up the work of Vygotsky in some detail. For now, we can simply offer the examples of passing and implementing fair housing legislation, eliminating the not-in-my-back-yard (NIMBY) phenomenon that continues to limit housing options for individuals with disabilities, eradicating other forms of stigma and discrimination both inside and outside the mental health system and revising disability and social welfare policies so that they provide incentives, as opposed to the current disincentives, for people returning to paid employment.

3.11 Summary of lessons learned

From this review of the work of Dix and Addams, we suggest the following lessons:

- People do not always have to be removed from their current life circumstances in order to receive assistance in addressing and overcoming their difficulties.

- People can be assisted in managing their own difficulties and lives, rather than to have those difficulties, and their lives as a whole, taken over by others.

- What one person is likely to find helpful in learning how to deal with a mental illness are the same kinds of things another person would likely find helpful were that person in the same life situation. To figure out how best to help, the most useful thing a helper can do to start is to ask the person what kind of assistance he or she thinks would be useful in dealing with his or her current situation.

- When the person in need does not know, or will not say, how he or she can best be helped, then it is most effective for the helper to put him- or herself in that person's shoes as best he or she can in order to identify what would be useful to him or her in that life circumstance, and then to offer that form of assistance to the person in need.

- One key thing that people often need is the opportunity to be active in their own lives and to be contributing positively to the lives of others. When these opportunities do not exist, and when people have disabilities or limitations which impede their taking advantage of existing opportunities, practitioners can participate in creating new opportunities that take these limitations and needs into account.

- The promotion of recovery, especially among people with severe and persistent illnesses, often requires interventions that extend beyond individuals and their families to the levels of the community, the city, the state, the country and even the globe.

Lessons to avoid repeating:

- Extracting people from their current life circumstances in the hope of relieving them of the personal responsibility for addressing those circumstances can be detrimental, inculcating a sense of impotence, helplessness and uselessness in the people involved.

- Extracting people from their current life circumstances also potentially replaces their existing difficulties with a whole new set of difficulties, the resolution of which may not prepare the person any better for dealing with his or her original difficulties.

- Assistance may be more difficult to accept and utilize when offered out of a sense of pity or charity than when offered in support of the person's own sense of responsibility for and active role in determining his or her own life.

- A person should not be viewed as being either a person needing help or a helper; rather than being mutually exclusive, people are most often in both roles at once. In fact, it may be easier to accept help from others if one feels that one is giving help as well.

4

The Everyday and Interpersonal Context of Recovery

4.1 The birth of psychiatry as a community-based practice

With the work of Addams, and the model of Hull-House, as our backdrop, we return to the topic of recovery and the discipline of psychiatry. By 'community-based' we do not mean to refer to community psychiatry per se, as that is a distinct discipline which has its own history, both chronological and conceptual. While there are some areas of overlap, not all of community psychiatry has been recovery-oriented, and not all of recovery-oriented practice would fall under the purview of community psychiatry. For our present purposes, we are referring instead to the conceptual shift that occurred with Adolf Meyer and his successors when *clinical* psychiatry first became liberated from the asylum. Since for Meyer, psychiatric difficulties – which, as we have said, he referred to as 'problems in living' – first arise at the interface between the person and his or her immediate social environment, it made no sense for him to extract this person from his or her environment in order to address these difficulties. The difficulties might very well disappear, but only to re-emerge again once the person returned to his or her ongoing life, as would inevitably happen. This is the conceptual shift introduced into clinical psychiatry with Meyer, and this is the point of departure for the present chapter.

This chapter will differ from the others in this volume in a couple of ways that deserve introductory comment. First of all, a significant part of this chapter is written in the first person from the perspective of someone, John Strauss, whose professional development was directly influenced by two of the protagonists whose work we will be discussing. Second, the third protagonist in this chapter will be John Strauss himself, as his work and career represent a natural evolution of the work of Meyer and Sullivan and bring this line of thinking up to the present day. We asked John to summarize his own career and research contributions within this

The Roots of the Recovery Movement in Psychiatry   Larry Davidson, Jaak Rakfeldt, John Strauss
© 2010 John Wiley & Sons, Ltd

context, and he reluctantly obliged. Even if John were not standing on the shoulders of these two giants, his work would have warranted space in this volume, given its significance in re-introducing the notion and possibility of recovery into clinical psychiatry in the early 1970s.

By the 1970s, Meyer and Sullivan's influence had faded into the background of 'common sense' – had become part of what we take for granted as obvious in psychiatry – while simultaneously being (dis)regarded as passé. By this time, the relevance of psychodynamic and psychotherapeutic approaches to serious mental illness was beginning to be questioned, organic and neurobiological models were on the rise and Kraepelin's legacy was permeating those aspects of American psychiatry that had been reluctant to give up on 'the chronically mentally ill'. At the same time, Laing (1967) was leading efforts to establish alternatives to mainstream psychiatry and Szasz (1961, 1974) was refuting its legitimacy. John's voice was one of the few at the time to draw the field's attention back to the person with the illness and his or her prospects for recovery through a combination of medication, social support, personal resilience and effort and an increasing array of psychological and social interventions. The work John carried out in collaboration with Will Carpenter and others in the 1970s and 1980s gave this notion of recovery mainstream credibility and provided empirical, scientific support for the consumer/survivor/ex-patient movement that was emerging at the time. To many people, John represents the closest thing there is to a 'father' of the contemporary recovery movement (not to take anything away from the fathers and mothers of the consumer/survivor/ex-patient movement, such as Judi Chamberlin, Joe Rogers, Sally Zinman or Howie the Harp, or of the field of psychiatric rehabilitation, such as William Anthony and Robert Paul Liberman).

We are fortunate to have John's first-person account of the exciting time in clinical psychiatry when he was first in training, a time during which the boundaries of the field appeared to be wide open and investigators were encouraged to pursue a diverse range of interests in trying to come to a better understanding of the nature and treatment of serious mental illness. We begin this chapter with John's perspective on his early experiences in the 1950s, and then turn to a brief description of the research John carried out with his various colleagues over the years, before turning back to the work of Meyer and Sullivan. We suggest that the work they initiated, and which John carried forward, remains as relevant today as it was when it first appeared – nestled between the demise of 'moral treatment' around the turn of the century and the closing of hospitals a half-century later, which we take up in the next chapter.

4.2 Beyond the illness paradigm (by John Strauss, part 1)

Even more than in the rest of medicine, the mental health (or mental illness) field has struggled with its core identity. Is it 'just' another branch of medicine? Does it have to prove itself part of medicine by being more rigorous, more biological, more 'scientific' than the other branches? Or does it exist of necessity, even more than the rest of medicine, in some intermediate location, with the potential to be a major link between the arts as reflective of the 'human condition' and traditional science?

A major psychiatric textbook of the twentieth century describes the work of Adolf Meyer in a way that can be viewed from this more general context. 'In the first decade of this century, Adolf Meyer, protesting against the organic and nosological rigidity of nineteenth century psychiatry, advanced the revolutionary idea that mental illness was a failure in the adjustment of the person to his situation' (Spiegel and Bell, 1959, p. 115). That simple sentence, and the work of Meyer itself within the broader context of the field of psychiatry, raises many questions about the very nature of our efforts. In this section, I describe some of the work of Meyer and Harry Stack Sullivan, who followed in a somewhat similar orientation. Having been raised, psychiatrically speaking, within the context of these two leaders in the field, I will also describe more concretely what that experience was like and what orientations it generated.

So where was Adolf Meyer coming from? Why was he, for a time, so successful? I will only describe briefly here the work of Meyer since it seems to me that in some strange way it was his attitude towards the mental health field and his influence on others who became leaders, through his teaching even more than his writings and specific ideas, that had such a tremendous impact, at least for a time, on American psychiatry. For those who care to read more about him I can recommend especially Lief's (1948) *The Commonsense Psychiatry of Dr. Adolf Meyer*, 'Adolf Meyer and the development of American psychiatry' by Lidz (1966) or any American textbook of psychiatry written in the 1950s or 1960s, such as the *American Handbook of Psychiatry* edited by Arieti (1959).

In his writing about what he called 'psychobiology' – thus mixing psychology and biology – Meyer emphasized the importance of many psychiatric problems being examples of excessive reactions that would, were they less exaggerated, be normal. This emphasis – far more than the neologisms he created such as 'ergasias' and 'parergasias' – led to a shift of focus in much of American psychiatry from defining supposed disease entities (as did Pinel or Kraepelin) to what a person was trying to accomplish or avoid. This orientation towards adaptation and maladaptation touched a receptive place in the American psyche – or at least some American psyches – relating psychiatric problems to 'problems in living' rather than existing exclusively as isolated diseases. Such an orientation provides a basis for considering improvement through living and adaptation rather than exclusively waiting for doctors to find the cure.

Meyer emphasized biology, biography and the social milieu in his teaching. For example, he emphasized the importance of work as well as physiology in understanding people and their problems. It is not surprising, therefore, that he is considered one of the founders of occupational therapy. Meyer promoted extensive interviewing and psychotherapy even with people diagnosed with '*dementia praecox*' – the term for schizophrenia still in use during much of his life. He was professor of psychiatry in the major American medical centres of Cornell and Johns Hopkins and was a president of the American Psychiatric Association, and through these positions had a tremendous impact on the field.

To understand Meyer's impact, it is first necessary to understand what the field looked like when he entered it. Meyer was born in Switzerland in 1866 and remained there throughout his medical and neuropathology training. At the time, European medical schools were organically and diagnostically oriented, focusing primarily on identifying and classifying supposed diseases and syndromes. In those schools, for example, it was customary for major figures such as Emil Kraepelin – who admittedly had contributed greatly to the psychiatric thinking of the time – to demonstrate to his students how a catatonic patient did not feel any pain when you stuck a needle into his hand. Most of these schools focused almost entirely on the careful examination, description and diagnosis of patients (who were presumed to have illnesses) with little attention to personal life factors, social situations or even treatment, since treatment was considered ineffective in the face of these 'organic' conditions. Little, if any, consideration was given to the difficulties the person might identify him- or herself, the strengths that he or she might have alongside of the symptoms and deficits or the role the person might play in dealing with the illness. Without exaggeration, it is reasonable to say that it was during this period that the identification of the person with the illness (which, as we have seen, had already preceded Pinel) was given scientific credibility. No longer indiscriminately referred to as 'lunatics' or 'maniacs', people with serious mental illnesses began, for the first time, to be referred to by their (presumably medical) diagnoses. People became 'catatonics', 'hebephrenics', 'paranoiacs' and 'manic depressives'. With the work of Bleuler (1950), we can then add to this list 'schizophrenics'.

It is true that people outside of psychiatry may also be referred to at times by their diagnosis, such as 'diabetics', 'asthmatics' and even as 'the broken leg in Room #236' (Flanagan and Davidson, 2007). It is customarily understood, however, that this form of medical shorthand does not call into question, or eradicate, the humanity of the person with the illness or the broken leg. Even if we decry the dehumanization of medicine as a whole, as some do, this still does not result in our viewing 'diabetics' as somehow less human than others. It does seem, though, that the European schools of thought in psychiatry in the late nineteenth century had lost any remnant of Pinel's compassion for those 'very talented persons' whose highly developed sensitivity left them vulnerable to attacks of 'madness', attacks which he pointed out were neither permanent nor complete.

Meyer's orientation, on the contrary, implied that there was often hope for improvement, for change in the person's condition, not merely from some medication now or in the future, or from purely psychological interventions, but from the person's own actions as well. Meyer, in fact, was heavily influenced by the beliefs of the British neurologist John Hughlings Jackson (1958), who emphasized the unity of the mind and body in his work but then went beyond this to include the importance of the social environment. All of these factors were allowed room in Meyer's theory of mental illness and recovery because he viewed the phenomenon of mental illness itself to have biological, psychological and social dimensions, predating Engel's (1977) formal introduction of the 'biopsychosocial model' of illness and health by over half a century. What had appeared to Meyer's professors in Switzerland to be an organic disease, and what was at the time appearing to Freud to be a developmental fixation, appeared to Meyer to be a given individual's difficulty in adapting to his or her current life situation. This difficulty can stem from any component of this dynamic person–environment transaction, including the person's biological inheritance and make-up, his or her early childhood and family experiences, his or her personality characteristics and attributes, his or her social relationships and any number of possible aspects of the nature of the situation itself, ranging from its social, cultural and political context to its unique significance and relevance for the person. If such a comprehensive and multifaceted approach to understanding mental illness is what current more sophisticated approaches to psychiatric research are aiming for (e.g. as in the case of post-traumatic stress disorder), then this represents not so much a 'common sense' approach to science (as it might seem) as a continuation of Meyer's legacy.

In some ways, it is possible to view the work of Harry Stack Sullivan as extending this more holistic orientation introduced by Meyer. Sullivan's 'interpersonal' emphasis goes even further in the direction of what at the time might have seemed like a uniquely American approach, focusing on one's life, personal action and possibility for change rather than exclusively on one's origins or biology. Like Meyer, who talked and wrote about ergasias and parergasias, Sullivan too developed many neologisms that by now have been mostly forgotten. But it seemed common at the time for writers in the English language to translate many concepts such as Freud's from an indigenous language (e.g. *ich* and *es* in German, *moi* and *surmoi* in French) to Latin or Greek words. Perhaps Meyer and Sullivan believed they too had to appear fancy in this way, and thus more neologisms were generated. For Sullivan it was words like 'parataxic', 'self-dynamisms' and 'sublimatory reformulations'. Although such terms did, of course, have useful meanings within the conceptual structures of those authors, they have been dropped probably because they proved more bizarre and confusing than useful.

In terms of his thinking, Sullivan shifted the focus from the isolated individual and his or her internal psychic or biologic processes to the interactions and experiences of that individual with his or her world. Thus Sullivan in his 'interpersonal' view of psychiatric problems wrote and spoke extensively about empathy, validation, security, power operations and adaptation. These concepts could be applied to the person with a mental illness, but also to those around him or her, including the treating personnel. Clearly, the orientations of Meyer and Sullivan provided a basis for thinking more broadly about the nature, origins, evolution and improvement of psychopathology than was true either for the more traditional biological or psychoanalytic models of thought that were dominant at the time.

The works and thinking of Meyer and Sullivan are not widely taught at present. There are probably many reasons for this, and certainly one is that the possibility of improvement or lack thereof in serious mental illnesses has always been a major issue for the field. Kraepelin (1921), in defining *dementia praecox* (which subsequently came to be called schizophrenia), placed in that category symptomatically diverse conditions because he believed that all of them shared an invariable downhill course and thus reflected a common pathological process. This view came to dominate clinical psychiatry to such a degree that when, for example, as part of the International Pilot Study of Schizophrenia, Will Carpenter and I (Strauss and Carpenter, 1972) sent a leading American psychiatric journal our first report using rating scales (for which we had established the reliability) and sophisticated statistical analyses showing a wide variation in the outcome of people with schizophrenia diagnosed by many systems, it was rejected. One of the reviewers stated blankly and without evidence: 'This cannot be true.' We then submitted the report to another leading and even more scientifically demanding journal, where it was published. But the degree to which the 'necessity' of non-improvement was held to, and the doggedness of that belief even to this day, notwithstanding the fact that all of the many studies from around the world have now demonstrated the diversity of outcome, are certainly trying to tell us something, perhaps more about our field than about the nature of serious mental illnesses.

In spite of over 30 studies carried out in over 30 countries over the last 30 years, all of which show a wide range of outcomes in schizophrenia, many professors in the United States and elsewhere are still teaching their students that schizophrenia is an invariably chronic illness, a so-called brain disease, and that patients with this illness will have to take medication all their life and will be permanently restricted in their abilities, activities and social lives. And many psychiatrists are still telling their patients: 'You have an illness called schizophrenia; you will have it all your life; it is like diabetes. You will have to take medication all your life, and there will be many things you will never be able to do.' One still hears that reported by people in the United States, and a few weeks before finishing this chapter I heard the same thing stated by a young person in Paris who also reported, understandably enough, how devastated he was at hearing that 'information'. It was fortunate for him that now he found himself in a setting where those around us in the seminar (where I met him) were perplexed, since many of the people in that centre, the Atelier de Non-Faire organized by Dr Di Girolamo, also had received the diagnosis of schizophrenia. Many were not on medication, many were doing quite well and were involved in a wide range of life endeavors and, in fact, were running the centre.

At times, the acceptance of the possibility that people with serious mental illnesses can improve and even participate actively in that improvement, as suggested especially by Meyer, have appeared to relate to the national characters of a particular country and also to the attitudes of the period in which the beliefs exist. In a discussion of schools of psychiatry and their ties to national traditions and attitudes, Redlich and Freedman (1966, p. 23) state the following:

> In the United States, the strong interest in dynamic psychotherapy
> is explained, at least in part, by the typically optimistic American
> belief that man can be and should be helped to actualize himself and

> overcome weaknesses, by a characteristic sense of social justice which
> holds that wrongs committed during infancy and childhood for which
> the individual is not responsible should replace the irrational ... For
> example, the psychobiological school of Adolf Meyer today really no
> longer exists, but it has influenced and enriched American psychiatry.

This is certainly one way of viewing our field from an international point of view. There were certainly 'optimistic' centres of psychiatry in other countries than the United States, but perhaps they were never so pervasive. Now, however, perhaps this characteristically American optimism and eclecticism has diminished significantly in this country and flourishes more in other centres. 'Voice hearers' organizations originating in the United Kingdom and the Netherlands, the existence of Soteria treatment centres in Switzerland and Germany and an interest by many psychiatric organizations internationally in subjectivity and the active role of people with serious mental illnesses in the improvement process is more widespread in many countries in Europe, for example, than in many parts of the United States. In the United States, however, perhaps the gathering interest in the recovery movement is a sign of shifting times for national attitudes in this country towards mental health.

4.3 Growing up inside Meyer's 'common sense' psychiatry (by John Strauss, part 2)

Now, I hope I have done at least part of my duty as a writer of this chapter by trying to provide a general idea of the role of Meyer and Sullivan in clinical psychiatry. Having attempted that, I want to write now more from the inside, my understanding and first-person experience, since they have had a tremendous impact on me personally and on many others in the field – whether we recognize Meyer and Sullivan as sources of that impact or not. Although I realize that may put some readers off (as it would have me, a few years ago), such a first-person approach has the potential for providing a clear point of view and a context for the reader's reflection that may otherwise be difficult or even impossible. Terry Krupa, an outstanding occupational therapist and a good friend of mine, said to me several years ago: 'Isn't it strange how scientific articles are written in the third-person as though the author as a person weren't there?' There are, of course, reasons for doing that which are important, but the advantages of such apparent objectivity may conceal important aspects of subjectivity (e.g. why the author has picked that topic, what he or she has left out in the presentation). So I choose here to write in the first person with the advantages and disadvantages that such an approach entails and hope the reader will not judge me too harshly for this.

First of all, it feels very strange to me to be writing about Meyer and Sullivan. It feels like a person trying to write as if one were a fish (I suppose) writing about the water in which he or she has always lived. As the ideas of Dilthey (1977) imply, we are all 'inside' a particular perspective or way of thinking, whether it is a 'mental illness is a brain disease' perspective or a 'psychiatric disorders are reactions to early childhood experience' perspective or some other. The strange thing then is realizing one way or another that you were brought up in it and then trying more objectively to figure it out. When I was coming up in psychiatry, from my first official contacts with the field as a medical student and then as a psychiatry resident, the basis of all around me *was* Meyer and Sullivan.

In reading for this chapter, I pulled down an old copy of the *American Textbook of Psychiatry* (Arieti, 1959) that I had taken when the Connecticut Mental Health Center had dissolved its library and given away all its books to make way for an additional conference room. There, under 'Meyer' in the index, was 'Wendell Muncie'. 'Hmm,' I thought, 'a vaguely familiar name.' I looked up his chapter on Meyer in the textbook and found it beautifully written and informative. That name, Muncie, still seemed more familiar than his just being the author of such a piece. I searched it through Google. Wendell Muncie Award. Hadn't I won that award or got second place or something? I searched further through Google under several headings and found nothing other than the information that Adolf Meyer had been a hero and mentor for Muncie. Then I thought to look in my CV. There, under awards, sure enough, 1966, I had won the Wendell Muncie Award of the Maryland Psychiatric Society for my first paper, the study of schizophrenic thought by using the tests of Piaget that I had learned when I was his student in Geneva. Meyer and his teachings and his students were all around me in my early experiences in psychiatry.

The first *Diagnostic and Statistical Manual of Mental Disorders* published in 1952 by the American Psychiatric Association Committee on Nomenclature (1952) – which was the one used in my earlier days in the field, describes 'reactions': 'Schizophrenic Reaction', 'Depressive Reaction' and the like. That was Adolf Meyer. In contrast, European psychiatry during and preceding that time was seen in the centres where I trained and by the people I knew as hopelessly and typically autocratic, rigid, dehumanizing, retrograde, stuck in the nineteenth century and before and only about hypothetical brain disease. 'Mental illnesses are brain diseases'; that was Griesinger (1882), nineteenth-century German old-school beliefs. There was also Freud, of course, but as popular as he was in the United States, he was still often seen as outside the established medical field of psychiatry. No, American psychiatry was from Adolf Meyer with the attention he had paid to the person and the social context as well as to the 'disorders'. So, Sullivan came from the Meyer tradition and in the places I found myself, Yale Medical School and then McLean Hospital (the Harvard psychiatric hospital in Belmont, Massachusetts), even later at the Intramural Program of the National Institute of Mental Health and the Washington School of Psychiatry, the air I breathed and the water I drank, so to speak, were Meyer and Sullivan. That was what psychiatry was. That was what mental disorders were. Patient evaluation, case conceptualization and treatment stemmed from that.

When I did my first psychiatric rotation in medical school at the Veteran's hospital, I was 'given' a patient, Mr W. (I still remember his name, and him.) I was told: 'Spend some time with him. Don't read his record; just get to know him.' So, not knowing exactly how to proceed, I suggested to Mr W. that we talk (I asked the usual questions, of course; 'How did you come to the hospital?' etc.). And then after a while, when I had got through some of that, I suggested that we go down to the hospital cafeteria and have coffee. We did, and over the six weeks of my rotation we did that a lot. Of course, I had seminars and lectures and 'worked up' a bunch of patients, but I don't remember any of that. All I remember is Mr W. He was a nice guy and we talked about life and the work he had done and, I guess, about his symptoms (I remember he had auditory hallucinations and delusions of persecution) but the symptoms were such a small part of our conversations I don't remember much about them.

And then, over time at McLean (in the Boston area, which was at the time at the heart of orthodox psychoanalysis) and after, I learned that, well, McLean was a bit different. In fact, most of the leading psychiatrists at McLean were refugees from the Washington Psychoanalytic Society (hard to realize now, but in those days, in the 1960s, much of American psychiatry was psychoanalysis and many department chairs were psychoanalysts). Sullivan, and then Fromm-Reichman, were from that area, and I was told the Washington group was sometimes getting thrown out of the American Psychoanalytic Association because they refused to follow the rules and adhere to the doctrine as required.

What did I know? The people at McLean seemed good to me, sensible, knowledgeable. We treated people with schizophrenia and other severe disorders with psychotherapy three times a week, an hour at a session, with medication when required, and with 'milieu treatment'. At McLean 'milieu treatment' was not just a term for group activities on the inpatient ward; we took the patients' environment seriously, or at least much more seriously than most facilities at the time, and tried to use it to foster improvement. Although it was suggested that we have the therapy sessions in our offices, if we thought it better, it was all right to walk around the grounds with patients while we talked. When I was the resident at the Day Treatment Center, I even remember seeing a patient in psychotherapy and then after lunch, which we doctors and patients often ate together, occasionally doing dishes with the same patient. That's just how things were: natural, and no big deal.

And then when I went from my residency to a post as clinical associate at the National Institute of Mental Health, in Bethesda, Maryland, just outside the psychiatrically 'notorious' Washington DC, my boss insisted that we do home visits on our patients. I resisted this 'waste of time' as long as I could, but then was finally required to do one and discovered that when you see a patient outside of a treatment setting, that patient, even if he or she were 'a schizophrenic', might not be at all what you had seen in the hospital, but a competent, socially cool, person, even inviting you to have coffee! Imagine! Who knew?

I think all this was part of the Adolf Meyer and Harry Stack Sullivan legacy. Sullivan was also an early leading figure in the Washington School of Psychiatry, where I was soon to take a seminar in community psychiatry led by Bert Brown, the head of the National Institute of Mental Health. So, to me, that was what psychiatry was, the wide river in which I found myself. What a pleasure! That meant that biology, sociology, linguistics, family theory, psychoanalysis, history, anthropology, psychology and statistics, and the people who practised those disciplines, and even ordinary life experience, all had input into how we thought and what we did. That milieu found interest in other leaders in our current of psychiatry and psychology, such as Maxwell Jones or Carl Rogers, no problem. That was the same Carl Rogers who described himself as being influenced by such leaders in the field as Alport (1937) and Maslow (1966). Our current in the vast ocean was just biopsychosocial! Such was the common-sense psychiatry of Meyer.

The Commonsense Psychiatry of Dr. Alfred Meyer was, in fact, the name of a book, the standard collection I was told, of Meyer's work. It had been edited by Lief (1948). Somehow, I already had a copy of it. I had bought it along with *Conceptions of Modern Psychiatry* (Sullivan, 1940) and *The Interpersonal Theory of Psychiatry* (Sullivan, 1953), both by Harry Stack Sullivan (*Schizophrenia as a Human Process* (Sullivan, 1962) had not yet been published) at the annual '20% off' sale at Whitlock's bookstore in New Haven. Even in medical school, I had thought I might want to be a psychiatrist and those were the kinds of books one bought.

It was not until joining the World Health Organization International Pilot Study of Schizophrenia after those first two years in Washington DC, when I began meeting leading psychiatrists from the other eight centres, that I realized that the 'old' European psychiatry – with its frequent emphasis on diagnosis and a narrow version of the medical model – was still alive and well. It is that model which has since swept over American psychiatry with such a vengeance that now many European centres are more open to diverse views regarding psychiatric disorders and treatment than are we Americans.

So who were these guys Meyer and Sullivan? Were they hopelessly gooey in their approach to psychiatric 'disorders' and 'reactions'? Was Griesinger (of 'mental illness is brain disease') along with the other nineteenth-century Germans really right after all? Well, maybe they were. It was certainly hard to define the concepts used by Meyer and Sullivan operationally and reliably, or to measure the things they talked about. But with this background in mind, let's try to take another look.

Adolf Meyer was born in Switzerland in 1866 and died in Baltimore in 1950. He is listed as 'American Psychiatrist' in the *Encyclopaedia Britannica*. His interests were: training, psychiatric social work, community psychiatry, common sense, strengths and weaknesses, and the present life rather than past background and complexes. Harry Stack Sullivan, in contrast, was born in the United States in 1892 (just seven years before my father) and died while at a conference in Paris in 1949. His students and followers included Horney (1937), Fromm (1941), Erikson (1950) and even leaders in psychiatric/sociological epidemiology, such as Leighton (1959). Many of these people are now being rapidly forgotten. These pioneers can be seen as having taken up strands of the work of Pinel and Esquirol in revolutionary France, who focused on treating mental patients increasingly as people, of Tuke in England, regarding providing more healthy and normal living contexts for people with mental disorders, and of Freud, regarding the psychological lives of people with mental disorders.

Meyer and Sullivan expanded on these ideas in theory, practice and psychiatric education both within psychiatry and in society more generally. So at the end of the nineteenth century, while Kraepelin was working in Germany and – all his positive contributions to the field aside – was sticking a pin in the hand of a catatonic patient to show students how such a person does not respond to pain, Meyer, and later Sullivan, was emphasizing that people with mental illness are people existing in important social contexts. What Meyer and Sullivan sacrificed in diagnostic and descriptive reliability, they gained in recognizing the humanity of individuals with serious mental illnesses. They also contributed to a more complex science of the mental health field as well. Has current biological psychiatry lost much of that crucial complexity by continuing to pursue the more purely biological model of the nineteenth century? I think so. In the struggle for our field to become a truly human science, we have yet to learn how to put the two – the complexity and subjectivity of the human being living in a social context and the objectivity of traditional science – together.

All in all, it seems to me that the most important contribution of these pioneers, at least the most important to me, was certainly not their neologisms or even the other specifics of their theories. I believe that their most important contribution, and one more easily lost than we notice, was their attention to patients as people, the psychological and social aspects of people's lives, people's skills as well as their problems but also people's subjectivity, their desire to live a full life, their efforts to do so and the meaning of their lives and of their surroundings. Equally as important was the general ambiance provided by the work of Meyer and Sullivan and how they took seriously people with psychological problems as people living in the world. As difficult as this atmosphere is to specify in traditional scientific terms, it is no less important. In a 2007 lecture to a department of psychiatry in Paris in which I focused on many aspects of patients' subjectivity and their surroundings, some of the residents coming up to me afterwards made some of the most beautiful comments I had ever received. They said: 'We didn't know psychiatry could be like that.' Well, it can, and Meyer and Sullivan were some of the most important figures in showing how that is possible.

So what light did Meyer and Sullivan shed on processes of 'recovery' or improvement? Sullivan's thesis that people with schizophrenia are far more human than otherwise and that working with them as such could lead to improvement was such a quiet and beautiful, not to mention profound, idea that it shaped much of American psychiatry and the mental health field more generally for almost a century. There is still a titanic struggle between this view now mostly in the minority, and that dogged view that 'schizophrenia is a brain disease, it is a disease like diabetes, people will have it all their lives and need to take medication all their lives and there are many things they will never be able to do'. This latter argument in its certainty and apparent scientific strength is still dominant, untroubled by the data from studies carried out around the world, without exception showing that the outcome of schizophrenia is in fact extremely diverse, that many people with schizophrenia improve significantly and some completely and that they can often do pretty much everything that anyone else can do and can often stop taking their medication. In much of the mental health community, much that has sounded like hard science continues to dominate, and much that has been seen as mushy sentiment and blind hope still struggles for recognition. But at least in some ways Meyer and Sullivan, in spite of the scientific inadequacies of their work, have turned out to have been correct all along. What a strange world we live in.

The psychiatric world of Meyer and Sullivan seems so distant from the world of *DSM-III* (American Psychiatric Association, 1980) and *IV* (American Psychiatric Association, 1994) and of contemporary 'scientific' psychiatry. Why do these two worlds have so much difficulty in arriving at a rapprochement – the world of professionals who really know the people with whom they work and their life contexts often so distant from the world of scientists with their numbers, reliability of data and replicable results? One world tends to be fuzzy and difficult to pin down; the other has clear data that seem to be so far from the complex reality of people who actually exist. Meyer and Sullivan succeeded in breaking away from the harsh, dehumanized rigidity of so much of nineteenth-century psychiatry but failed to provide a structure that was amenable to traditional methods of scientific inquiry. Subsequent scientific inquiry found a way of generating numbers, reliability and replicability. Are we as a field doomed to repeat eternally this reflexive repetition of going from one extreme to the other, or will we some day be able to construct a field that is a human science, that is both human and scientific? Why do we as scholars and investigators seem so incapable of dealing in depth with the whole phenomenon?

I had not fully realized until writing this chapter how much these pioneers had influenced my own work in this field, from my very first paper on hallucinations and delusions being on a continuum with normal functioning (Strauss, 1969), to my later work (Strauss, 1994b) on the person with delusions as a person, to my more recent work on *Le concept de la maladie mentale* (Strauss, 2007). I probably will not live to see the promised land, where science and humanity, objectivity and subjectivity, come together with the complexity that would be involved, but these pioneers have certainly contributed to the evolving idea I have of what it will look like.

4.4 Subjectivity and the person (by John Strauss, part 3)

At this point, Larry asked me to write: 'But how did the work of Meyer and Sullivan influence your work and what resulted from that?' I will start with the story of how to cook a carp, changing the story a bit to fit this question.

A long time ago, I was told by my father the story of how to cook a carp. You get a large carp, clean it and stuff it with all kinds of good things. Then cook the carp for two hours. Then take it out of the oven, add more good things to the stuffing and cook it for another hour. Then take the carp out of the oven, remove (and eat) the stuffing and throw the carp away.

For me, the metapsychology of Meyer and of Sullivan, their theories of parataxic distortion and the like, the things I had to learn in college about their contributions to abnormal psychology, are like the carp. I don't see how they contributed much to our understanding or to the field more generally. They seem more like what many people of their era in our field needed to do to be heard given the huge lexicon of neologisms generated by the English translations of Freud. The 'stuffing', however, that Meyer and Sullivan provided in huge and beautiful amounts, although difficult to define precisely, heavily influenced American psychiatry and my life and work as part of that.

How to describe that much more complex and wonderful 'stuffing'? Well, it contrasts both to the 'rigor' of psychoanalysis, which gave a clear structure and method (the couch and the interpretations), and to the rigor of descriptive psychiatry, which gave the basis for developing more reliable terminology. The approaches of Meyer and Sullivan also contrast to the rigor of biology, which gave a traditional scientific approach to understanding the workings of the brain and the broader neuroendocrine systems. But the work of Meyer and Sullivan provided the air of freedom. They provided the freedom to observe and be with patients with a minimum of judgement and preconception. They provided the freedom to see people with psychiatric problems, even the most severe and long-standing psychiatric problems, as people. They and their followers provided the crucial freedom to see people with psychiatric disorders through sitting behind them as they lay on a couch, or through their bodily fluids or brainwaves, or through the methodological magnifying glass for looking at symptoms and functioning provided by descriptive psychiatry. Because of the work of Meyer and Sullivan and their followers, it was all right to listen to people as they lay on a couch, or to examine their bodily fluids or brainwaves, or to define their symptoms more clearly, but it was also okay to take a walk with that person, wash dishes with him or her, just talk with them as you would any other person, about their work, their life, their hopes or fears or the trivia of being in the world. And it was okay, even essential, to include all those things in one's thinking about mental health and illness.

Ah, but that's too vague, I tell myself. Yes, it is not sufficient, all that, but it is absolutely crucial. When I read in Kraepelin's (1921) textbook of psychiatry that patients with '*dementia praecox*' have an organic disease with an inevitable downhill course, but that sometimes, if the person continues to work, the course is not downhill, I admire him for his wonderful powers of observation even when the observations contradicted his theory. I am also amazed that Kraepelin apparently didn't notice that his observation did contradict his theory. I was equally amazed while recently attending a conference about neuroplasticity by leaders in the field. In several presentations, there were extensive discussions about the ways in which experience could change major aspects of brain structure and function. Applications of this knowledge to help patients with serious mental illnesses were described. At the same time, in the introduction to the conference, we were told that these were brain disorders, biological disorders. Does that mean that experience can influence the brain in the course of these disorders but not in their origin? How do they know that? The openness of Meyer and Sullivan to a wide gamut of processes and interaction with patients helped to avoid the number of narrow orthodoxies (whether from aberrant ego–id–superego development or 'mental illness is a brain disease') that have so distorted our field and led to a perversion of what are purported to be scientific approaches. This is true not only for our practice and research but also, of course and unfortunately, for our training as well (Andres-Hyman, Strauss and Davidson, 2007; Strauss, Staeheli-Lawless and Sells, in press).

So, what to do with this great gift of freedom to be with, to look, to explore, that Meyer and Sullivan have given us? Well, as Yogi Berra said: 'You can observe a lot by just looking.' When, during my psychiatry residency, a supervisor I had, Paul Howard, the associate director of McLean Hospital at the time, would ask me about the patient I was describing: 'What's she doing?' I would become quietly furious. Here was a young schizophrenic woman who didn't like to talk much and I needed to have some 'material' from which to make interpretations. And when I would complain about her tendency not to talk very much, Dr Howard, who was a pretty quiet person himself, would only say: 'What is she doing?' I would tell him (e.g. she was participating in music groups, shopping in a big city, etc.) and he would then ask: 'Did she ever do that before?' And I would reply: 'No' but then quickly get back to my litany of complaints about her talking so little and what could I do about that. Years later, I realized that Dr Howard was teaching me one of the great lessons, but I couldn't hear it until years later. What the young woman was doing was important too, not just what she was or wasn't saying.

I would add to the idea that you can observe a lot by just looking that 'you can learn a lot by just being with'. A few years ago, I was hanging out in a Paris psychiatric hospital to see how they did things, and a nurse said she was going to Ikea with two patients to buy decorations for the Christmas party and invited me to go with them. I accepted, and as soon as we left the hospital everybody changed. I was no longer the distinguished professor from America but had become the slightly dim-witted member of the group, since although I speak French pretty well it was certainly not as well as the three of them. But they were very kind and understanding to me. Driving to the store, the nurse whose car it was became the chauffeur. When we arrived at the store, a huge monster of a building, the nurse/chauffeur and one of the patients and I were totally overwhelmed. The other patient knew the store well, however, and said to the nurse: 'Just give me the list and I'll find the things.' So he became the leader.

Yes indeed, 'you can observe a lot by just looking', but it is so hard to look and then register what you see. I guess any artist could tell you that. And the degree to which unrecognized presuppositions or theories can render you almost blind is almost beyond belief. 'Experience can affect the course of disorder but has nothing to do with aetiology' indeed! If you haven't shown it, you don't know it.

So little by little, and with much help from those ideas formed by Meyer and Sullivan, I think I have been taught to observe more, to try situations for learning about people with serious mental illnesses that don't fit the usual research paradigms and to notice and register things that don't fit the usual limitations that we put on what we hear and see. This often happened more by chance than by foresight. A bit tired of doing only 'outcome' studies, a research group of which I was chief decided that we would try to learn about the trajectory, or course, of disorder as well. Do people get better or worse or stay the same in a straight line over time, or what? And if they do have ups and downs, is there some way of understanding that? The obvious thing to do was to do serial follow-up assessments of people over several years. So we submitted a grant application to do that, but it was turned down because the time series analysis required to analyse the results was not possible with the small number of subjects we planned to see. One way or another, we managed to carry out the study anyway. The review committee had been right about the impossibility of using various approaches to time series analyses for our data. Their correctness was a great disappointment for us. We did find a wide range of 'outcomes' that people experienced over the period of our study, but that of course was nothing that had not been shown by our earlier work and, by now, by the work of many others as well.

But we did seem to be learning a great deal, even though what we were learning was not possible to analyse statistically. When I sat down one night on my living room floor with the graphed trajectories of our participants' courses over the numerous follow-ups all around me, I could find not one that represented a straight line. Every last one had major ups and downs! Since we had come to know our participants at least a certain amount, and since all of us were clinicians as well as researchers, it had become possible to get very strong impressions about what those ups and downs might have represented. From those strong data-based impressions we described what we thought were 'Longitudinal Processes in the Course of Psychiatric Disorder' (Strauss *et al.*, 1985). These processes included phenomena such as 'woodshedding', which one of us (Paul Lieberman) suggested from his college experience as a disc jockey. In the world of jazz, he noted, there is for many performers a period when they retreat from public performance to the figurative 'woodshed' to develop new forms of their music out of the public view where they can make mistakes freely without fear of repercussion. Many of our follow-along participants described (without using the term) just such experiences in their efforts to recover from a severe psychotic episode. Another 'process' we hypothesized was the 'low turning point' (Rakfeldt and Strauss, 1989), described in more detail at the end of this chapter, in which people hit a kind of rock bottom before pulling themselves together to improve. Other findings still less definitive were also fascinating and often very moving. The efforts people made to get better, to continue to lead productive lives, the young man who returned to college time after time, each time followed by the recurrence of hallucinations, each time with his trying to learn a little more about how to get through it and making progress in those attempts.

In another analysis of our data, Tyson (1989), for her medical school thesis, studied in depth our research protocols from two participants to explore possible connections between development and mental disorders. Her analysis suggested that in those people, while the disorder seemed to interfere with some developmental issues, it actually assisted others, and that 'the strength of normal development is such that it can continue despite the presence of disorder, or even be furthered by the necessity of having to cope with the disorder' (p. 87). For me personally, the necessity from our data to push us to turn more to first-person reports of our participants' experiences and to our own impressions even if we didn't have statistical findings in certain areas was a stimulus to look at our research findings in new, more qualitative and subjective ways.

But I think another thing we found out with these serial follow-up (or follow-*along*) interviews was unanticipated, although it is so obvious in retrospect. If you see a person many times over a few years (we always had the same person do the repeated interviews with a given participant) he or she gets to know you a little, and then she or he starts telling you things you never asked, or even thought to ask. 'Dr Strauss,' one lovely woman said to me with a bit of impatience during our fourth or fifth re-interview when I asked her yet once again: 'Given your problems in thinking clearly [that she had once again described] how are you able to work as a secretary in that busy confusing office setting?' 'But, Dr Strauss, as I've told you several times before, when I'm in that setting I *have* to organize myself.' She *had* told me many times before, but I had never registered it; I mean, who would think that anyone with a serious mental illness could have a major role in helping herself?

Another person with schizophrenia asked me after several follow-up interviews early on in our research: 'Why don't you ever ask me what I do to help myself?' I imagine it was because I reckoned that could never be an important consideration – I mean, who would? After she asked me that, we started to ask people that same question routinely and published a paper about it (Breier and Strauss, 1983), and I began using it clinically. 'Is there anything you can do to help yourself (e.g. with the disturbing voices)?' And if the person replied 'No', I continued by telling him or her that I knew other people with that problem and asked whether he or she would be interested in hearing what that person had found helpful so that he or she could try such strategies out. As I became more and more involved in the consumer/survivor/ex-patient movement later in my career, I would describe this as playing the 'middleman role' between two or more people in recovery, learning what worked well for one person so that I could offer that suggestion to others experiencing similar difficulties.

Unfortunately, difficulty for the professional in grasping the subjective experience of the person is not limited to me. Several years ago, Larry and I were invited to give an extended workshop on schizophrenia in Madison, Wisconsin. Not being too sure what we had to teach that major centre of community psychiatry, Larry and I decided that we would start out with a demonstration interview, where I would take the role of a psychotic person coming to treatment and he would be the admitting doctor. The time came and not having talked with each other more specifically about the interview, there we were in front of about 150 professionals, many very competent in working intensively with people with schizophrenia, and we started the mock interview. 'What brings you to the hospital?' Larry asked me. 'I started hearing voices when there was no one there and they were really terribly disturbing,' I replied. Larry then proceeded to go down what seemed to me to be a mental checklist of questions: 'What did they say? When did you hear them? Were they the voices of men or women?' and so on. It rapidly became clear to me that Larry didn't care the least bit about me, that he was completing a mental checklist and that my feelings, my experience, were of no interest to him, 'my doctor'. Rapidly, I became furious, though I tried not to show it because, after all, I needed him for my treatment, for my medication or whatever else was required, but I seethed. After a few minutes of this, I couldn't manage it any more and said to Larry and the audience that I wanted to stop the exercise.

Larry and I were and are good friends, but in that situation he was treating me, a person who was in obvious distress, as though I were a billiard ball. (He explained during the discussion that he had decided beforehand to demonstrate the currently accepted, 'objective approach'.) When I described to the audience my fury and my sense of helplessness in that situation, they thought I was kidding! Many people spoke up and said they saw nothing wrong at all and that they couldn't believe I had such feelings. Wow!

A few years later, I was giving some lectures in Stokmarknes, Norway and decided with a wonderful psychiatrist I had met there that we carry out an intake interview in front of a group of students. We did so, and it went beautifully. We stopped every few minutes to discuss with the students his questions and attitude and my responses and feelings. Two years later, in Tromsø, Norway, that psychiatrist and I decided to do the same thing, this time in front of a group of professionals and some people with serious mental illnesses and their family members. But since he had already 'interviewed' me a couple years previously, this time it would be a follow-up interview. Again, there was an audience of about 150 people and he began asking me questions about how I was doing since we had seen each other last. I replied that I still heard the voices, although they were not so bad now. We continued and after a few minutes he asked me what I was doing now. I told him I was working at McDonald's and that it wasn't a great job but it was better than nothing. He then asked me about friends and family, but within a few minutes I found I no longer wanted to talk with him. Here I was, an invited speaker, an 'expert American' in front of a large audience and after a few minutes I had nothing further I wanted to say. Very disconcerting! So we opened it up for a discussion of the interview and its premature termination.

Several people from the audience asked me (very politely) what went wrong, implying, I think, that I was simply being difficult. I didn't know. This embarrassing situation continued for what seemed to me to be a horribly long time. Then someone from the back of the room raised his hand and said: 'I'm a patient here and that has happened with me and my psychiatrist too.' Then a person near the front of the room raised her hand and said she too was a patient and she too had had the same experience with her doctor. All of us in the room discussed this situation further and gradually it became clear to me that I had wanted to discuss my job at McDonald's further but that 'my psychiatrist' just went on to another topic. (I had been a bit dismissive in my response of 'it was better than nothing', and so had given him little indication that I wanted to talk further about my job. To a more empathic listener, though, that interchange could have been taken to be a kind of clue that

I actually wanted more in my life than to work at McDonald's. The interviewer had not responded to my demoralized affect, but only to the explicit content.) We three 'patients' tried to describe what we felt and why we became so resistant so that the rest of the people in the room could understand. But they never did! Unlike the situation of the interview with Larry, I didn't think in the least that it was 'my doctor's' fault, only that there was a major problem in our interaction. But even with the help of the other 'patients' in the room we couldn't get anyone else to understand. That was sad. Subjectivity, experience, is not always so obvious even to the kindest and best-trained professionals.

This problem with subjectivity, empathy and seeing the person as an active, creative agent in practice, theory and science has another and closely related branch as well. I will write about it here only briefly. Bernard (1865), the father of modern physiology, believed that to understand the pathological it was essential to understand normal function. More recently, Canguilhem (1966) has pursued further the question of the relationship between normal and abnormal functioning, the complexity of that relationship, unwarranted assumptions we make about it and the tendency to see the abnormal as having no close connection to the normal.

Several years ago, I happened to be in the Netherlands when two colleagues, Marius Romme and Sandra Escher, had recently been on Dutch television to invite people who heard voices when no one was around to come to a meeting in Utrecht. Since I happened to be in the country at the time of the meeting, they invited me to attend. I did. The meeting was held in a building that was not connected to medicine or psychiatry and there was a large crowd of, it seemed to me, over a 100 people. There were a couple of lectures which a helpful person who had been assigned to me translated for me. They were all right, but nothing striking. Then the attendees broke into groups to meet in smaller breakout rooms. I went to one of these and was amazed at the discussion. Some people said, as I would have expected, how they heard voices and that the voices were ruining their lives. Others, though, said things like they had heard voices all their lives, that the voices were wonderfully helpful and that it was difficult to understand how someone could get through life without hearing voices. It was not apparent that these people had any bad effects from the voices at all. In fact, I then recalled that during certain follow-up interviews some participants in our research had talked about their voices as though they were not at all part of a problem (one person heard the singing of Barbra Streisand, her favorite singer, and very much appreciated that experience). Are there 'normal' or even 'helpful' voices?

Once again, I believe that in our tendency to narrow our conceptual point of view and our opportunities for a range of learning experiences, we gain more certainty but lose the possibility of knowledge about what this mental illness thing is all about. We tend to isolate in our theory and in our experience our exploration of the relationship between the pathological and the normal and thus to impede the possibility for understanding either. As I noted above, this is true not only for our practice and research but also for our training as well (Strauss, Staeheli-Lawless and Sells, in press).

4.5 Blending science and art in a human science (by John Strauss, part 4)

'Every night I think that maybe this time it will turn out differently.' That was the response of the outstanding actress Merritt Janson, who had just played the role of Liza in the play adapted from Dostoevsky's *Notes from Underground*. She said that in response to my question during the talkback: 'How do you manage to play such an intense and sad role night after night?'

Following Larry's asking me to describe how the work of Meyer and Sullivan influenced my work, I wrote the above last few pages without problem, but then got stuck. It seemed to me that the freedom I have felt the last couple of years to let my intuition lead me wherever it wanted in my work, and my subsequent plunge into trying to develop a more human science of psychiatry using the arts and traditional logical science, had no connection with the work of Meyer or Sullivan. I have pursued the idea of two kinds of knowledge bolstered by the work of some European philosophers (e.g. de Biran, 1805) and the strong feeling that the 'knowledge' from experience and the arts is in many ways different from traditional rational scientific endeavors and that somehow both need to be included if we are to have a field that is scientific while not excluding the data that come from the richness of subjective experience. The comment above by Merritt Janson would be a poignant example of that latter. It would be absolutely stupid to make a statement such as the one she made – from a traditional scientific point of view. I mean the damn play is all written out. She and the cast and the director all know that. The lines are scripted. The plot is set. Obviously, her statement is patently idiotic. And yet, of course, it is incredibly beautiful and not stupid at all.

This problem of logic and whatever we're going to call this other stuff – subjectivity? creativity? feeling? whatever – I had noticed several years ago when reading *La Gradiva*, a composite publication with the novella by Jensen of that name followed by Freud's (1907) analysis of it. When Freud starts his analysis, he notes the beauty of the story (which it absolutely has), but then puts that aside to make his analysis of the plot. But, it seemed to me in reading Freud's commentary, how can you put aside a major and important part of a work, analyse the plot and ignore a huge amount of the data, that is its beauty?

So I've been trying to figure that out in my thinking, my writing and my presentations: how not to drop one or the other part of the science–subjectivity whole. 'But what has that to do with Meyer and Sullivan?' I asked myself. My answer over several days was 'nothing'. Sorry, Larry.

Then, while showering after a workout at the gym, I thought: 'That's not true at all. Great teachers don't just provide the content of knowledge; they also give you the tools and the encouragement to try to go further.' It has seemed sad to me that very bright people like Kraepelin, the leaders of the neuroplasticity conference and Freud himself, all noticed this 'logic–feeling/experience' problem, but perhaps in order to be true to their dominant ideology had to let it drop. What Meyer and Sullivan gave to me, I think, was certainly the freedom to try to figure things out, but also the perspective to look at a large part, perhaps the whole, of the picture, and the licence, even if I couldn't do any better, to think, talk and write in a relatively fuzzy manner if that was what I needed to include the whole picture, all the data, in my work and thinking. And it didn't come naturally to me to try to be more open. The smaller, neater, grossly incomplete picture is very seductive. After all, it gives a sense of knowledge and clarity even if these are not warranted by the data.

Just exactly to counter that premature sense of closure, it is not for nothing that many of our greatest people and teachers have told us again and again: 'Listen to the patient, doctor. He's telling you the diagnosis' (from Osler, one of America's leading physicians), or of course: 'You can observe a lot by just looking.' And, for me personally, how many patients have tried to help me: 'But Dr Strauss, as I've told you before, when I work in that [confusing] place, I *have* to organize myself.' Or: 'Why don't you ever ask me what I do to help myself?' And so many more, like the woman with bipolar disorder with whom I was doing a follow-up interview who told me the past year had been really good for her. Since I knew she had been hospitalized a few times over that period and assumed this was the famous manic denial, I asked her (very neutrally, I hope): 'Why was it so good?' She replied: 'Well, I was in a very abusive marriage and I was finally able to get divorced.' (Chalk up another one for Osler and Yogi Berra.)

What people do to help themselves, the interdigitation of normality and pathology-related experiences, the perplexing role of 'illogical' experiences and explanations ('Every night I think that maybe this time it will turn out differently'), even beauty – very, very complicated, very confusing. But very, very, real and very important.

I think that Meyer and Sullivan helped to provide me with the licence to look wherever I might learn something and the tools for how to go about that involving the wide range of patients, of human experience, which for me have been tools of incredible value. I feel I have learned a lot, even if it does not fit easily into most contemporary psychiatry. The workshops I lead on writing creatively about clinical experiences, the writing I do combining scientific questions and information with efforts at expressing things subjectively and 'creatively' as well, these are ways of proceeding which to me seem obvious and crucial if we are ever to have a human science, a field that does not exclude half of the data or distort it to fit a procrustean model. Meyer and Sullivan said that looking at the whole picture, at the human condition in its complexity, is okay. They tried also to be scientific in the narrow sense, and in my view failed at that. But it's up to us, then, to welcome what they gave and to take it further.

What does this have to do with improvement? I can't prove it, but I think it has everything to do with improvement. Our research, and the research of others since, has found that there are a vast array of factors that influence course and improvement in serious mental illnesses. These include the importance of previous levels of function in different life domains; the nature of the person's problem; the surroundings and relationships of that person; his or her urge and efforts to get better; the help he or she gets, whether through medicine, encouragement, understanding, hope, point of view or confidence from those around them; and so much more that we don't yet understand. We learned both that many people with serious mental illnesses experience significant improvements over time, no matter how disabled they had been, and that we knew extremely little about what predicted or contributed to such improvements. Finally, we learned that to understand better both the trajectory of illness and of the person's recovery we would need to attend to many more factors and issues than those that had fit neatly into either existing models of disorder or of science. We would need to do a lot more looking and listening, using whatever tools that we could find that would help us to do so more effectively.

In one presentation to a mixed audience of psychiatrists, nurses and people with serious mental illnesses, I was talking about the work Jaak Rakfeldt and I had done on what we came to refer to as 'the low turning point' (Rakfeldt and Strauss, 1989), a phenomenon we had noted in our follow-up interviews. Some people who are doing better report this kind of experience: 'One day I looked around me at all those sick people on the ward and I decided I could do better than that' and then they did. That is a relatively common report. I was giving a lecture about that to the group and someone at the back of the room, obviously a troubled person with a serious mental illness, asked: 'But how do you know when you've reached the low turning point?' That question broke my heart, but both that question and my, and others', efforts to find the answer I think would have been an acceptable tribute to the work of Meyer and Sullivan.

4.6 From a psychiatry based in death to a psychiatry based in life

> The emphasis on the living patient became the central characteristic of the American movement destined to reach its culmination in mental hygiene – Adolf Meyer's 1928 Presidential Address to the American Psychiatric Association. (Meyer, 1928, p. 12)

In addition to John's personal account of the energy and optimism he encountered when walking into the largely Meyer/Sullivian-dominated psychiatry of the 1950s, the magnitude of the shift in clinical psychiatry that is embodied in Meyer's career is probably best appreciated through his own account. In 1928, Meyer had the opportunity to present the Presidential Address to the American Psychiatric Association. He used that opportunity both to look backwards, over his 35-year history with the organization, and forwards to what he hoped psychiatry was by that point coming to be (i.e. 'mental hygiene'). His account is one of contrasts, but also provides useful clues as to what he thought needed to be encompassed by a psychiatry that was worthy of its name. Our inclusion of passages from this speech is not meant solely to give the reader an appreciation of the historical evolution of the field during this important transitional period, but also to lay some foundations for an adequate conceptual approach to recovery.

To begin with perhaps the most dramatic example, and the one from which we derived the title for this section, Meyer suggested in his speech that the institutional psychiatry he had encountered at the beginning of his career was characterized by two prominent streams, both of which had limited psychiatry to the study of death rather than of living people. The first aspect of institutional life in the late nineteenth century, as we know from our previous chapter, was the over-crowding and under-staffing of what had become by then large and primarily custodial state 'hospitals'. Writes Meyer:

> Psychiatry was then, as it still is in many places, largely an institutional and legal task. Under the rise of state care it had for some time been gathering from the almshouses and detention houses the persons who proved to be impossible in the community but who were nevertheless in need of more promising treatment than that of retaliation or mere exclusion. Psychiatry could deal with *individuals* only to a slight extent. It had but scant room for an interest in the life-problems of specific persons. (Meyer, 1928, p. 2)

Meyer reports that when, in 1895, he 'received an invitation to try my hand at work with 1200 patients, at the Worcester Lunatic Hospital', he was given 'a staff of only four co-assistants'. After a year of struggle and avid lobbying, he was finally able to secure the services of 'four additional junior men assisting the senior assistants' (Meyer, 1928, p. 9), thereby doubling his staff. This was the extent of the staffing he had to manage a hospital of 1200 patients.

According to Meyer, though, his incredulity at the scope of the responsibilities to be handled by so few people was not widely shared by the field itself. This was, in part, because the role of the doctor was severely limited in these hospitals to attending to the physical or medical diseases, conditions and needs of the patients; there was, in other words, little properly *psychiatric* work for the psychiatrists to do. This was, in part, because mental illnesses were once again viewed (as they had been in Pinel's day) to be largely incurable diseases. The remaining staff were occupied with the largely custodial tasks of keeping the hospital operating, because there was nothing else that could be done for the patients. This state of affairs is reflected in a story Meyer tells about his early days in the field:

> In Kankakee, in 1893, there were six assistant physicians to *2200* patients and one of these, temporarily acting superintendent, proudly claimed that he could do all the medical work alone if necessary.
>
> In Worcester I became the fifth member of the staff of four attending to 1200 patients and *600* admissions a year, myself supposed to be free from routine. I obtained the doubling of the staff, whereupon one of our medical visitors asked me: 'How do you keep the boys busy?' I never had any worry on that point. (Meyer, 1928, p. 16; italics in the original)

The view that mental illnesses were incurable and that people afflicted with them could summarily be written off as no longer having a life worth living extended to the nature of the scientific activities undertaken at the hospitals. This brings us to the second aspect of hospital life in the late nineteenth century with which Meyer was concerned. Apparently, very little of the research being carried out at the hospitals had anything to do with the patients per se or with their care. The scientists working out of these institutions did not concern themselves with the people admitted there, with their day-to-day functioning, with their treatment or rehabilitation (of which there was very little) or even with their symptoms and impairments. The prominent scientists of the day were concerned rather with the patients' bodies, and primarily *after* they had died. This was during a period when, in Meyer's words, 'real science in medicine was identified with the deadhouse and the use of the microscope and a few other instruments, and when the *life* aspect of pathology in medicine generally had just barely begun to assert itself' (Meyer, 1928, p. 2; italics in the original). Science at the time was primarily a science of death rather than a science of life, and the same was true for a psychiatry which at the time was modelling itself after medicine. Most hospital administrators or doctors were more interested in investigating the tissues and cells of former patients than they were in addressing the needs of the patients who were still alive.

This recognition led Meyer to decry the state of the science of the day and its lack of relevance to the presumed work of the 'hospital' as a place for people to receive care. For example, he described one of the few men who he considered to be making scientific advances in this era of hospital psychiatry as a scientist who 'for a long time remained the seeker of salvation in post-mortems, more as a collector of material than as a formulator of principles which might in turn have affected the work with the living' (Meyer, 1928, pp. 3–4). He recalled another prominent psychiatric pathologist of the time, of whom he writes:

> I well remember, as an example of the diversity of expectations from a laboratory worker of those days, a task waiting for him on the shelves: a collection of desiccated feces to be analyzed chemically by him (the aim being to find the disease in pure culture). (Meyer, 1928, p. 8)

Although he too was convinced of the importance of the biological dimension for psychiatry – emphasized in his concept of 'psychobiology' – Meyer had little confidence that studies such as these would shed much light on as complex a phenomenon as mental illness. In fact, Meyer eschewed any theoretical framework that remained one-dimensional, regardless of the dimension in question. His criticism of post-mortem studies and studies of faecal matter was equally relevant to behaviorism and psychoanalysis, even though they purported to offer more psychological and social explanations. In fact, he was so convinced of the multifaceted, complex nature of human life and mental illness – which he conceptualized within the context of human life – that he joked that the challenge facing Albert Einstein was favorable in comparison. He writes:

> Anyone who thinks that Watson's accounts of behaviorism should cover all that arises in our field, will have ... difficulty. Those who imagine that all psychiatry and psychopathology and therapy have to resolve themselves into a smattering of claims and hypotheses of psychoanalysis and that they stand or fall with one's feelings about psychoanalysis, are equally misguided. I sometimes feel that Einstein, concerned with the relativity in astronomy, has to deal with very simple facts as compared to the complex and erratic and multicontingent performances of the human microcosms, the health, happiness and efficiency of which we psychiatrists are concerned. (Meyer, 1928, p. 25)

What did he propose in the place of such one-dimensional theories? 'We simply have to grant', suggests Meyer, 'that a psychiatrist has to have a truly comprehensive knowledge of the human organism and also of its functioning in complex personal and social relations, past, present and future, and objective and subjective' (Meyer, 1928, p. 26). As we saw in Strauss' prose preceding this section, this is, of course, easier said than done. But Meyer was not persuaded that complexity should be used as an excuse for a psychiatry that had become largely based on the examination of dead bodies. This type of science he refers to as 'psychiatry without psychiatry ... like human life without a goal; or a book without a topic, or effort without a purpose' (Meyer, 1928, p. 22). At another point he suggests, in relation to this period, that 'one is tempted to say: Never was there more psychiatry with so little psychiatry in the ordinary sense of study of mental disease as seen in life' (Meyer, 1928, p. 13). For Meyer, it was precisely 'life' that was primarily at issue in developing a psychiatry worthy of its name. A psychiatry of the 'deadhouse' would not only be of no use in the running of a mental hospital but also of little use in helping us to understand how mental illnesses develop in the context of the person's everyday *life*. This is where Meyer chose to focus his attention.

He gives credit in his Presidential Address to a previous Presidential Address given to the American Psychiatric Association, this one in 1894 by Weir Mitchell (the same psychiatrist who recommended her first European trip to Jane Addams), one short year after the association had changed its title from the Association of Hospital Superintendents to the American Medico-Psychological Association. This meeting, 'in the midst of reasonable satisfaction with existing conditions and developments', writes Meyer, 'brought something of a storm in the form of the memorable Philadelphia address of Weir Mitchell' (Meyer, 1928, p. 5). What was memorable about this address, in addition to its 'rhapsodic' quality, was that it was the first critique of psychiatric hospitals that Meyer had heard to come from within the field itself. There had been numerous critiques of the field prior to this, but none by so prominent and respected a psychiatrist and none (in Meyer's experience) that had set the bar so much higher for what could and should be expected from the field. He writes:

> To me, Weir Mitchell's address was a spur in more than one way. So far most of the scrutinizing of the status of psychiatric work seemed

> to be coming from the outside, as during the strife between the New York neurologists and the giant who held the fort at Utica (Dorothea Lynde Dix had been interested largely in the attitude of the legislators). I sent to Governor Altgeld a copy of the speech of Weir Mitchell and urged a move from within, making the suggestion that even more profitable discussion might come from the workers themselves. The resulting printed public document led to the first open examinations for internships in state hospitals. (Meyer, 1928, p. 6)

With this inspiration, Meyer set off on the task of constructing the field of (American) psychiatry almost from scratch. Not only did he turn away from investigating dead bodies and faeces, but he also eschewed the other achievements for which psychiatry had come to be known, especially, in this case, in his native Europe. He found, that is, little of utility in diagnosis:

> Current practice in general medicine uses hard and fast diagnostic, prognostic, etiological and descriptive and explanatory 'pathological' terms, and wants to force us to use for our far more multiconditioned and complex field that which works to perfection in the simple patterns and problems but may not be so simply applicable in our own field. Diagnosis and disease concept, in the form of a one-word diagnosis, does not work. (Meyer, 1928, p. 28)

Here, too, psychiatry was trying to emulate medicine to its own detriment. People cannot be reduced to one-word concepts. There is much more to human life than a particular condition a person may suffer from and, in the case of psychiatry, it is not clear that it is a condition at all. After all, the psychiatrist comes to the conclusion that it is a condition only by excluding all of the data that pertain to the person's overall life, including his or her social relationships and personal history. But these were precisely the things, the things related to the person's life, in which Meyer was most interested. As he concludes: 'To me, the facts of each case were more important than the assumption of as yet problematic disease-processes' (Meyer, 1928, p. 10).

In order to build a psychiatry based in life, Meyer found it useful to return to the same basic approach that had been adopted by Pinel, that is the approach of observing, recording and analysing facts. In Meyer's case, the facts of most interest were those that pertained to what he felt he needed to describe as 'the living patient'. 'Although I was engaged under the name of pathologist,' he writes, 'I had become more and more determined to make the living patient the centre of my interest' (Meyer, 1928, p. 9). The psychiatrist, he argues, should take 'pains to digest what we know of man as we know him from actual, reasonably wide experience, and what we know of psychiatry as we meet it every day' (Meyer, 1928, p. 8). As long as people were to be retained in hospital settings (which Meyer was soon to turn away from), psychiatry should concern itself with observing and understanding 'the living patient' within its midst. While this insight might have seemed obvious to Pinel given his medical training, it had since been lost within the culture of the large custodial state hospitals, and it took Meyer to bring the field back to the principle of unbiased observation. At the time of his Presidential Address, more than 30 years after Mitchell's, he was able to confidently state that:

> We are getting to closer quarters with the facts that count; with a frank determination to study the facts that constitute nature's experiments on man, and to study them as we find them without bewildering and confusing preoccupations. (Meyer, 1928, p. 19)

The 'bewildering and confusing preoccupations' we can imagine to have come as much from psychoanalysis and behaviorism as from post-mortem studies, given that neither superegos nor conditioning can be considered observable facts of everyday life. It is the case, however, that the facts of everyday life occur at multiple levels of organization, including at the biological and physiological level, and at the interpersonal and social level as well. While the individual person, 'the living patient', could be considered one unit of analysis for psychiatry, it was not the only one to be considered. Some aspects of life could be determined by genes, others by environmental factors and others still by social factors. Psychiatry would need to be conversant with all of these levels and domains of study. Writes Meyer:

> Today we use this critical common sense as 'controlled experience with the experiments of nature' first and last, and solid training and proficiency in the entire field of intensive study of the various levels of integration, structural and functional – with total function (psychobiology) and part functions (physiology) – and physico-chemical, individual and social. We work with the facts contained in the life history and family history and the results of our examinations, with the individual assets and maladjustments, and the individual and social adjustments open to us. (Meyer, 1928, p. 24)

Given his dissatisfaction with the hospital-based psychiatry he inherited, and his growing interest in everyday life, the environment and social factors, it is perhaps not surprising that Meyer left the hospital environment to create what he refers to as 'extra-mural psychiatry'. Influenced also by Clifford Beers' autobiography (*A Mind that Found Itself*, first published, in part owing to Meyer's insistence, in Beers, 1908) and Beers' ideas that came to shape in the form of the 'Mental Hygiene movement' (Meyer's terms), Meyer was involved in the opening of the first outpatient mental health clinic: the Henry Phipps Psychiatric Clinic at Johns Hopkins, in 1913. While he began his career in mental hospitals, as everyone did in those days, he quickly came to see the limitations they posed, not only on the person's chances for treatment and recovery but also on any chances the scientist might have of learning about the nature of mental illness. Beginning as early as 1904, and in partnership with his wife, Meyer began to expand the scope of his practice beyond the boundaries of the hospital; 'the return to the community', he writes, 'began to receive more practical attention'. Then, in 1905, he continued, 'to head off an antiquated patronizing after-care scheme, we offered home-visiting and obtained probably the first psychiatric social worker' (Meyer, 1928, p. 17). From there, the progression further and further into the community was inevitable:

> In harmony with my dynamic conceptions of most mental disorders, I had to reach out, in my actual work, more and more toward a broader understanding of the patients, which led me to a study of the family settings and by and by also of the place where the individual first becomes a member of the community, the school. I might also have looked to the church, but since that was too much split up, there seemed to be less hope of achievement. (Meyer, 1928, p. 16)

Since we have had occasion to consider the backgrounds of Pinel, Dix and Addams, and the ways in which their life experiences might have influenced their thinking and practice, it only seems fair to wonder what in Meyer's life might have given impetus to his dissatisfaction with the reigning views of mental illness and treatment of his day and led him to shift to consideration of 'the living patient'. After all, Meyer was in fact trained as a neuropathologist, not a psychiatrist. What could have led him to such a perspective on the people languishing within the hospitals in which he had worked? We have no need to wonder about this for long, however, as Meyer gives his own explanation in his customary matter-of-fact and 'common sense' style. He writes:

> No doubt the interest became more insistent when my coming to this country helped with many other factors to precipitate a serious depression of three years' duration in my own mother, who had always appeared as one of the sanest persons in my experience and who recovered against the expectations of my old teacher, giving me many an opportunity to incorporate well-known human facts in my more strictly medical thought of the time. (Meyer, 1928, p. 21)

He remained convinced of the humanity of the person with the mental illness, and the person's possibilities for recovery from it, because he had seen his own mother go through both processes. Despite being consigned by his own mentor – who at the time was considered an internally renown expert on mental illness – to chronic, debilitating depression from which there presumably was no cure, Meyer's mother recovered on her own after three years. We recall that Pinel lost a good friend to mental illness, and that both Dix and Addams had their own experiences of mental illness and recovery. As we will see throughout the remainder of this volume, this kind of personal exposure to mental illness, either in oneself or in a loved one, appears to be one of the core commonalities of these proto-recovery advocates. While not surprising, this fact is perhaps worth noting and lends additional credibility to the forms of peer support and other peer-delivered services that are currently coming to maturity as part of the recovery movement. Apparently, they have deep roots in the lives of many major figures in the history of psychiatry, figures whose own illnesses or experience of illness in their loved ones has seldom been an acknowledged part of their legacy.

4.7 Problems in everyday living and their resolution

> The main thing is that your point of reference should always be life itself and not the imagined cesspool of the unconscious. (Adolf Meyer; cited in Perry, 1982, p. 237)

One of the possible explanations offered for why Meyer's work is no longer taught in medical schools – above and beyond his use of inelegant neologisms – is that he offered neither a comprehensive nor even a coherent conceptual framework for his views. The majority of his influence appears to have come through his teaching and through his students' ability to digest his overall approach to understanding and responding to patients' difficulties and making the key elements of the approach their own. This, too, was apparently in line with Meyer's teaching, as he actively discouraged his students from becoming disciples, encouraging them rather to take from his work what worked for them and abandon the rest, as they digested his teaching and then went on to construct their own models and theories. This was one way of characterizing his own approach to the people from whom he had learned himself, from Kraepelin to Freud. In this way, Meyer stands out as an unusual figure, along with Jane Addams, as someone who strove to live his life and carry out his work in ways that were consistent with his own stated values.

In developing his own pragmatic approach to psychiatric research and practice, Meyer was certainly influenced by the work of American philosophers William James and Charles Pierce, as well as by his friendships with John Dewey, George Herbert Mead and Charles Cooley – the same 'Chicago group' with whom Addams had also associated. According to Theodore Lidz, who was one of Meyer's students, and Eugen Bleuler's son Manfred, who was himself a leading psychiatric researcher in Meyer's native Switzerland, the roots of Meyer's foundation in pragmatism ran further back and deeper in his own family tree. In researching his family history, they found out that Meyer's grandfather had been a follower of an eighteenth-century Swiss folk philosopher, Jakob Gujer, who was better known as Kleinjogg, and that the Meyer family had joined, through marriage, with the Kleinjoggs (Lidz, 1966, p. 323). In the following description of Kleinjogg's approach to farming, Lidz recognizes many of the themes and key elements of Meyer's eventual approach. Lidz writes:

> Kleinjogg had practiced and taught an instrumental approach to farm-ing, observing what worked and what did not work, and trying out

new ways that seemed to make sense rather than blindly following tradition, as did other peasants. He fostered communal activity and teamwork. At first he was hated and considered a menace for departing from ways that had become sacred through long usage; but when his techniques bore results he became a revered and widely renowned person whom Goethe, Pestalozzi, and other great men visited. Kleinjogg's basic concerns were with how people could be healthy and happy. He demonstrated that joy could be obtained from useful work and the ensuing accomplishment, and he emphasized that children became happy and skillful adults only through the example of parents. (Lidz, 1966, p. 323)

It was not only Pussin and Pinel who associated farming and work with recovery, and not only Butler and Freud who thought that the roots of mental illness were laid in early childhood experiences and family life. But like Kleinjogg, Meyer both departed from some of the sacred beliefs of the psychiatry he was taught and developed new techniques that bore results.

For an account of these techniques, we will have to rely on the descriptions of one of Meyer's many influential students. We return to an account given by Lidz as part of an Adolf Meyer Lecture presented to the American Psychiatric Association in honor of Meyer's 100th birthday (he had actually died 16 years earlier in 1950). According to Lidz, the first major step Meyer took in departing from the sacred cows of the institutions in which he initially worked was simply to talk with the patients, and to listen to what they had to say, to listen to what they had to say, that is, without interpreting it solely as manifestations of their illnesses. 'He became interested in talking to patients about their lives and found that they seemed to explain much of why they had become ill' (Lidz, 1966, p. 324). When contrasted to representing either brain lesions or the unfettered rambling of the unconscious, considering patients' stories as valid and valuable clinical material in and of itself was truly revolutionary. It meant that the person was still very much there, despite the ravages of the presumed 'illness', and that the person could still play a role in understanding and dealing actively with his or her own difficulties (rather than ceding this function entirely to the psychiatrist). Writes Lidz:

> The life stories of patients seemed to make sense; their experiences seemed to clarify why they were disturbed and suggested ways of helping them. Bolstered by pragmatism, [Meyer] could cease looking for 'something else' to explain their mental disorders. As a neuroanatomist and neuropathologist, he knew that what he found in a brain might explain disorganization of thought and behavior, but it could never explain a life story or show how to remedy it. He grasped the need for a genetic-dynamic understanding of mental disorders in terms of the unique biography of each individual. He had the right to trust his common sense and he taught his colleagues to trust theirs. (Lidz, 1966, p. 326)

As Lidz suggests in this passage, this open and direct approach to involving the person in understanding and addressing his or her own difficulties was at the heart of what Meyer meant by 'common sense'. Continues Lidz:

> What he meant was that psychiatrists must be willing to use data about a patient's life in its own terms, not persist in seeking something behind and beyond experiences. He had found psychiatrists neglecting the obvious, the 'common sense', because the scientific tradition insisted that they must seek causes in the brain cells, physiology, or biochemistry; or because they must cure the 'mind' that they could not locate rather than seek to modify the patient's life and behavior. (Lidz, 1966, p. 326)

It was because it was the patient's life which primarily interested and concerned Meyer – rather than the causes of his or her difficulties which lay in someone's imaginary constructs – that he eventually gave up the disease and diagnostic language altogether and instead introduced the phrase 'problems in living'. Meyer demonstrated this shift even in the most severe cases of psychosis, as he did when he gave a lecture on this topic at the same meeting at Clark University where Freud and Jung first presented their psychoanalytic theories to American psychiatry and psychology. After congratulating Freud and Jung on their fine, groundbreaking work, which Meyer valued in particular for the efforts they were making to understand human experience and behavior in meaningful, if symbolic, terms, Meyer insisted that: 'We are, I believe, justified in directing our attention to the factors which we see at work in the life-history of the cases of so-called *dementia praecox*' (Meyer, 1910, p. 403). By factors 'we see at work', Meyer was asking his audience to put aside, at least temporarily, their conviction in the importance of what was going on behind the scenes (in the brain or the unconscious) in order to simply look and listen to what was going on in the light of day. We can recall here Strauss' mention of Yogi Berra's comment that: 'You can observe a lot by just looking.'

Meyer the pragmatist was intent upon applying this method as a 'natural experiment' and seeing to what degree and in what ways it was able to bear fruit. He was, that is, willing to put his ideas to the test. By adopting this common-sense approach, he then came to identify at least two possible sources of solutions to his patients' problems. The first, perhaps obvious, source would be to help the patient change his or her behavior. While such an idea might have been obvious to Pinel or even Tuke, this goal had long been lost in the large custodial hospitals that were simply warehousing presumably incurable cases. What also was different about Meyer's sense of this source of solutions was that the patient was him- or herself involved in identifying the solutions, as were the doctor and other staff. All of the answers did not have to come from the staff, but could, and preferably would, come from the patients themselves, especially once they had come to a fuller understanding of the nature of their difficulties through dialogue with the psychiatrist. The doctor, in Meyer's view, did not do things *on* or *to* the patient to fix him or her, like a surgeon, but rather helped the patient to figure out what he or she needed to do differently to escape from, address adequately or otherwise overcome their current situation.

In this respect, we might think of Meyer as applying Jane Addams' democratic and person-centred approach to resolving the problems that others were viewing at the time as mental illnesses. The most innovative feature of Meyer's approach, in comparison to the figures we have discussed thus far, however, was in where he located the second possible source of solutions. In addition to helping the patient to change his or her own behavior, Meyer discovered that he could change or modify the patient's social and physical environment as well. While he appreciated – along with Pinel, Tuke and Dix – that the environment likely contributed to the person's difficulties, his solution was not to remove the person from the environment (to place him or her in a hospital) but rather to help the person change the environment along with him- or herself. As Lidz describes, for Meyer psychiatry 'could try to help patients to achieve more workable and useful solutions to problems, and it could seek to modify the circumstances in which they lived' (Lidz, 1966, p. 327). Lidz suggests that this innovation was part and parcel of Meyer's deep roots in pragmatism, as we will see in the next passage. Even if this were an accurate attribution of Meyer's brilliance to the influence of American philosophy and culture, it was nonetheless a radical idea at the time and was in large part responsible for his founding, along with Lev Vygotsky, whom we discuss in Chapter 7, the disciplines of occupational science and therapy. Of this aspect of Meyer's work, Lidz writes:

> The essence of pragmatic, pluralistic thinking is that through the ingenuity, thought, and effort of man, the face of nature can be altered to man's needs. Such concepts stand at the core of the American tradition. Such ideas obviously turn away from the idea of a completed world which man seeks to know so that he can fit himself into it, or ideas of a given truth we must uncover, or even of those evolutionary concepts which maintain that everything unrolls in a predetermined and irrevocable manner. (Lidz, 1966, p. 325)

In anticipating other ideas yet to come, we will return to this notion of the denial of 'a completed world' when we get to our Chapter 6 discussion of Martin Luther King, Jnr and Gilles Deleuze. They took this argument further, and connected it to a social and political agenda that promoted human and civil rights at the level of a society. While Meyer and his co-founders of the Mental Hygiene movement, along with Harry Stack Sullivan, ended their careers focusing on societal solutions to what they had come to view as primarily societal problems (e.g. mental illnesses could be prevented by proper mental 'hygiene'), this level did not form the major focus of their attention prior to the Second World War. It was, understandably, in the wake of the atomic threat that the focus on the societal level became intensified.

For the majority of his career and teaching, Meyer's belief in the incompleteness of the world and the ability of humankind to change the world played out at the level of the individual and his or her immediate social environment. The family was thus one of the more important components of this picture, especially for children and youth, but then so were the other social institutions and settings in which people lived out their lives, including the school, the workplace, the faith community, the sports team and so on. These were the environments in which the person was expected to function, and the environments that could be altered to better suit the person's character, needs and strengths. As Lidz describes:

> Although Meyer did not disregard the potential importance of unknown hereditary factors, he refused to accept the prevalent pessimism about combating hereditary conditions. Pragmatically he focused on what could be worked with: change the environment, alter habit patterns and ways of thinking, help the patient solve or resolve problems. See what works and what does not work; mobilize the patient's assets, and they may suffice to counterbalance his deficiencies. Meyer was a meliorist, interested in improvement when he could not cure; and he taught that every patient should somehow be better off because of his relationship to the psychiatrist. (Lidz, 1966, p. 327)

Lidz's mention of 'assets' in this passage is neither incidental nor insignificant. In fact, one of the most important contributions that Meyer made to psychiatry, and consequently to recovery, in our humble opinion, was his focus on strengths. We have seen this in minor ways in both Pinel and Addams, where identifying and eliciting strengths was described as a way to ignite a person's involvement and improvement. It was not until Meyer, however, that the notion of personal assets and strengths assumed a central role as a theoretical construct. His view of the role of strengths in practice was very similar to that of Pinel and Addams. Pay close and careful attention to the person, identify with the person what motivates, what interests and what he or she is passionate about, find what gives the person a spark and then build on that to shore up the healthy functioning aspects of the person and to extend that strength to the weaker or more disrupted functions. With Meyer, this technique or strategy used perhaps intuitively by his predecessors came to be a major component of his conceptual framework. It was primarily through the mobilization of assets, as Lidz describes, that people's problems could be solved; this constituted, in fact, the main thrust of Meyer's approach to treatment and recovery. Rather than viewing the identification of strengths as a nicety that compassionate clinicians might use in developing rapport or in enabling them to check off areas on a list as being 'unproblematic' or 'unremarkable', he insisted that it was one of the doctor's primary functions, an 'obligation' as he describes it in his article 'The life chart and the obligation of specifying positive data in psychopathological diagnosis' (Meyer, 1919), to assess strengths as well as symptoms and areas of difficulty. Only then would a clinician have the chance to grasp a comprehensive picture of the whole person, including how that person functioned in his or her various life domains.

What would the clinician do with such data? Just as he had done in his own research and teaching, the clinician would then identify which patterns of behavior, or 'habits', worked for the person and which did not. Those that worked well would be shored up and built upon to address the areas in which the person's habits were not working well. In terms of those patterns which were not working well, either the person needed to create and adopt new habits or he or she needed to alter or modify the environment in which those habits were not working well. Either the habit could be made more adaptive or the environment could be changed to better accommodate or suit the existing habit. Once again, it is important to stress that this was Meyer's view not just in terms of what we might consider 'neurotic' or less serious mental illnesses, for which psychotherapy has long been shown to be effective, but also for the more serious mental illnesses with which this book is concerned. To return to the Clark conference at which Meyer had spoken about 'The dynamic interpretation of *dementia praecox*' (Meyer, 1910), this was his view of the difficulties and the solutions to be found for individuals with psychotic disorders as well. Given his commitment to a pragmatic approach, Meyer left this open to empirical verification. Only if, as Lidz suggests, 'Meyer acted on his unproven belief that schizophrenic patients could be helped through altering their milieu and modifying their habits of thinking could the fact be demonstrated' (Lidz, 1966, p. 325). And this was precisely what Meyer's practice and teaching did in fact demonstrate.

The 'problems in living' experienced by those individuals others would have diagnosed as having schizophrenia can be understood as stemming from the disorganization of the person's habits, a poor fit between the person's habits and his or her environments and/or the need to develop new habits that are more effective in those environments. As a result, Meyer focused most directly on how the person spends his or her day, in what environments and on what those environments demand of him or her. Once understood, these same domains would be the focus for intervention as well. Even when still working within a hospital setting, the patient's everyday life within the hospital milieu was his focus. It is from this basis that he, his wife and a few of their acquaintances developed what came to be called 'occupational therapy'. Meyer had known that in European asylums and in an increasing number of American hospitals as well, the staff had found 'occupation' to be 'a substitute for restraint'. As he writes in 'The philosophy of occupation therapy': 'This represent[ed] the attitude of many hospital men of the time. Industrial shops and work in laundry and kitchen and on the wards were the achievements of that program – very largely planned to relieve the employees' (Meyer, 1922, pp. 1–2). Patients worked in the hospitals primarily to have something to do, to relieve the employees of required tasks and, at least in the United States, to generate a profit – something we will return to in Chapter 6. But Meyer found work to have a similar effect to what Pussin and Pinel had described at the beginning of the development of '*traitement moral*', to have, that is, a therapeutic, or healing, or beneficial impact on the patient's functioning. For Meyer, this was because how people choose to spend their time is what gives their life a sense of meaning and purpose, and a purposeful, meaningful and productive use of that time is what gives people pleasure and enjoyment, what makes life worth living. It was 'the proper use of time in some helpful and gratifying activity', Meyer writes, that appeared to be 'a fundamental issue in the treatment of any neuro-psychiatric patient' (Meyer, 1922, p. 1).

To express this view of the centrality of purposeful activity in human life Meyer found the notion of 'work' to be too narrow and to be confined to productive labor carried out in the marketplace, a notion which he felt had been distorted by industrialism. The ideal of material success had generated a false notion of the value of human activity, 'bringing with it a kind of nausea to the worker and a delirium of the trader living on advertisement and salesmanship' (Meyer, 1922, p. 8). Meyer's further comment that 'The man of today has lost the capacity and pride of workmanship and has substituted for it a measure in terms of money; and now his money proves to be of uncertain value' (Meyer, 1922, p. 8) could not be any more true then than it is today. To move away from these distortions, he suggested the term 'occupation' to cover not only what one does to earn a living, or to have a career, but also all of the other things people *do* to have a life. The emphasis was on human activity, whether that activity produced something tangible or not. In performing an activity, people were to find the intrinsic meaning and enjoyment that made the activity worthwhile. To capture this broader notion, he took what he described as a 'new step' to introduce a 'freer conception of work . . . a concept of free and pleasant and profitable *occupation – including recreation and any form of helpful enjoyment as the leading principle*' (Meyer, 1922, p. 8; italics in the original). It was involvement in these types of activity that Meyer found to be both compensatory and healing in the case of serious mental illnesses.

When initially running a hospital, this focus on activity dictated Meyer's approach to management. The contrast between this approach and that, for example, of the Tukes becomes quite evident in passages such as:

> A pleasure in achievement, a real pleasure in the use and activity of one's hands and muscles and a happy *appreciation of time* began to be used as incentives in the management of our patients, instead of abstract exhortations to cheer up and to behave according to abstract or repressive rules. The main advance of the new scheme was the blending of work and pleasure. (Meyer, 1922, p. 3; italics in the original)

As we saw above, Meyer's emphasis on the importance of time in this passage is reflected throughout his work. Understanding how people spend their time and assisting them in spending their time happily and in constructive, enjoyable activities constitute the two major tasks of psychiatry. Time in this sense is not simply clock time or chronological time, it is rather time as the fundamental symbolic medium for action, with the movement of the hand on the clock analogous to the beating of the heart as the blood flows through an organism's body. It is important in understanding Meyer's synthesis of mind and body in 'psychobiology' to see how these two flows, of time and of blood, are considered equally essential to the functioning of the organism. He writes:

> Our body is not merely so many pounds of flesh and bone figuring as a machine, with an abstract mind of soul added to it. It is throughout a live organism pulsating with its rhythm of rest and activity, beating time (as we might say) in ever so many ways ... Our conception of man is that of an organism that maintains and balances itself in the world of reality and actuality by being in active life and active use, i.e., using and living and acting its *time* in harmony with its own nature and the nature about it. It is the *use* that we make of ourselves that gives the ultimate stamp to our every organ ... Just as in the medical aspects we have come to value an appreciation of the exceedingly *simple* facts of basal metabolism (that is, the simple measure of the amount of CO_2 we produce), so the simple fact of employment of time has become an important measure and problem for physician and nurse ... The formulation in terms of habit-deterioration of even those grave mental disorders presenting the serious problem of *terminal dementia* made *systematic engagement of interest, and concern about the actual use of* TIME *and work an obligation and necessity.* (Meyer, 1922, pp. 4–5; italics in the original)

One gets the impression that Meyer felt it necessary to insist on the obligatory and essential nature of this concern about time because of the difficulty involved in communicating this central aspect of his perspective and his work to others. It is as if he could not state strongly enough just how important and core to the work of psychiatry this concept was that he had to continue to emphasize and insist on its value. If we take him seriously and at his word, then perhaps it is not so difficult to appreciate just how much of a challenge this was for him at the time. Indeed, it is most likely not that much less difficult today to convey the importance he attributed to how people use their time than it was a century ago. Imagine, for instance, trying to train psychiatric personnel to take the equivalent of 'vital signs' of a person's mental health the way medical staff currently take vital signs in relation to a person's physical health. For Meyer, this would be an appropriate analogy for a person's activity level, including the meaningfulness and enjoyable nature of the activity. An elevated temperature, a rapid heart beat or low blood pressure can indicate that someone's physical health is compromised. In the same way, a lack of activity, engagement in alienated activity or being forced to perform activities under the authority or coercion of others rather than by the person's own free choice can all indicate that a person's mental health is compromised. And in the same way that physical health can affect mental health, Meyer was convinced even more so that mental health affected physical health. This is what we take him to mean by 'It is the *use* that we make of ourselves that gives the ultimate stamp to our every organ.'

4.8 Opportunity and occupation

> Our rôle consists in giving *opportunities* rather than prescriptions (Adolf Meyer, from the first article in the first issue of the first volume of the *Archives of Occupational Therapy*; Meyer, 1922, p. 7; italics in original)

With this background, we can now take up the question of what implications Meyer's emphasis on time and activity has for recovery-oriented practice, as well as how Sullivan expanded on his efforts. First, we can argue that this emphasis on time and activity suggests a central role for what Meyer termed 'performance' in both the creation of psychopathology and its treatment. By performance, he meant simply the carrying out of an activity; not, as we now might think, a performance that is put on for or is to be judged by others, but in a more purely functional sense. This sense of performance was to occupy the role that would be given to insight in later forms of psychotherapy; the emphasis in Meyer's approach to care was on what people *do* rather than on what they are aware of or what they think. In fact, for Meyer thinking was simply one category of doing, and a form of doing that was much less important than other forms of doing that were more enjoyable or productive. Thinking could be important to the degree that it constituted planning for future action, but even in this case it was the activity itself that was crucial, not any particular mental content. He writes:

> This growing conviction that personality is fundamentally determined by *performance* rather than by mere good-will and good intention rapidly became the backbone of our psychology and psychopathology. It became a fair task for our ingenuity to *obtain* performance wherever it had failed to come *spontaneously* and thereby to serve the organism in the task of keeping itself in good form. (Meyer, 1922, p. 6; italics in original)

The only way to assist someone in developing new or more adaptive habits was to encourage the person to act in new ways, repeatedly, over time. This requires ingenuity because it is not enough simply to tell the person what to do. For one thing, you may not know what the person needs or wants to do differently. But even more importantly, the new activity that is performed solely in response to another person's demands will not have the characteristic of freedom that Meyer thought so crucial to healthy functioning. It therefore is not the doctor's role to prescribe new behaviors, as one might prescribe medication. It is not for one person to tell another person how to live. It becomes a 'fair task' for one's ingenuity when one accepts that the best one can do is to offer the person opportunities for trying out new behaviors and perhaps inviting the person to try on certain things for size, so to speak. For the performance to be meaningful, and for the new habits to develop in a sustainable way, it has to be the person him- or herself who decides on and engages in new activities. Just as a coach cannot throw a pass for a quarterback or sink a three-point shot for a point guard, the clinician cannot undertake or perform the activity for the person. Nor can the clinician put in the significant time and effort required to practise these behaviors sufficiently to ensconce them as new habits.

It is for this reason that we opened this section with the quote from Meyer that: 'Our rôle consists in giving *opportunities* rather than prescriptions' (Meyer, 1922, p. 7). One key difference between coaching football and basketball on the one hand and being a recovery-oriented clinician on the other is that the clinician's role is to encourage and assist the person in performing those activities that he or she wishes to perform, not those that the coach identifies for the person to perform in order to play a certain game 'well'. Athletic coaches have content expertise; they know the game they coach inside and out. In the case of recovery, we can hope that clinicians have 'reasonably wide experience' (to use Meyer's terms), but we cannot assume that clinicians know more about life in general, or about the specific kind of life a given person wants to lead; and, as we noted above, it is a crucial aspect of this life that it is actively and freely chosen by the person him- or herself. While this point was suggested by Pinel, Meyer accords it more centrality in his approach to care. Reclaiming the person's freedom to choose to lead the particular life which he or she will find personally meaningful actually provides the foundation for recovery in Meyer's view. It is upon this foundation that all other efforts towards recovery become possible, and within this context that the identification and use of strengths becomes a crucial, and necessary, component.

In what is perhaps one of the first American attempts to lay out guidelines for a form of psychotherapy, Meyer describes his approach as follows:

> It takes, above all, resourcefulness and an ability to respect at the same time the native *capacities and interests* of the patient. Freedom from premature meddling, and tact in avoiding false comparisons or undue expectations fostering disappointment, orderliness without pedantry, cheer and praise without sloppiness and without surrender of standard – these may be the rewards of a good use of personal gifts and of good training. (Meyer, 1922, pp. 7–8; italics in the original)

This is not to say that clinicians never make suggestions or try to steer their patients in one direction as opposed to another. Especially in cases of more serious mental illnesses, it may even be necessary for clinicians to become directive, but even then the suggestions should come from what the clinician has been able to learn about the patient as a unique individual, the person's interests and strengths, and what the clinician thinks the person would choose on his or her own had he or she the requisite confidence, self-regard and energy. As he writes:

> It is not a question of specific *prescriptions*, but of opportunities, except perhaps where suggestions can be derived from the history of the patient and a minute study of the trends of fancy and even delusions

> reveals the lines of predilections and native longings – yet even here
> the physician would only exert his ingenuity to adapt *opportunities*.
> (Meyer, 1922, p. 8; italics in the original)

Meyer's focus on *native* longings and capacities cannot be over-emphasized. He clearly saw the role of the clinician as helping the person to become who he or she was 'meant to be', who he or she would become in the absence of barriers to his or her development, were the environment fully supportive of healthy habits and meaningful pursuits. This is different from the disciplinary approach of the Tukes, as they appeared to think that they knew how people in general should behave and they left little room within the retreat for the individualization of care. Meyer, on the other hand, encouraged 'freedom from meddling' and 'orderliness without pedantry', wishing instead to offer the person multiple opportunities to pursue his or her own ideal, confident that life experience will be the best teacher of what works for the person and what does not.

Although Meyer pointed out that change and recovery could come about through modifications of the person's environment, he gave less attention to this component of care at the level of the individual. Meyer's focus on changing the environment appeared to come later in his career, as part of the Mental Hygiene movement, and was concerned instead with social, cultural and societal change for the benefit of the entire population. It was up to Harry Stack Sullivan to begin to experiment with changes to the person's environment, at first within the context of the mental hospital and then later within the community context. Sullivan's most salient addition to Meyer's basic approach was to recognize that the doctor – patient relationship provided one more window onto the person's difficulties and functioning and therefore also provided one more – and for Sullivan the central – opportunity for growth, development and recovery. It is true that Freud had been the first to focus intensively on the relationship with the psychoanalyst and the patient through such mechanisms as transference and counter transference. And it is true that Freud viewed this relationship as offering a key mechanism for therapeutic change. But it was Sullivan who first applied this insight to the care of individuals with psychotic disorders (whom Freud thought inappropriate for psychoanalysis) and Sullivan who first applied this insight in a broader, more reality-based and concrete way. For Freud, the psychoanalyst was not supposed to exist as a person for the patient, but rather as a blank screen upon which the patient would project unconscious content. For Sullivan, the clinician was not only to be considered a fellow human being, but it was the nature of their interpersonal relationship as being a genuine interaction between two people that was thought to be curative.

One way to contrast the clinical approaches of these figures is to suggest that while Meyer stood outside of the person's immediate social world in order to observe his or her activities and habits objectively, and Freud attempted to penetrate into the person's subjective world as if by stealth, Sullivan was content to view himself as simply one other person in the patient's social world – albeit a hopefully useful one – who both observed the person's activities and habits and participated actively in them. To capture this dual role, Sullivan described his approach as 'participant observation' and was keen to use his own subjective experience of the person to shed light on the nature of the person's objective difficulties and strengths. Sullivan, in other words, viewed himself as a subject (as doctor) interacting with another subject (the patient) within the context of an intersubjective world. If, through this relationship, Sullivan could identify and assist the person in correcting the distortions and maladaptive habits that interfered with their enjoying a fully human and reciprocal relationship, these improvements could then generalize to the person's life as a whole. Learn how to relate to me and you will learn how to relate to other people in general. The advantage of relating to me first is that I am trained and experienced in terms of being able to create an environment that will elicit and build on your strengths and accept and ameliorate your difficulties.

4.9 The interpersonal context of recovery

Sullivan first developed this approach as chief of an inpatient unit at Shepard and Enoch Pratt Hospital in Baltimore in the 1920s. He chose to specialize in the care of young men with psychotic disorders, which, as we mentioned in our introductory chapter, he attributed to having had his own 'schizophrenic break' around the age of 17 years old, leaving him with a heightened sensitivity to other young men going through similar experiences. His conviction in the value of such sensitivity as a prerequisite to effective care and cure extended to his innovative practice of hiring men who had recovered from psychosis to return to his unit as attendants (another early precursor to peer support). In stark contrast to the Kraepelinian perspective that was still dominant at the time, his experience with this unit led him to conclude that 'schizophrenia is an illness of excellent prognosis' (Sullivan, 1962, p. 288).

Despite his extraordinary success with his young patients (he reported a recovery rate of around 80%), like Meyer, Sullivan left the hospital setting after accumulating about a decade's worth of experience. Anticipating the criticisms of inpatient care that would come 30 years later from Goffman, Basaglia and others, Sullivan quickly ran up against the limitations of caring for people in institutional environments that do not represent the realities the person will have to face upon discharge. Writes Sullivan, if improvement

> is made solely on the basis of the particularly favorable institutional environment, with repression of hopeless features of the social situation awaiting him outside, a recovery of a tenuous and unstable kind may be accomplished – the prospect being for prompt relapse. (Sullivan, 1962, p. 15)

Thus, while Sullivan was convinced of the importance of the therapist having a keen sensitivity to the person's struggles and of fostering a therapeutic relationship in which these struggles were accepted, understood and addressed, he did not view the hospital as the only, or even as the preferable, place in which to offer such care.

As a result, he spent the majority of his career providing, and teaching, intensive outpatient psychotherapy for individuals with serious mental illnesses. The majority of efforts made since to provide psychotherapy to people with serious mental illnesses, whether inpatient or outpatient, stem from this early work of Sullivan, including the cognitive-behavioral approaches currently under development that we mentioned in our Introduction (e.g. Kingdon and Turkington, 1994; Fowler and Garety, 1995; Chadwick *et al.*, 1996).

Of what did Sullivan's psychotherapy consist? Recalling that many of his predecessors had spent the majority of their time doing post-mortem studies, it is perhaps not that surprising that the first principle upon which Sullivan insisted was that 'from the start' each of his patients was to be 'treated as a *person among persons*' (Sullivan, 1962, p. 285; italics in the original). He insisted on this principle not only because individuals with serious mental illnesses had been, and were continuing to be, treated as other than human in the large custodial state hospitals, but also because it was only through genuine human contact that progress would be possible. In this regard, he appeared to be in agreement with Jane Addams' view of the emphasis on reciprocity within the American ideal of democracy. As Helen Swick Perry, Sullivan's editor and biographer, points out: 'His observation of people from the beginning was within the framework of a democratic society. There was an acceptance of the basic dignity of mankind' (Sullivan, 1962, p. xxv). As he had himself been one, it is understandable that he would extend this dignity to people with serious mental illnesses, and that he would go so far as to insist that any potential treatment be offered based on this important foundation.

What then? In agreement also with Meyer, Sullivan argued that one way of according his patients the dignity they deserved as 'persons among persons' was to view them as active and goal-directed agents in determining their own lives. A student of philosophy as well as of psychology, sociology, anthropology and psychiatry, Sullivan was impressed by what he called:

> the obvious fact of *teleology* as a characteristic of things mental. As McDougall has put it, 'Purposive activity is the most fundamental category of psychology' . . . In attacking the problem of understanding and treatment of schizophrenia, the element of motivation seems logically fundamental to all others. As Dr. William A. White has said, 'We must understand what the patient is trying to do'. (Sullivan, 1962, p. 8; italics in the original)

This was one of the first guidelines for the psychotherapist: strive for an understanding of what the patient is trying to do, both in his or her life in general and, as a result of Sullivan's unique contribution, what he or she is trying to do in relating to the psychotherapist specifically. What is the patient trying to accomplish in his or her relationship with me? And once we understand what the patient is trying to do, we can begin to wonder about why he or she is trying to do precisely this and not something else.

This question was to be answered by exploring the person's previous life experiences. It could be reframed as: 'What experiences led up to or contributed to the patient's desire or need to accomplish whatever it is the person is trying to accomplish at this time and in this place?' For from Sullivan's perspective, all human behaviors, thoughts, attitudes and beliefs were derived from, or produced by, his or her life experiences up to this point. A second guideline for psychotherapy was the assumption that 'the gamut of behavior and thinking, usual or unusual, "normal" or psychotic, can be explained very largely on the basis of the individual's experience' (Sullivan, 1962, p. 11). Having a condition like psychosis did not suggest that the person was somehow fundamentally different from others, either by birth and body (e.g. lesions in the brain) or by personality composition (e.g. pre-Oedipal). It merely meant that the person had had different experiences from others *up to this point*. The person was still capable of having other, more 'usual', experiences, and to the degree that he or she was offered the opportunity to do so, such as in relation to the psychotherapist, he or she would naturally become less schizophrenic.

Although perhaps implicit in Meyer's view of schizophrenia, Sullivan was the first to put forth this promising new theory of the development and treatment of, and recovery from, serious mental illnesses. Perry chose to title her collection of Sullivan's essays on understanding and treating psychosis *Schizophrenia as a Human Process* (Sullivan, 1962) because this was Sullivan's core assumption about the nature of serious mental illnesses. They represented merely the effects of exaggerations or extreme or unusual forms of *human* experience. He writes:

> Schizophrenic thinking shows in its symbols and processes nothing exterior to the gamut of ordinary thinking, including therein that of reverie and of dreams. Even its extraordinary symbol situations have parallels in the extravagances of dreams. Neither is its occurrence explicable on the basis of any novel cognitive processes. It is, as a whole, a peculiarly inadequate adaptation of the cognitive processes to the necessities of adult life. (Sullivan, 1962, p. 92)

Situating psychotic experiences within the range of human experience had profound implications related to a number of theoretical issues. For example, it attributed to a society, or to a particular culture, the power to determine what was to be considered 'usual' or 'normal' as opposed to what was unusual, extreme or 'abnormal', and, as a result, what was to be considered unhealthy and pathological and therefore in need of treatment. The socio-cultural context determined the parameters of what was to be considered adaptive or maladaptive. What we currently define as 'schizophrenia' stands out as unusual or extreme because it represents a particularly maladaptive constellation of behaviors for this particular society. One could imagine, however, a culture in which such individuals would not be considered to have a pathological condition, but might instead be considered to have a heightened sensitivity to experience that could pose some advantages.

Our view of schizophrenia cannot be separated from the social context in which it is identified as such. It can only emerge within an interpersonal context. Writes Sullivan:

> There could not be a meaningful use of the term schizophrenia in regard to a man who had grown from birth into adolescence in utter detachment from any person or personally organized culture. Again, it is possible so to organize a society that the living of its persons, normal to each other, would be regarded as schizophrenic by psychiatrists who studied any one of its members in sufficiently alien surroundings. In brief, schizophrenia is meaningful only in an *interpersonal context*; its characteristics can only be established by a study of the interrelation of the schizophrenic with schizophrenic, less schizophrenic, and non-schizophrenic others. A 'socially recovered' schizophrenic is often still psychotic, but is certainly *less* schizophrenic than is a patient requiring active institutional supervision. To isolate the *non*-schizophrenic individual, however, is no small problem. (Sullivan, 1962, pp. 276–277; italics in the original)

Sullivan's quip about the difficulty of identifying 'the *non*-schizophrenic individual' would be picked up later and exploited by some of the more radical members of what became the interpersonalist tradition, such as R.D. Laing and Gregory Bateson, as we will see in Chapter 6. Sullivan's basic point was simple, however. The ideal of a fully mentally healthy individual, a person who was perfectly well adapted to any and all contingencies life might throw at him or her, a person who had had no difficult, problematic or damaging experiences simply did not exist. Everyone has habits that are more or less adaptive, everyone has vulnerabilities and everyone has areas both of function and of dysfunction (we recall here Pinel's emphasis on the preservation of areas of health and competence in the midst of 'madness'). To insist that a person aspire to or achieve another person's ideal of perfection in order to be considered 'recovered' was both unreasonable and unscientific. We are all more or less schizophrenic; the point of treatment is to reduce those areas of difficulty that get in the person's way of achieving the kind of life he or she wishes to lead. Other aspects of schizophrenic experience, such as a heightened sensitivity to stimulation, may prove to be adaptive or advantageous in certain settings (e.g. in the arts, in architecture, etc.). Experienced and effective clinicians can help people retain the habits and strategies that work for them and shed or change those that are maladaptive in relation to what they are trying to achieve. The habits and strategies do not exist in themselves or in a vacuum; they cannot be separated from the contexts in which they were developed and in which they are currently being used.

In the case of the 'inadequate adaptations' to which Sullivan referred in the above, he discovered that it often was the case that the habit or strategy had in fact become divorced or separated from the context which had originally stimulated its development. When placed back into the context which gave it birth, so to speak, the habit or strategy appeared no longer to be as extreme or unusual as it had by then appeared to be. It might have made sense as a response to the original situation, but to have outlived its usefulness, the way in which the hypervigilance associated with post-traumatic stress disorder is no longer as useful as a survival strategy once the person leaves the battlefield. In cases such as these, it proves useful to explore and identify the experiential origins of the habit or strategy and to reconsider its utility within that original context. As William Alanson White might have suggested, it is useful to try to understand what the patient was trying to do in that original situation when he or she developed the habit in question. Putting people back in touch with those experiences reminds the person of his or her previous agency and of his or her previous efforts to adapt as best he or she could given the circumstances, thus re-awakening in the person a sense that it is now possible for him or her to decide and to act differently. It suggested to patients that even though they had developed what Sullivan referred to as 'inadequate adaptations' to adult life *up to this point*, they were still quite capable of developing more adaptive processes and strategies, still capable of establishing new habits, were they given adequate and appropriate opportunities to do so and perhaps the kinds of encouragement and support they were not given in the past. Sullivan summarizes the two major components of his psychotherapy as follows:

> These are, firstly, a retrospective survey of the experiential basis of tendencies that conflict with the simple adaptation of the person to others with resulting growth to a more adult character; and secondly, the provision of experience that facilitates the reorganization of the undeveloped or warped tendencies such that adaptation becomes more successful. (Sullivan, 1962, p. 283)

More succinctly stated, Sullivan suggested that the clinician and patient together explore and identify those habits or strategies that were not working for the person at the present time (in achieving whatever he or she was trying to achieve), trace those habits or strategies back to the original experiences which gave them shape and perhaps even required them and then pursue and participate in new and different experiences (first within the doctor – patient relationship and then in other spheres) through which more adaptive habits and strategies can be developed in their place. Some of the more promising cognitive-behavioral psychotherapies being developed today basically follow this same process. Identify the anomalous experiences or challenging situations in which the person first developed the symptoms and impairments they are currently experiencing, reconsider with the patient (within the context of a therapeutic relationship characterized by 'collaborative empiricism') how he or she made sense of those experiences at the time and then entertain the possibility that other explanations or responses are possible – at least at the present time even if they weren't when first experienced. On this basis, the patient can try alternative ways of making sense of and responding to the key situations in question in order to try those that offer the best fit.

One of the common habits that individuals with schizophrenia appeared to suffer from in Sullivan's experience was the conviction that they were inferior to others and incapable of social relationships with people outside of their families. In such cases, which again Sullivan saw as ubiquitous among this population, the doctor–patient relationship provided the obvious and first context in which to question this habit and to encourage new experiences that would facilitate a reorganization of the person's self-concept and view of others. A key theme of psychotherapy was therefore, in Sullivan's terms, 'helping in the re-development or development *de novo* of self-esteem as an individual *attractive* to others' (Sullivan, 1962, p. 285; italics in the original). Outside of such readily apparent or tangible themes, the therapist and patient were left with the challenge of identifying idiosyncratic areas of difficulty and tracing their origins back in the person's own life experiences. Sullivan cautioned therapists from coming to quick conclusions or making their own interpretations of such themes, perhaps in response to the psychoanalytic excesses of the day. At best, the therapist can make suggestions of possible themes or issues, but it must be up to the patient to appropriate those that fit and abandon the rest. Writes Sullivan:

> During this phase of the work, the patient may or may not grasp the dynamics of his difficulty as they become more apparent to the physician. Interpretations are never to be forced on him, and preferably none are offered excepting as statistical findings. In other words, if the patient's actual insight seems to be progressing at a considerable pace, it can occasionally be offered that thus-and-so has, in some patients, been found to be the result of this-and-that, with a request for his associations to this comment. (Sullivan, 1962, p. 288)

We close this section and chapter with this caution, as the tendency for therapists to try to remake patients in their own images is likely to be as problematic today as it was a half-century ago. Sullivan regarded such interference by the therapist to be not only unhelpful and distracting the patient from the real work to be done (i.e. becoming him- or herself) but also as a betrayal of the trust the patient had placed in the therapist and to be ultimately destructive. He clearly had strong convictions on this issue, as revealed in the following passage:

> It is emphasized that interpretations and other suggestions thrust upon the patient without close regard to the life situation from which the psychosis resulted, and painstaking studies of indices to the actual conflicts which necessitated the upheaval, in themselves represent a destructive dilettantism which jeopardize any success which might otherwise result from the psychosis; and thus tend to determine an unfavorable outcome. Observations are plentiful which suggest that the catatonic is frequently the victim of psychological homicide perpetrated by attendant, nurse, or psychiatrist who forgets that his duty is to understand and assist, not to tinker and amuse himself . . .

the reformer element, who 'know' how life should be lived, and what is good and bad, if they must do psychiatric work, should keep far from the schizophrenic. (Sullivan, 1962, pp. 18, 289)

One contemporary critique of the field of psychiatric rehabilitation is that it has, perhaps unwittingly, inherited this 'reformer element' from the days of moral treatment, moving the paternalism and coercion that were evident in the writings of Samuel Tuke, and presumably in the practices of his grandfather and his colleagues, from the retreat into the rehabilitation programme (Lilleleht, 2002). And the continued use of the 'level system' described in Chapter 2 in some psychiatric rehabilitation programmes can be seen as evidence of the legitimacy of this critique. It is important, therefore, to take note of and heed Sullivan's caution. Psychiatric practitioners have no privileged claim to knowing how life should be lived, or what is good and bad. When they forget this fact, and lose the humility that is warranted in the face of life's unpredictability and complexity, then they are at risk perhaps not of committing psychological homicide but of adding to the person's already heavy burden rather than lightening and sharing it.

4.10 Summary of lessons learned

From this review of the work of Meyer, Sullivan and Strauss, we suggest the following lessons:

- Mental illnesses will be better understood, and perhaps better treated as well, within the everyday and interpersonal context in which they develop and in which they manifest themselves. People do not necessarily have to be extracted from this context in order to receive and benefit from effective care.

- Mental illnesses, like life itself, are most likely multifaceted and multidimensional phenomena that involve biological, psychological and socio-cultural components. We have yet to discover or develop an adequate way to identify and understand the relationships between these different components.

- Before looking behind or beyond the phenomena of mental illness as they are experienced in everyday life in order to discover their causes, there is much that we can learn about their nature and impact by observing them, recording those observations and describing and analysing what has been seen. This includes eliciting, listening to and understanding individual's life stories or narratives in their own terms.

- Having first-person experience of mental illness, whether in one's own life or in the life of a friend or loved one, can be used advantageously in shedding light on the nature of mental illness, especially on the fact that it is an aspect of human experience and does not reduce the person afflicted to a sub-human or alien existence.

- Pragmatism can be a useful approach to psychiatric research, teaching and practice. This is, of course, a pragmatic statement in and of itself, especially in areas of science in which so little is known or understood; identifying those things that work and those things which do not can be a credible place to begin one's investigations.

- People can make progress by identifying and building on their own personal assets and strengths.

- A central focus of recovery-oriented care is on how people spend their time on an everyday basis in natural community settings. Related key questions for practitioners to consider are: 'What is this person trying to do in his or her life?' 'How can I (and others) be of assistance in helping this person to move towards his or her own goals and aspirations?'

- Mental illnesses are defined as such within a social and cultural context. As a result, they need to be treated within such a context as well. The practitioner–patient relationship may be an especially valuable medium for identifying and beginning to address the person's concerns and needs.

Lessons to avoid repeating:

- Improvements that are brought about in artificial and institutional settings that do not replicate the person's natural environment seldom are sustained once the person leaves that environment, leaving the person vulnerable to relapse.

- Assessing and focusing on problems, diagnoses and difficulties in the absence of an equal focus on strengths can leave the person feeling demoralized and helpless.

- As people with serious mental illnesses often enter mental health care feeling inferior, demoralized and unattractive to others, practitioners need to avoid compounding these beliefs and feelings by treating the person as less than an equal.

- With an appropriate degree of humility, practitioners should avoid giving people with mental illnesses the impression that they are experts on how a person should live his or her life. They should be mindful that people need opportunities to act and try things out more than they need prescriptions for how to act (which they inevitably won't follow).

5

Closing the Hospital

> Mental hospitals institutionalize a kind of grotesque of the service relationship. (Goffman, 1961, p. 369)

5.1 The failure of the asylum

Many forces came together in the mid-1940s and 1950s to begin to sound the death knell of the asylums Dorothea Dix had worked so hard and so passionately to build. Although many students leave professional schools in psychiatry, psychology, nursing, social work, occupational therapy and even psychiatric rehabilitation spouting the conventional wisdom (e.g. in textbooks and encyclopaedias) that asylums were closed as a result of the introduction of psychiatric medication (to which readers of this volume will hopefully now *not* add themselves), this is both a gross over-simplification and, more importantly, historically incorrect. In fact, chlorpromazine was not introduced to the United States until 1954. Efforts to expose the harsh and inhumane realities of what asylums had become, and calls for their closure, can be found throughout the prior half-century. State mental hospitals were no sooner built than criticisms of their size, the quality of their care and their therapeutic function started to appear.

As early as 1866, Dr Butler had complained that large hospitals 'harmed patients by denying them personal attention and caused them to be treated like a mob in which they lost their human attributes,' while in 1874 Dr Jarvis 'pointed out that all the state's mental hospitals had been enlarged to accommodate far more patients than the original plans allowed' (cited in Bockoven, 1956, p. 177). In 1879, Bockoven writes, 'the first direct attack on mental hospitals and their medical officers was made by William A. Hammond in a paper, "The Non-Asylum Treatment of the Insane".' This paper concludes that 'the medical profession (outside the hospital) is, as a body, fully as capable of treating cases of insanity as cases of any other disease, and that in many instances sequestration is not only unnecessary but positively

The Roots of the Recovery Movement in Psychiatry   Larry Davidson, Jaak Rakfeldt, John Strauss
© 2010 John Wiley & Sons, Ltd

injurious' (Bockoven, 1956, p. 182). In 1894, one of the leading psychiatrists of the day, Weir Mitchell, declared that 'upon my word, I think asylum life is deadly to the insane' and in 1899, Sanborn issued a pamphlet entitled 'A Remonstrance in the Name of the Insane Poor Against Crowding them into Hospital Palaces or Asylum Prisons' (cited in Bockoven, 1956, p. 182).

One notable example of impassioned criticism of asylum life which made its way into popular culture was the book *A Mind that Found Itself* published in 1908 by Clifford Beers (at the encouragement of Adolf Meyer). Beers had been hospitalized for a serious mental illness and survived the treatment he received in the hospital to expose the horrors he had encountered there. In conjunction with Meyer (see Chapter 4) and prominent American philosopher, psychologist and educator William James, Beers then launched the Mental Hygiene movement in the United States. These and related efforts coalesced shortly after the end of the Second World War, initiating what has come to be called the 'de-institutionalization movement'. This movement was aided only secondarily by the new medications, which were framed initially not as treatments or as curative agents but rather as chemical lobotomies, used, that is, not to restore the person to health but rather to subdue, sedate and tranquilize him or her into being a cooperative patient.

Equally important to the de-institutionalization movement were media portrayals of life inside the asylum. The now-classic novel *The Snake Pit*, about the dreadful conditions found in asylums at the time, for example, was published in 1946 and then turned quickly into a hit Hollywood movie starring Olivia de Havilland, garnering several Oscar nominations and awards in 1948. At the same time, many principled people who had served as conscientious objectors during the war had been placed in state hospitals as the site for their community service. They came together following the war to publicize the conditions they had witnessed and to lobby for reforms (Johnson, 1990). As a result, President Truman signed the National Mental Health Act into law in 1946, establishing the development of community-based care for mental illness as a national priority, five years before chlorpromazine was even discovered in France and eight years before it was introduced to the United States.

Perhaps most important, however, was the fact that the buildings which housed the state hospitals were nearing their 100th birthdays and were falling into disrepair. Once-stately facilities located on pristine campuses scattered around the countryside across the United States (and some European and Asian countries), these buildings were now over-crowded and rapidly becoming dilapidated. Governors and state governments across the country were becoming increasingly worried about the costs of maintaining and rehabilitating these old facilities, viewing the economic burden of sustaining what had become fairly large institutions as exorbitant and beyond their means. In fact, in the United States the first meeting of the National Council of Governors took place in 1954 and had as its primary focus the question of what to do about state mental hospitals. It was at this meeting, and in its aftermath, that the de-institutionalization movement was officially born.

Why and how had the asylums failed? Many reasons have been, and can be, given to account for what came of Dorothea Dix's mission to make 'moral treatment' available to every person suffering from a mental illness regardless of the person's ability to pay. Practitioners of moral treatment, as we have seen, had insisted that 'retreats' be limited to about 200 people at any given time, as that was the maximum number that they thought could be attended to in a personal way. By the 1940s, however, state hospitals had increased in census from an initial few hundred to several thousand, with increases in staffing lagging far behind. For example, according to Bockoven, 'during the 1830s, there were, on the average, two doctors and 15 attendants at the Worcester State Hospital. During the 1930s, there were, on the average, 14 doctors and 336 attendants.' With the census increasing 10-fold and the doctor-to-attendant ratio going from 1 : 7.5 to 1 : 24, it should not be surprising that the recovery rate would go from 45% in 1833 to 4% in 1933 (Bockoven, 1956, pp. 182–183). Asylums had become 'dumping grounds' for anyone who was problematic or unwanted by the community, admitting increasing numbers of immigrants, people with developmental or physical disabilities and the elderly, many without any signs of a mental illness. The State of Connecticut, as only one small example, established three state hospitals to serve its population of roughly 3 000 000 people. At its peak, the largest of these facilities housed 9000 patients. Wholesale dumping, over-crowding and under-staffing certainly played into asylums becoming little more than warehouses for discarded human beings.

If that were all there was to the story, though, one could make the case that what is needed are well-funded and well-staffed institutions that could live up to Dix's ideal of making moral treatment available to anyone and everyone who needs it. In this case, the only obstacle to recreating asylums would be financial in nature, with the argument hingeing on a society's political willingness to give priority, and adequate funding, to addressing the needs of its citizens suffering from mental illness. And there continue to be some mental health advocates who take this position, calling for a return to institutionalization as the only conceivable response to the failures of the de-institutionalization movement (of which there are many; some of which we describe in Chapters 5–7). This clearly was not the vision of the US President's New Freedom Commission on Mental Health, however, as that vision was of 'a life in the community' for everyone. It also is not the vision of the recovery movement with which that commission and this volume are concerned (Davidson, 2007a). One of the important lessons we have learned over the previous 200 years is that putting someone in a mental hospital is not an effective way of affording that person a life in the community. The remainder of this chapter will explore some of the more important reasons why this is so.

5.2 Erving Goffman and the presentation of self

We mentioned above the attention mental hospitals had attracted from conscientious objectors and the popular press and media in the 1940s, following on from decades, if not a couple of centuries, of former hospital patients exposing the inhumane treatment they had experienced while presumably receiving 'care' for their condition. A decade or so later, mental hospitals began to receive a similar kind of attention from within the mental health field, a field which at the time was broad enough to include researchers from sociology, anthropology and social and organizational psychology. The first of several such books to appear, Stanton and Schwartz published their seminal description of Harvard's McLean Hospital in 1954 under the title: *The Mental Hospital: A Study of Institutional Participation in Psychiatric Illness and Treatment*. With Stanton being director of the hospital at the time, this book was far from being an exposé or critique, but rather framed the institutional dimension, structures and processes of the hospital in terms of psychological, social and group dynamics (drawing heavily from psychoanalysis). They did note, however – as the title suggests – that the institution played a role not only in treating the illness but also in the experience and expression of the illness itself. By focusing on the culture of the institution and on its role in shaping and maintaining the illness, this study opened the door to far bolder and more critical approaches.

Perhaps the boldest, most critical and most influential of these investigations was carried out by Erving Goffman, the noted American sociologist who had been trained in the symbolic interactionist perspective of George Herbert Mead at the University of Chicago and went on to become considered the most important sociologist of his generation. Goffman's now classic text entitled *Asylums: Essays on the Social Situation of Mental Patients and Other Inmates* was published in 1961 and suggests, by its very title, the critical turn such studies had by then taken (i.e. mental patients being considered 'inmates'). The publication of *Asylums* – published in the same year as Thomas Szasz's *The Myth of Mental Illness* – marked a dramatic shift in how mental illness and its treatment were to be viewed by society. While not going nearly as far as Szasz to pronounce mental illness a myth or empty social construction, Goffman was impressed by the degree to which an institution and its all-engrossing culture limited and shaped, if not strictly determined, human interactions, behavior and eventually even a person's own internal sense of identity. His observations and descriptions of these processes suggested that many of the more bizarre, alien and problematic behaviors of mental hospital patients were due more to the culture in which they were forced to live than to any illness which might have warranted their being brought to the hospital in the first place.

These observations, later confirmed and lent more scientific credibility by leading British schizophrenia researchers John Wing and George Brown in their book entitled *Institutionalism and Schizophrenia* (Wing and Brown, 1970), led to the labelling of this phenomenon as 'institutionalism'. So persuasive was the evidence for this phenomenon and its devastating effects for people receiving treatment within such settings that any advocate for the preservation or re-establishment of asylums for the care of individuals with mental illnesses will now first have to demonstrate how such an asylum could be run without recreating the conditions for this 'second illness' (Franco Basaglia's term for institutionalism) to emerge.

In order to understand fully the nature of institutionalism and its effects it will be useful first to back up and describe briefly the evolution of Goffman's thought and work on this topic. In his first important work, *The Presentation of Self in Everyday Life*, Goffman (1959) describes what he calls a 'dramaturgical perspective' on the social processes involved in the construction of a sense of self and personal identity. In the preface to this book, he writes:

> I mean this report to serve as a sort of handbook detailing one sociological perspective from which social life can be studied, especially the kind of social life that is organized within the physical confines of a building or plant. A set of features will be described which together form a framework that can be applied to any concrete social establishment, be it domestic, industrial, or commercial. The perspective employed in this report is that of the theatrical performance; the principles derived are dramaturgical ones. I shall consider the way in which the individual in ordinary work situations presents himself and his activity to others, the ways in which he guides and controls the impression they form of him, and the kinds of things he may and may not do while sustaining his performance before them. (Goffman, 1959, pp. xi)

Consistent with his symbolic interactionist training, Goffman goes on to suggest that identity does not develop from 'inside' the person, from any kind of privileged access I may have to who I am or who I may become. Rather, identity and one's sense of oneself (or of one's self) is a product of our social environment and a result of the interactions we have with others and how those others view and treat us in return. We learn about ourselves primarily by experimenting or improvising, by trying on roles, by performing or presenting ourselves to others and then by internalizing the feedback we receive from them and from the effects of our behavior on others. We come to see ourselves as individuals – and as individuals of a certain type, with certain traits and characteristics – by differentiating ourselves from and in relation to others.

We will return to this kind of perspective in Chapter 7, when we take up the action theory and activity analysis of the social, cultural and cognitive developmental psychologist Lev Vygotsky. This perspective may seem foreign at first to students or practitioners of American origin, who have grown up within a highly individualistic culture that emphasizes competition and personal achievement based on a kind of Lone Ranger/John Wayne model. It would not be surprising for their approach to seem alien to Americans. Goffman, although born in Canada, was of Ukrainian dissent and Vygotsky was born and raised in Belarus. In a related, if possibly tangential, point, it also is no accident that there have been criticisms of the characteristically American view of recovery (i.e. that it is seen as a uniquely personal journey) from advocates and investigators from other cultures (Deegan, 1988). There are most likely aspects of recovery that are unique to each person, such as Deegan's concept of 'personal medicine' (Deegan, 2007) which refers to those things that I do and value that are important to me and that can counteract, or give me motivation to battle, an illness. For me, this may include playing with my children, listening to Mozart and doing yoga while for you it may include walking, talking to friends and praying. But surely, there are aspects of recovery that are shared by many people and/or that may be specific to a certain culture or subculture. Prayer and faith may be more important in predominantly Christian societies like the United States, for example, while meditation and yoga may be more important in predominantly Buddhist or Hindu societies. Recovery is equally, if not more, a social process as a personal one.

While this may pose challenges for individualistic societies, understanding the social nature of recovery – and its antithesis, chronicity – is extremely important if we are to appreciate the limitations, as well as the contributions, that can be made by organizations, agencies and institutions devoted to treating mental illness and promoting mental health.

5.3 The hospital as 'total institution'

Asylums (Goffman, 1961) consists of four interrelated essays on the processes and consequences involved in being admitted to and 'treated' within the context of a mental hospital. A follow-up work on *Stigma: Notes on the Management of Spoiled Identity* (Goffman, 1963) followed people labelled as 'mental patients' out into the community to consider the broader ramifications of their having been given this particular identity in a society which discriminates against people with mental illness. But in *Asylums*, Goffman is mostly absorbed with the details of having been admitted to a mental hospital and the nature and effects of the process he described as 'institutionalization'. Given that many people in the early 1960s continued to live out the remainder of their adult lives within such institutions, such a focus certainly seemed warranted.

The first essay in *Asylums*, 'On the characteristics of total institutions', is a general examination of the nature of social life in these establishments, drawing heavily on the two main examples that feature involuntary membership: mental hospitals and prisons. Despite the fact that their explicit social functions differed (i.e. treatment versus punishment), Goffman found mental hospitals and prisons to be much more alike than dissimilar, therefore choosing to describe residents of mental hospitals as 'inmates' rather than as patients. In this essay, the schemes developed in detail in the remaining papers are stated and their place in the broader whole suggested. The second essay, 'The moral career of the mental patient', considers the initial effects of institutionalization on the social relationships the individual possessed before he or she became an inmate. The third essay, 'The underlife of a public institution: a study of ways of making out in a mental hospital', is concerned with the attachment the inmate is expected to manifest to his iron home and, in detail, with the way in which inmates can introduce some distance between themselves and these expectations. The final essay, 'The medical model and mental hospitalization', returns to the professional staff to consider, in the case of mental hospitals, the role of the medical model and its assumptions in presenting to the inmate the so-called facts of his or her situation. This fourth essay contains a powerful indictment of the claims made that mental hospitals actually help, rather than primarily hurt, the individuals in their care, and we will have reason to return to it after introducing the work of Basaglia later in this chapter.

We begin, however, with the concept of 'total institution'. Goffman describes them as follows:

> When we review the different institutions in our Western society, we find some that are encompassing to a degree discontinuously greater than the ones next in line. Their encompassing or total character is symbolized by the barrier to social intercourse with the outside and to departure that is often built right into the physical plant, such as locked doors, high walls, barbed wire, cliffs, water, forests, or moors. (Goffman, 1961, p. 4)

These are the establishments that Goffman describes as total institutions, and it is their general characteristics and their effects on their inhabitants that he explores. A basic social arrangement in modern society is that the individual tends to sleep, play and work in different places with different participants, under different authorities and without any overarching plan. The central feature of total institutions, according to Goffman, can be described as a breakdown of the barriers ordinarily separating these three spheres of life. First, all aspects of life are carried out in the same place and under the same central authority. Second, each phase of the member's daily activity is carried on in the immediate company of a large batch of others, all of whom are treated alike and required to do the same things together. As a result, any autonomy or freedom to make one's own choices, pursue one's own interests or associate with people of one's own choosing is denied. Third, all phases of the day's activities are tightly scheduled, with one activity leading at a prearranged time into the next. This sequence of activities is rigidly imposed upon inmates from above. Finally, the various enforced activities are brought together into an overall plan, presumably designed to accomplish the goals of the institution.

The second essay then describes the sequence of changes that people admitted to such institutions, in this case mental hospitals, undergo. For this purpose, Goffman chooses the term 'career'. The moral career of people involves a sequence of changes in how they are regarded by others and, as a result, in their way of conceiving of themselves. Goffman notes that changes in people's moral careers occur within the confines of all institutional systems, whether it be a social establishment such as a mental hospital or in the complex of personal and professional relationships in any other formal or informal organization. The self, then, for Goffman, can be seen as something that resides in the arrangements prevailing in a social system for its members. Rather than the self being the private property of the people to whom it is attributed, a person's sense of self dwells in the complex pattern of social control and social connections between him or her and the people around them.

Traditionally the term 'career' has been reserved for occupations or professions. Goffman uses the term in a broader sense, however. For Goffman, career refers to all of the social strands that weave through people's course in life. Moreover, the value of the concept of career is its two-sidedness. The first side is linked to the internal issues that are held dearly and closely, such as people's images of themselves and their felt identity. The second side refers to the official positions, jural relationships and lifestyle, and in particular to people's publicly accessible and institutionally embedded roles. The concept of career, then, allows for the movement back and forth between the personal and the public, between the self and its significant social contexts.

In Goffman's analysis, the 'career' of the mental patient falls into three phases. The first is the period prior to entering the hospital. This he calls the 'pre-patient phase'. The second is the period within the hospital, which he refers to as the 'inpatient phase'. The third is the period after discharge from the hospital, or the 'ex-patient phase'. As we noted above, in this work Goffman deals only with the first two phases.

An individual often begins a 'pre-patient' career with social relationships and civil rights, but then ends up at the beginning of his or her hospital stay with very little of either. The moral aspect of this portion of the career typically involves experiences of abandonment, disloyalty and embitterment as a result of the person having been placed in such an institution by others, most often family members with whom he or she had shared trust and affection. Pre-patients come into the institution with conceptions of themselves made possible by the stable social arrangements in their home worlds: they are spouses, children, parents, students, workers, Democrats or Republicans and so on. Upon admission to the hospital, they are often stripped of the supports provided by such social arrangements, both physically and symbolically. Inpatients then experience a series of abasements, degradations, humiliations and profanations of self, during which the self is systematically, if often unintentionally, mortified. Inpatients undergo radical shifts in their moral careers, which are composed of progressive changes that involve their beliefs concerning themselves and the significant others in their lives.

Goffman maintains that an important feature of the pre-patient career is its 'retroactive quality'. This means that people's life histories are revised in light of their newly received psychiatric diagnostic label. In the process of doing an anamnesis (a psychosocial history), mental health staff routinely seek out incipient symptoms of mental disorder and then trace them forward from the patient's childhood into the present. In order to make sense of the current situation, the patient is made to recast all of his or her past life as that of a pre-patient with some insidious mental illness progressively developing and leading up to his or her present state of involuntary confinement. Often, patients must accept other people's views that they are sick. In the case of serious mental illness, this almost inevitably involves coming to accept that their self-images were 'false', while the views of them held by the staff are 'true'. When this happened, Goffman considered this to mark the 'conversion' to a mental patient identity.

Upon entering the hospital, inpatients may very strongly feel the desire not to be known to anyone as someone who has been reduced to such circumstances.

Consequently, inpatients may avoid talking to others; they may stay by themselves so as to avoid ratifying through social interaction their new lot in life. They struggle to refuse accepting the status and role of mental patient. But, after a while, this struggle comes to be too difficult and they give up this over-taxing effort. The all-consuming culture of the institution overshadows and negates their best efforts and, in the words of the staff, they eventually 'settle down'. Through it all, according to Goffman, inpatients experience the process of a 'stripping and mortifying' of their former social self. They are no longer respected as individuals, no longer accorded privacy, dignity or the sense of self-worth that came from their previous relationships and status, no matter how flawed or inadequate these might have been.

Once on a locked and supervised unit, inpatients quickly learn about the limited extent to which a conception of self can be sustained when the usual setting and supports for it have been suddenly removed. Once patients 'settle down', the outlines of their fate tend to follow those of other segregated establishments: jails, concentrations camps, monasteries, work camps and so on. In such places, inmates spend their lives on the facility's grounds, marching anonymously through regimented days in the immediate company of a group of like-situated and anonymous others. Inpatients are discredited in many ways. One way is by being moved from ward to ward based on their 'progress' or their 'regression' (recall here the 'level system' introduced by the Tukes). Through this process, the self loses it stability and becomes something that is controlled by others from without. The self is built up and broken down, until inpatients come to experience this as some sort of an absurd game. Ironically, in Goffman's view, inpatients seem to gain a new plateau of freedom through this process and what he calls a 'moral loosening' ensues. He offers examples of moral loosening such as a 'marriage moratorium' (during which it becomes acceptable to have sex with other inmates or staff) as well as now having licence to act out in bizarre ways that would never be tolerated in the outside world. In his famously sardonic and understated style, Goffman writes:

> The moral career of the mental patient has unique interest, however; it can illustrate the possibility that in casting off the raiments of the old self – or in having this cover torn away – the person need not seek a new robe and a new audience before which to cower. Instead he can learn, at least for a time, to practice before all groups the amoral arts of shamelessness. (Goffman, 1961, p. 169)

Anticipating perhaps that naïve readers may assume such moral loosening and amoral activities are due to the mental illness rather than the institution, Goffman describes the various 'career contingencies' that appear to have led to people being hospitalized during the 1940s and 1950s. These contingencies included: (i) socio-economic status, (ii) visibility of the offence, (iii) proximity to a mental hospital, (iv) amount of treatment available and (v) community regard for the treatment given. In addition, Goffman lists several of the specific career contingencies that might be linked to extraneous events, such as: (i) a man is tolerated until his wife finds a lover, (ii) an unmanageable teenager is tolerated until she has an affair with an older man, (iii) an alcoholic is sent to the hospital because the jail is full and (iv) an elder is tolerated until the family moves into a smaller apartment. Given the fact that the number of people with serious mental illnesses residing outside of the hospital at least equals, if not vastly outnumbers, those on the inside, Goffman concludes that inpatients suffer not from a mental illness per se but rather from these types of career contingencies. If institutionalization and its effects were due entirely to mental illness, then many more people would be in hospitals and, of these, very few would ever leave. As we will see later in this chapter, a similar argument was made by Franco Basaglia in defending his closure of asylums in Italy. Most people with serious mental illnesses live outside of asylums. What puts people into and keeps them in such settings must be other than the illness itself.

Our primary interest here, though, is on what happens to people once admitted. Were the mental hospital effective in treating the conditions for which it was built, and/or in caring for the patients placed there, these particular contingencies might not be so relevant. If I can treat and eliminate the illness with which you have been afflicted, then it does not really matter what particular event or coincidence brought you to seek help, or to my attention, at this particular time. But Goffman found nothing in the mental hospital which he studied – which, we may note, was at the National Institute of Mental Health in Washington DC, and thus presumably represented the state-of-the-art treatment of the day rather than a poorly funded and neglected state hospital – that resembled care or cure. People did not appear to benefit at all from their confinement in such a total institution, but rather to lose what resources and strengths they had when they first arrived. While they came from a social context in which they occupied various roles and had some sense of a personal identity, these aspects of their lives were systematically stripped from them as their sense of themselves was negated, pathologized and mortified, leading to what Goffman termed a 'disculturation'. With little of significance or meaning with which to replace what they had lost, people became absorbed into the mass, or herd, of inmates who were shepherded around the institution from one regimented activity to the next, shuffling indiscriminately from one sterile, impersonal room to the next, passing their time and wasting their lives away under the close and continuous scrutiny of the staff. Rather than curing or reducing the illness, this process led to role dispossession, skill deterioration and demoralization and rendered people less capable of managing life in the outside world. In addition to disculturation from their previous roles and identity, acculturating inmates to life in a total institution prepares them only for remaining within the institution. It does little, if anything, in preparing them for the contingencies they will face once again upon discharge.

Goffman concludes from this investigation that taking a person with a mental illness out of his or her life context, admitting him or her to a mental hospital and then returning the person to the same life context was like taking a drowning man out of a lake, teaching him how to ride a bicycle and putting him back into the lake. This analogy falls short of capturing the horrors and tragedy of the institution, however, as people being brought to mental hospitals never had a desire to learn how to ride a bicycle, nor are the skills they 'learn' there useful in any other context. Goffman's outlook is not entirely bleak, though, as he discovered, and describes in the third essay in this collection, how some people manage to survive even the most dehumanizing of these institutions. A final lesson for recovery can be gleaned from these insights on the resilience of the human spirit.

In the third essay, 'The underlife of a public institution: a study of ways of making out in a mental hospital', Goffman concludes that while every social establishment imposes official expectations as how its participants should act, and how they should be, in virtually all instances there remain examples of how people decline to accept or act in accordance with this official view. For example, where enthusiasm is expected, we often find apathy; where attendance is required there is absenteeism; where robustness is valued, illness prevails. Goffman writes:

> We find a multitude of homely little histories, each a movement of liberty. Whenever worlds are laid on, underlives develop ... One strives to retain some self-hood beyond the grasp of the organization. This recalcitrance is not an incidental mechanism of defense, but rather an essential constituent of the self ... It is always against something that the self emerges. (Goffman, 1961, p. 305)

In this sense, passive submission and total acquiescence is not the only option. Inpatients may also, Goffman suggests, 'play it cool' or merely 'colonize' the institution. They may view their submission and acquiescence as necessary, if temporary, roles to play. Rather than 'settling down' as desired by staff, they may decide just to 'play the game' in order to gain discharge. In such cases, they do not accept viewing themselves as mental patients at all, but rather come to view the institution and the staff as agents of social control (which, of course, they are, at least in part). Others may, for a variety of reasons, view life on the inside of the institution to be preferable to life on the outside. Such people may become pseudo-staff and participate in the control and coercion of others. Thus, there are different modes of adjustment and adaptation to the hospital. In and among these various forms lie possibilities for enacting more proactive and empowered roles even while living in a total institution.

In other words, the capacity of total institutions to reshape inmates may, at least in some cases, be limited. Since, in Goffman's view, 'it is always against something that the self emerges' (Goffman, 1961, p. 320), it has been possible for people not to become entirely absorbed or engulfed by the institution but to define themselves, at least in part, in opposition to the institution, even while remaining within it. In one of his more poignant statements, Goffman observes that: 'Our status is backed by the solid buildings of the world, while our sense of personal identity resides in the cracks' (Goffman, 1961, p. 320). We are never only or entirely how we are defined by others. We are always more than this, and it is always possible that in the future we will be different from who we have been in the past. If people can survive and reclaim a self-determined and meaningful life following confinement to concentration camps,

POW camps and prisons, then they can survive and reclaim a self-determined and meaningful life following extended hospitalization for a serious mental illness. We just should not look to the hospitalization to help with, to contribute positively to, this process. As Goffman trenchantly showed, it is in the cracks, not in the bricks and mortar, of the hospital that the person's sense of personal identity survives. Having eluded the grasp of the total institution, the human spirit can still be found there and, like a smouldering ember under the ashes, given the proper circumstances, it may be rekindled once again to glow and to grow. This was the hope and the inspiration for the work of our next thinker and doer: Franco Basaglia.

5.4 Franco Basaglia and the Italian mental health reform movement

If it took Goffman and his colleagues to document the process of institutionalization and its contribution to the phenomenon of chronicity pervading the asylum, it then took the Italian psychiatrist Franco Basaglia, his wife and his colleagues to take the bold step of closing the asylum altogether, firm in their belief and resolve that chronicity could be left behind along with the institution which gave it birth. They believed, in other words, that asylums were unnecessary and that people with serious mental illnesses could live safely and productively in the community as long as they were provided appropriate and effective care and support. In a fashion reminiscent of Pussin's unchaining of the inmates of the Bicêtre in 1789 based entirely on the hope that they would not be violent if they were not themselves treated in violent ways, Basaglia and his colleagues demonstrated a leap of faith in the 1960s in imagining that serious mental illness would look very different, and be much less disabling, once separated from the horrors of what had by then become disabling – while remaining violent – institutions.

While it is true that Basaglia's efforts followed along after initial efforts towards de-institutionalization in other parts of the world (particularly the United States, England and France), his efforts were directly influenced by the work of Goffman and his contemporaries and were unique in several important respects that make them worthy of discussion. To this day, in fact, Italy remains the only country on earth that has a law abolishing all insane asylums and prohibiting any new ones from being built. This 1978 law was a direct result of the advocacy efforts of the Democratic Psychiatry movement (*Psychiatria Democratica*) founded by Basaglia and his colleagues and continues to stand alone after 30 years as a singularly visionary assertion of the right of individuals with serious mental illnesses to live in the community. In this respect, 'the Law 180', as it has come to be called by both proponents and detractors alike, predated the vision of 'a life in the community' of the US President's New Freedom Commission on Mental Health report issued in 2003 by 25 years. More importantly, however, it enshrined this vision in law, giving it much more authority, weight and clout than a Presidential commission which could only issue recommendations. Even the 1999 *Olmstead Decision* by the US Supreme Court – which made it illegal to confine someone with a mental illness to an institution against his or her will based solely on the lack of available community-based resources – falls well short of the Law 180. As Basaglia had anticipated, and argued, as long as mental hospitals remained standing and open, reasons would be found to justify placing and keeping people there. This remains true in the United States to this day, with tens of thousands of people continuing to live significant portions of their adulthood, in many cases the remainder of their adult lives, within the locked confines of state institutions.

Finally, Basaglia's conviction that asylums needed to be abolished entirely – rather than, for instance, being reserved for those individuals considered the most seriously disabled – is only one of several examples of the ways in which he was able to benefit from visiting like-minded colleagues in the United States, France and England. By the time Basaglia had risen to a position of influence in Italy, he had been able to observe some of the early de-institutionalization strategies being implemented by the Americans, French and English. In addition to being blessed with a keen intellect, a tremendous capacity for compassion and empathy, and a considerable amount of personal charisma, Basaglia apparently was a very astute observer. As a result, he was able to anticipate many years ahead of time that these well-intended approaches to creating alternatives to the traditional asylum were bound to fail as long as they stopped short of according all people with mental illness their fundamental birthright to community inclusion. We will describe the centrality of this birthright as a foundation for, rather than as a reward of, recovery in detail in the remainder of this chapter, as this remains one of Basaglia's principal contributions. We mention it here as a final reason for our selection of the Italian mental health reform movement as the most important of the various de-institutionalization efforts in terms of its conceptual, and practical, contributions to the recovery movement.

5.5 De-institutionalization the Italian way

Italian psychiatry had had its own Pinel, a physician named Vincenzo Chiarugi (1759–1820), who – the same year Pussin was introducing the use of '*traitement moral*' within the Bicêtre – was busy reforming the philosophy and operation of the St Bonifacio Hospital in Florence. Inspired by the values of the Enlightenment and consistent with the principles being articulated by Pinel, Chiarugi insisted that residents of asylums be treated first and foremost as individuals deserving of respect (Burti, 2001, p. 41). His efforts were likewise limited in their effectiveness, however, and by the time Basaglia took over as superintendent of his first mental hospital in the Italian town of Gorizia in 1961 he was faced with an asylum as appalling in its treatment, or lack of treatment, of its residents as the worst of the so-called snake pits in the United States.

Prior to taking up the post of superintendent at Gorizia, Basaglia had occupied an academic position as a research scientist at the Neuropsychiatric Clinic at the University of Padua for 13 years. During these formative years, he had been influenced both by the phenomenological approach to psychiatry being developed by the students and followers of Edmund Husserl and Martin Heidegger (e.g. Minkowski, Binswanger, Strauss) and by the existentialist school of thought sweeping France and being articulated by Jean-Paul Sartre and his contemporaries (Camus, Merleau-Ponty, de Beauvoir). The concepts of these approaches – especially their central focus on subjectivity, intentionality and personal agency – were very influential in shaping Basaglia's thought and in contributing to his assessment of and response to what he found at the Gorizia asylum. While some of his critics suggest he was unprepared for the crass, degrading and vulgar realities of the asylum after spending his early career in a university clinic, we suggest instead that Basaglia's shock, dismay and determination in the face of these tragically inhumane circumstances represent the understandable and legitimate reaction of a thoughtful, principled and compassionate person who had become committed to viewing autonomy, agency and subjectivity as defining characteristics of human nature. It certainly is the case that Basaglia's reform efforts, even at this first hospital, went well beyond addressing simply the material and physical conditions of the asylum, as we will see below.

According to Scheper-Hughes and Lovell (1986), who introduced the English-speaking world to Basaglia in the 1980s, when he arrived at Gorizia, Basaglia:

> was revolted by what he observed as the traditional regime of institutional 'care': keys and locked doors only partially successful in muffling the screams and weeping of the patients, many of them lying naked and helpless in their own excreta. And he observed, with repugnance, the institutional response to human suffering: strait jackets, physical abuse, bed ties, ice packs, ECT and insulin-coma shock therapies to 'soothe' the terrified and the melancholy, and to strike terror in the difficult and the agitated. (Scheper-Hughes and Lovell, 1986, p. 160)

Like Goffman, what he found at Gorizia impressed Basaglia as being more of a prison than a hospital, although he was to come to recognize later in his career that even prisons accorded their inmates more rights and dignity than the typical asylum. As he wrote in 1980:

> The asylum is also an extraordinary observatory of behaviour patterns and the huge experimental laboratory where the lack of individual life, (i.e., lack of productive and rational life) is the excuse for the failure to apply ethical principles to the same extent as in medicine and, moreover, justifies the withholding, temporary or permanent, of individual rights to a greater extent than in the prison system. (Basaglia, 1980c, p. 20)

Since no treatment or rehabilitation was being offered there to justify the confinement of people who were said to be ill, Basaglia came to the eventual conclusion that there were only two functions served by the asylum, neither one to the benefit of the inmates.

The first function was to extrude individuals with mental illnesses from the community. While in principle, and as stated in law, this was due to the perception that people with mental illnesses were dangerous to the public and could not take care of themselves, Basaglia agreed with Foucault's analysis (Foucault, 1965) that this was more likely due to the fact that they were being punished for not being able, or willing, to join the workforce of industrial, and industrializing, capitalist economies. It is for this reason that he defines 'individual life' in the above passage as both rational and *productive*. People were placed in asylums – many of them immigrants, with intellectual disabilities, or simply poor, and without any observable signs of mental illness – not because of a mental illness but because of their failure to contribute their human labor to the production and enhancement of capital (cf. also Davidson, 1988; Warner, 1985). This is a point to which we will return in the following chapter.

The second, related, function of the asylum was to transform this mass of unproductive, recalcitrant or unwilling labor into a commodity that could then serve the capitalist economy, but in a different way. The hospital became a self-perpetuating institution which justified and sustained the employment of doctors, nurses and other staff while serving as a means of keeping the insane from undermining the work ethic of the broader population. Mental health consumer advocates came to this same conclusion separately in the United States around the same time, noting that the only reason to keep mental hospitals open is so that health care practitioners could keep their jobs. Despite sounding harsh, and suggestive perhaps of a simplistic conspiracy theory of sorts, this view has garnered considerable support from historians and sociologists, such as Parry-Jones (1971) and Scull (1981), who have written of various forms of 'trafficking' in what they came to call the 'lunacy trade'. This is not to suggest that individual doctors or nurses were aware of the social function they were performing by confining individuals to an asylum. The assumption is that they were caring professionals who thought they were tending to the sick as best they could. From the perspective of a philosophically informed, politically aware and keenly astute and thoughtful young and idealistic psychiatrist, however, the facts did not support this rationalization of the asylum. Basaglia saw little, if anything, in Gorizia that approximated therapy or care. Instead, as he writes:

> The hospital as a system seems to exist for itself, to be its own reason
> for being, in the sense that the intense activity within it seems to serve
> only to keep it going, otherwise aiming at nothing that might justify
> its function. (Basaglia, 1985, p. 44)

Having visited Maxwell Jones in the United Kingdom, Basaglia's first instinct was to reform the asylum along the lines of a 'therapeutic community'. Somewhat similar approaches were being developed in France under the title of 'institutional psychotherapy', having in common with the therapeutic community model the attempt to resurrect moral treatment and augment it with the recent advances made by the newly emerging psychodynamic psychotherapy. So, in addition to unshackling the patients, providing them with dignified and humane surroundings, prohibiting assaults and the use of violence and terminating the use of restraint, seclusion and shock treatments, Basaglia began to introduce what he at first considered therapeutic processes and structures into the hospital milieu (Scheper-Hughes and Lovell, 1986). Recalling Chapters 2 and 4, we might consider such an effort to be a combination of the best of what *traitement moral* and a Sullivanian-like relationship-focused psychotherapy could offer.

The present volume does not have a chapter on the therapeutic community model, however – despite the suggestions of some of our reviewers – because Basaglia very quickly came to realize that as long as these efforts were being made within the confines of the asylum they would be extremely limited in their efficacy. Goffman, as we have seen, had already pointed out that socializing a person to an institutional culture did little to prepare him or her for life outside of the institution; if it did anything at all, it was to further undermine what capacities and resources the person already had when arriving at the institution. With a background in existentialism and phenomenology, Basaglia took this insight a step further to explore the destructive impact of the asylum and its processes on the very 'personhood' of the person. Placing someone in an asylum not only lessened their chances for a full recovery but also robbed them of the very agency that they would need in order to recover.

Basaglia discusses this important and central point in the technical jargon of the schools of existentialism and phenomenology in which he had been trained (i.e. with terms such as 'personhood'), jargon which unfortunately is off-putting and difficult to understand, especially for English-language readers. As this is a crucial point in our presentation, however – and one of the reasons we chose to focus on Basaglia's work – we will attempt to translate his argument into more accessible language rather than simply skip over it, as many commentators have done. This is, in fact, the first of the two major contributions made by Basaglia that we will identify in this chapter. It has been our sad but consistent experience that this central aspect of Basaglia's work was one of the first aspects to be lost in the implementation of what came to be known in Italy as the 'Basaglia method'. As a result, it also has been an aspect of his work that has consistently been overlooked, misunderstood or dismissed by many commentators and critics. Without an appreciation of the central role of the subject as agent in recovery, and without an appreciation of the need for the community itself to change in order to accommodate some individuals with serious mental illnesses – the second major point to which we will come below – Basaglia's legacy dwindles down to his being simply 'the man who closed the hospitals'. Given what the hospitals had become by the 1960s and 1970s, this is of course an admirable and noteworthy feat. In Basaglia's case, though, it only refers to the tip of the iceberg.

Before turning to the reasons why Basaglia's initial efforts to reform the asylum failed, we do want to emphasize nonetheless the importance of one of the lessons of the Italian mental health reform movement, especially as it remains an elusive lesson even to this day. As Burti concludes:

> The bottom line is that Italy has shown in practice, for almost a quarter
> of a century, that it is possible to do away with the mental hospital
> and to provide a nationwide system of psychiatric care according to
> the principles of community mental health. (Burti, 2001, p. 45)

In the significant amount of time that has passed since the passage of the Law 180, psychiatry in Italy has functioned without access to a mental hospital, even for individuals with the most severe and disabling conditions. A variety of alternatives have been developed to support people with disabilities in community settings, and we will review some of these below, but the asylum as a place for people with mental illnesses to be confined for extended periods no longer exists. In this sense, Basaglia is indeed 'the man who closed the hospitals' – apparently for good. Most of the world outside of Italy, including most communities in the United States, have yet to take up this challenge and would benefit from knowing at least this much of the story; even though there is, as we have said, much more of the story to tell.

5.6 Bracketing the illness

To appreciate how radical, and ahead of his time, Basaglia was, it would be useful first to try to put ourselves in his shoes. Especially since some of his most original insights have yet to be fully understood, much less embraced, by psychiatry, we think it worthwhile to describe in some detail the perspective he brought to, and developed through, this work.

By way of offering some backdrop to these efforts, we should note that the mainstream of Italian psychiatry that Basaglia was entering in the late 1940s had a very clear concept of mental illness; it was, in his terms, both 'incomprehensible' and 'incurable'. This was the traditional view of psychosis that could be traced back to Kraepelin's (1904) landmark studies of '*dementia praecox*' at the turn of the century that had laid the foundations for the field of descriptive psychopathology. First Kraepelin and then later Karl Jaspers and others considered the psychotic state to be non-rational and therefore not understandable by 'normal' or 'sane' people, including psychiatrists. In addition, they considered psychosis organic in nature and, in the case of schizophrenia, to represent an irreversible, degenerative disease from which the person could not recover, but that would lead necessarily to premature dementia (the meaning of *dementia praecox*), disability and death. One could imagine that such a view would justify the existence of asylums, and perhaps even account to some degree for the horrors found there. Unfortunately, this view was equally born *from* the asylum and the horrors found there to begin with, the vast majority of psychiatrists practising when Basaglia entered the field never stopping to question which had come first.

Through his training in existentialism and phenomenology, however, Basaglia had come to question at least the assumption of incomprehensibility. Minkowski, Binswanger and other phenomenologically oriented psychiatrists had been actively attempting to describe and come to an empathic understanding of the subjective experiences of people with various forms of serious mental illnesses, including psychosis. In the United Kingdom and the United States, similar attempts had been and were being made by psychoanalytically oriented psychiatrists such as Harry Stack Sullivan (discussed in the previous chapter) and his contemporaries who worked with individuals suffering from psychosis within primarily private settings. One could imagine that after spending 13 years at the university clinic in Padua, Basaglia had honed his own therapeutic skills and eagerly awaited the chance to put them to use in Gorizia. Regardless of whether people with psychosis could eventually be cured, Basaglia came to the asylum in Gorizia intent on interacting with them and coming to understand their experiences through phenomenological and psychotherapeutic means. He found this more difficult than he had imagined, but not – as one might think – because of the severity of the illness. Rather, he found the asylum structure and culture to make genuine, empathic interaction with patients exceedingly difficult, if not impossible.

The primary focus both of phenomenological and of psychotherapeutic approaches to mental illness, especially in the first phase of treatment, is on the development of a trusting relationship between practitioner and patient in which the practitioner demonstrates to the patient a genuine interest in his or her experiences and perspective. People cannot be expected to let therapists – or phenomenological investigators, for that matter – into the private details of their everyday lives, including their perceptions, thoughts, emotions and beliefs, unless and until they have reason to believe that this person can be trusted and has their own best interests at heart. Basaglia found it extremely difficult to establish this foundation of trust, and to convince the patients that he had their best interest at heart, within the confines of the Gorizia asylum. One reason we have already touched on is the fact that, as Basaglia came to recognize quickly, the Gorizia asylum was not designed or operated in such a way that it could be described as existing for the benefit of the patients. It existed for the presumed benefit of society, and for the benefit of the individuals employed there, but did not appear to be helping the patients; people Basaglia, like Goffman, thought were more accurately described as 'inmates'.

In addition to extruding people from society and keeping them confined within a locked institution, the structures, culture and practices of the hospital seemed antithetical to establishing trust. As described above, people were routinely medicated, isolated, shocked and lobotomized, not in order to treat the illness (which, as we have said, was considered incurable) but in order to subdue them and make the milieu 'manageable'. They were, in effect, punished into submission. Such practices had the opposite effect on the patients from what Basaglia had wanted. Rather than inviting reluctant, suspicious and suffering people out from the shadows of their distress into a human connection with a caring other, these ways of exerting control pushed the person further and further away from the staff and further and further into his or her own private hell, from which any possibility of a return became more and more distant.

Basaglia used strong language to characterize what he viewed as a form of assault on the person and his or her autonomy and experiences, describing these practices as 'aggressive' and 'violent'. In response to such treatment, it was only understandable that a person would withdraw and eventually become numb to the ongoing abuses; abuses which destroyed his or her spirit or identity more than his or her body. As a result, the person, in effect, would disappear and eventually be replaced by the illness with which he or she had been labelled. Writes Basaglia:

> When the mental patient – alienated from life, suffering from the loss of relationship with others, and himself – enters the asylum, instead of finding here a place where he can free himself from the burden of others, where he can reconstruct his own personal world, he finds new rules, new structures that make him lose himself still more, and push him more and more towards objectiveness, until he identifies with them . . . Isolated, segregated . . . the patient seems to assume a value other than that of a man. (Basaglia, 1964, p. 2)

Rather than a unique individual with his or her personal strengths, interests, life-history, family and social context, the patient becomes quite simply, and nothing more than, 'a schizophrenic', 'a psychotic' or 'a manic depressive'. No longer a person with whose experiences, suffering and aspirations we may identify, and wish to explore, we find instead an alien body that is, and will forever be, incomprehensible to us. As Basaglia writes, perhaps the best that such a person can hope for is to become an interesting object of scientific scrutiny:

> By distancing the patient from our world, we are uprooting him from his real world, and turning him into an object which is isolated from its life-history, from its environment, and even from its own life. In fact, he is simply reduced to the state of an object by our aggression. This is why patients who have been taken out of their social context – where they still maintain some alternative (however fragile) which keeps them, through ties, in contact with reality – are stripped of all human factors. They are reduced, at best, to the status of an object for contemplation: an interesting case! (Quoted in Giannichedda, 1988, p. 255)

As Goffman had already shown, once inside an institution people are no longer viewed and treated as individuals but as instances of an abstract category; in the case of prisons, they all become criminals; in the case of a mental hospital, they all become ill. While it may be useful in other branches of medicine to determine the illness with which a person suffers in order then to provide treatment and care that is responsive, there did not seem to be the same relationship in psychiatry. Here, determining the illness became a kind of end in itself, if anything a way of justifying why the ill person was *not* receiving effective treatment or care. Even after the introduction of chlorpromazine and other psychiatric medication, the field had yet to develop any approaches that could be said to be truly therapeutic or curative; serious mental illnesses, after all, were considered incurable. As Goffman writes in the fourth essay of *Asylums*:

> Compared to a medical hospital or garage, a mental hospital is ill-equipped to be a place where the classic repair cycle occurs ... the problem of easing the patient's attitude to the world is confused and exacerbated by the problem of easing his attitude to involuntary hospitalization. In any case, the treatment given in mental hospitals is not likely to be specific to the disorder, as it is, in general, in a medical hospital, garage, or radio repair shop; instead, if treatment is given at all, a cycle of therapies tends to be given across the board to a whole entering class of patients, with the medical work-up being used more to learn if there are counterindications for the standard treatments than to find indicators for them. At the same time, the patient's life is regulated and ordered according to a disciplinarian system developed for the management by a small staff of a large number of involuntary inmates. (Goffman, 1961, pp. 360–361)

What possible function, then, could diagnosis serve within the context of such a hospital?

In Basaglia's view, it was used mainly as a way to introduce distance – rather than lessen the distance – between the practitioner and the patient, and this primarily to defend the practitioner from the patient's suffering and to rationalize his or her actions towards and abuses of the patient. It was clear that diagnosis did not lead to new understanding or more effective care; no advances or breakthroughs were being made in psychiatry at the time that would have justified this narrow focus on illness. Once again, as Goffman points out in his fourth essay in *Asylums* on the use of the medical model in institutional psychiatry:

> The nature of the patient's nature is redefined so that, in effect if not by intention, the patient becomes the kind of object upon which a psychiatric service can be performed. To be made a patient is to be remade into a serviceable object, the irony being that so little service is available once this is done. (Goffman, 1961, p. 379)

In one of his more controversial and least understood uses of phenomenological terminology, Basaglia tries to explain that this was because the field was operating backwards:

> Given the extremely reduced level of our knowledge in the area of mental illness (in particular schizophrenia, where we know the different ways in which it expresses itself, but virtually nothing regarding its aetiology), we cannot continue to 'set aside' the ill individual while waiting for a more profound understanding of what exactly it is he

or she suffers from, thereby increasing his or her suffering through internment and segregation. Instead, we should 'set aside' the illness as an empty definition and simple act of labeling, and seek to create the possibility of life and communication so as to nurture and free up elements which can provide us with indications for future investigations. If the illness continues to be masked by institutional illness, it will be impossible to escape from this total identification which prevents us from obtaining any possible understanding. (Basaglia, 1979)

Basaglia is suggesting several important points in this passage. What he here describes as a 'setting aside' of the illness in other places he frames as placing the illness 'in brackets'. Given the ways in which the illness was being used to introduce distance precisely where it should be decreased (i.e. in the relationship between the practitioner and the patient), he considered it essential for this labelling process to be curtailed or abolished altogether if there were to be any hope of ever connecting with the person. In addition, he saw the labelling process and its product, person-as-illness/object, to be more destructive to the person than the illness for which he or she purportedly was being treated. What he referred to above as the 'institutional illness' (the equivalent of 'institutionalism' in the English-speaking world) was so formidable and impenetrable, there was little chance for the practitioner to be able to identify or explore the so-called primary illness which was thought to be underneath. 'So,' Basaglia suggests:

> The psychiatrist has to bracket the illness, the diagnosis, and the syndrome with which the patient has been labeled if he wishes to understand him and, above all else, succeed in helping him, since the patient has been destroyed more by what the illness has been held to be and by the 'protective measures' imposed by such an interpretation than by the illness itself. (Basaglia, 1980c, p. 49)

This suggestion has been criticized by Basaglia's detractors as minimizing the mental illness or as a reflection of his wish to overlook or ignore the presence of the illness (as if that were possible); similar to criticisms of our own work, which have accused us of 'normalizing' psychosis. By reading that the illness was to be 'bracketed' or 'set aside', some critics have argued that Basaglia gave up on psychopathology and psychiatry altogether, or even that he was an adherent of the 'antipsychiatry' movement which at that time was beginning to spread across the Western hemisphere. He has, for example been compared to Thomas Szasz in the United States, who asserted that mental illness was an empty social construction, and to R.D. Laing in the United Kingdom, for whom psychosis was a quasi-religious inward journey of self-realization. But readers who are the least bit familiar with the phenomenological tradition will recognize Basaglia's use of the notion of 'bracketing' as one of the core philosophical and scientific tools introduced by Husserl in the process of founding phenomenology.

Husserl had been trained as a mathematician, and for him the notion of bracketing had a very clear and definite theoretical meaning and function. It was not used to deny the existence of something (e.g., mental illnesses don't exist) but rather to open up a more direct route to gaining insight into the nature of something by questioning our ordinary beliefs and assumptions about that thing, that is by no longer taking it for granted. By highlighting that which we take to be obvious, Husserl hoped to uncover the processes by which that thing comes to be perceived as it is. In this case, Basaglia considered the then popular psychiatric preoccupation with observing and counting the symptoms of mental illnesses (which some would suggest continues to this day) to be a distraction from attending to the real object of interest, which should have been the illness itself and its impact on the person standing before the doctor. The symptoms might very well have been real, and the diagnoses might very well have been accurate, but taken together these facts tell us very little about the nature of the 'illness' or the person, his or her life history, subjective experiences, social context and present needs. The symptoms and diagnosis should not be taken to be proxies for the person's own experiences and actions. When they were, the person him- or herself was no longer viewed as a person, no longer a subjective agent making his or her own decisions, but was transformed into nothing more than an object of scrutiny and manipulation by others – nothing more, as we quoted above, than 'an interesting case'.

In a highly insightful, if perhaps sarcastic, critique of the pursuit of many of his academic colleagues of the time – which, again, some would suggest is equally relevant today – Basaglia bemoaned the preoccupation of the psychopathologists which took them further and further away from the lived reality of the illnesses experienced by their patients by concluding that: 'Instead of questioning the fact that patients are objectified, they continue to analyse the various forms of their objectification' (Basaglia, 1987, p. 64).

5.7 'Freedom is therapeutic'

Having successfully bracketed, or set aside, the illness, what else, we may ask, is to be involved in questioning and presumably reversing, the objectification of the person? It involves first and foremost recognizing, valuing and validating the person's status as a sovereign subject who is in charge of his or her own life. It involves restoring to the person his or her own life history, family and social context, suffering and aspirations. It involves restoring the person's membership in society and the rights and responsibilities associated with it. In short, it means returning to who the person was, and what his or her life was like, prior to entry into the asylum. But then would it be possible to restore or preserve the person's status and role as a sovereign subject once he or she was admitted to the asylum? Would it be possible to provide treatment and care to the person for his or her mental illness within the context of the asylum? Basaglia thought not.

It is reasonable, of course, to ask why not. People can be hospitalized for other medical conditions, such as heart disease or cancer, without ceding their personal agency and autonomy to the hospital staff. Why should this necessarily be different in a mental hospital? It has been different in mental hospitals because in mental hospitals it has been precisely the person's judgement, decision-making capacity and actions that have been challenged, criticized and ultimately controlled. Setting aside the issue of incurability, one could argue that this challenging and controlling of the person's agency was intended only to be temporary, and that the goal of doing so was to restore the person to his or her 'right mind'. But Goffman and others had shown, and Basaglia had experienced, that the institution generated precisely the opposite effect. How can a person be expected to acquire and then to demonstrate improved judgement and decision-making capacity without making judgements and decisions? How can a person be expected to learn how to act differently without being allowed to act? How can a person regain use of his or her 'right mind' without using it? With mental illness, even if a temporary convalescence were required, like with a broken leg, it remained the case that the affected organ (i.e. the brain) had to be used again in order to be rehabilitated. There appeared to be no way to do so within the asylum structure.

In addition, if the illness were generated, even in part, by the person's life circumstances and relationships outside of the asylum, how could anything that happened inside of the asylum address those circumstances and relationships prior to the person's discharge, when he or she returns presumably to the same situation he or she was in prior to admission? As Goffman had quipped, and as more than three decades of behavioral research has since confirmed, taking a person with a mental illness out of his or her life context, admitting him or her to a mental hospital and then returning the person to the same life context is like taking a drowning man out of a lake, teaching him how to ride a bicycle and putting him back in the lake. This represented, for Basaglia, the fundamental flaw of the therapeutic community model. As he writes: 'We could attempt to do some therapeutic work, but this was not very logical while the situation in society as a whole remained unchanged' (Basaglia, 1980c, p. 26).

It would not be possible for patients to be treated and rehabilitated within the context of an institution and for them gradually to earn their freedom back as their clinical status improved, as the conditions which gave rise to the illness existed outside of the institution and the faculties that had to be exercised for the person to improve could not be exercised inside of the institution. In this respect, Basaglia's understanding of the central role of freedom and agency in human nature, in the nature of everyday life within a social context, and therefore in the nature of mental illness and recovery as well, was profoundly influenced by the existentialist school of thought, in particular that brand of Marxist existentialism being developed at the time by Jean-Paul Sartre. Within the context of the asylum, and as long as the doctors (and, by extension, the other staff) held the keys, their power was absolute. As long as they remained the determinants of the patient's everyday life, and as long as they controlled who was free to go and who had to remain, it was not possible for the patient to regain his or her sovereignty. As he writes: 'As long as they (i.e. the patients) accept liberty as a gift from the doctor, they remain submissively dominated' (Basaglia, 1964, p. 1). Such a 'submissively dominated' patient, such a person who allowed others to make his or her decisions, could not hope to recover independent functioning. It was only the tenaciously rebellious, resistant or refusing patient who stubbornly held on to his or her own power who could even hope for a return to independence, but then often at the price of being beaten, further segregated, restrained or lobotomized (one thinks of Jack Nicholson's character in *One Flew Over the Cuckoo's Nest*). Clearly, such a power dynamic could not be healing or therapeutic.

Basaglia therefore came to what at the time were the radical conclusions that all patients needed to be released from the asylums and that all asylums needed to be closed, permanently, conclusions he and his colleagues were able to translate successfully into the drafting and passage of a landmark federal law which stands, with only minor revisions, to this day. His perspective on this issue differed in a fundamentally important way from that of his British, French and American colleagues, leading to what we consider his first major contribution. This difference was his conviction that *freedom and the restoration of the person's agency and citizenship needed necessarily to precede, rather than come later as a result of, his or her recovery*. As he said in the talk he gave at the first international meeting of social psychiatry in London in 1964: 'The psychiatrist of today seems to have discovered, suddenly, that the first step towards the cure of the patient is his return to liberty of which, until now, the psychiatrist himself had deprived him' (Basaglia, 1964, p. 1). Later he was to summarize the challenge presented by this 'first step' as follows:

> What about the inmates? In place of their total dependence on the mental hospital, the aim was to re-establish their standing as members of society at large. Patients had to be given back their rights as citizens, both in legal and in economic terms, replacing the relationship of *custodia* by a contractual one. Moreover, this process of laying the unshakeable foundations of his membership of the social body was the first step, not the last, in the rehabilitation of the former inmate.
> (Basaglia, 1980a, p. 187)

Patients and staff of the asylum in Trieste, which was the first one that Basaglia was able to close successfully, accordingly adopted the slogan above of 'Freedom is therapeutic'. They also came to appreciate the other implication of this perspective, which is that any other potentially therapeutic measure or approach, regardless of how promising it may appear to be, will be rendered ineffective in the absence of freedom. As long as the person's decisions and actions are controlled by others, no matter how benevolent or well-meaning, the person will not be able to take the steps needed to address and recover from his or her mental condition. This is in part due to the fact that taking initiative, creating one's own ideas and making one's own decisions of whether, and how, to act on those ideas are essential mental capacities needed to function in society. To the degree to which these same capacities are undermined or inhibited, so is the person's progress. It is for this reason that Basaglia suggests that it is only 'when the movement for change in psychiatric institutions begins to perceive the patient as the principal protagonist in the transformation [that] the functions of the treatment staff become clearer' (Basaglia, 1964, pp. 182–183).

Recall that the patient needs to be viewed as the 'principal protagonist' from the very first step in his or her rehabilitation and recovery, not once he or she has been treated or cured by others. This then poses a significant challenge for the staff. How are they to view and treat the person as a sovereign agent, a citizen of the social body, when the person remains 'mentally ill'?

5.8 Avoiding the re-creation of the asylum in the community

How mental health practitioners view and treat people who are experiencing mental illnesses as citizens of their communities can be taken to be the central question of this entire volume, and will not be answered in its totality in this one section. A first, and very important, step towards an answer, however, is to understand that simply having a mental illness does not in and of itself deprive a person of his or her civil liberties and rights to begin with. In the United States, this is a conclusion that has to be inferred from the fact that federal and state statutes are very clear in articulating the limited circumstances in which, and under whose legal auspices, a person's liberties and rights may be curtailed (i.e. typically when the person poses a serious, imminent risk to self or others or has been formally determined to lack the capacity to take care of him- or herself by a judge). This conclusion was affirmed by the US Supreme Court as a 'common law' in its decision in *Union Pacific Railway Co. vs Botsford*, in which we read that:

> No right is held more sacred, or is more carefully guarded, by the common law, than the right of every individual to the possession and control of his own person, free from all restraint or interference of others, unless by clear and unquestioned authority of law.

In Italy, thanks to the strenuous lobbying efforts of Basaglia and his *Psychiatrica Democratica* colleagues, this principle was made clear through the mechanism of the Law 180 passed in 1978. Shortly before his untimely death, Basaglia summarized the major thrust of this law as follows:

> We need only reread the Mental Health Law to be convinced that what appears, in the eyes of many, to be a risky adventure, full of threats, merely inserts into the medical norm a civil and constitutional principle that should have been implicit, but was not: the recognition that all men and women, whether healthy or sick, have rights. (Basaglia, 1979, pp. 299–300)

A first answer to the core question raised above is thus: it is not a matter of treating 'mentally ill' people as citizens; it is a matter of recognizing that people are first and foremost citizens who may be experiencing, or who may have, mental illnesses. It is not for mental health practitioners to decide when someone is mentally healthy or in his or her 'right mind' enough to be accorded full citizenship. This is rather established as a birthright. The law is very clear about under what circumstances, under whose auspices and for how long a person may be denied these rights, but in all other cases the rights stand. This is, so to speak, the default condition. It is not up to the person with a mental illness to prove that he or she is deserving of freedom, but instead up to the mental health practitioner to justify any interference of, or imposition upon, a person's freedom. As Basaglia suggests in the passage above, while this may appear to be, or perhaps should have been, obvious, it has been anything but obvious in practice and has rather profound and far-reaching implications for how practice needs to change.

With respect to the difficulty and magnitude of the changes in practice needed, Basaglia showed exceptional, if tragic, foresight, predicting the situation which was to emerge in the United States and most of Western Europe 20 years later. He was concerned that, without the closing of asylums altogether, compassionate mental health practitioners would unknowingly recreate the asylum culture in community settings. As long as the possibility of confinement remained, practitioners would continue to view themselves as the ultimately responsible parties, and former inpatients, and even new patients, would continue to view their freedom and agency as contingent on the will of the doctor. With the spectre of the asylum in the background, even if it is said to be reserved only for the most seriously disabled, people with mental illnesses will remain 'submissively dominated' by the mental health culture. Their only possibility for full recovery will lie outside of the boundaries of the service system, no matter how permeable those boundaries may become. People who do not escape from or refuse to participate in community-based services can only achieve a 'shadow existence' or secondary class of citizenship in which their access and opportunities are restricted to artificial 'programme' settings that approximate or model themselves after, but never quite become, real life (Rowe, 1999). Wrote Basaglia at the end of his life, two years after the Law 180 was passed and over 20 years before the consumer/survivor/ex-patient movement, a number of anthropologists and sociologists in the United States, and eventually the US President's New Freedom Commission on Mental Health, were to decry the failures of the community support movement that had just been launched in 1976:

> Segregation is replaced by an emphasis on socialization under the supervision of an expert who constructs a network of sheltered relationships aiming at the recreation ... of models and living conditions resembling as closely as possible those of real life ... The course of these experiences, though rich in critical stimuli and practical suggestion, confines itself to the model of the institutional management of

the illness as its field of study and makes no attempt to define or determine its own specific goals. Even where . . . a relationship between the
productive world and the management of the institution *does* emerge
or (in France) the connection between the existence of existential
problems and social alienation is established, they only suggest new
areas where the expert may intervene or new treatment techniques
be applied . . . It is, though, still the doctor who decides which type
of admission is suitable for the patient to be admitted, with varying
degrees of urgency and permanency, to one of the range of available
institutions . . . Individual rights, which these regulations contribute
to guaranteeing, are enhanced therefore inside the institution itself
and entrusted to the doctor as a strictly medical problem. So, as far
as the norms are concerned, the declaration of principles becomes, in
practice, a recommendation to the doctor to ensure that sanction and
disorder are each accorded due weight. Yet, while the experiences of
alternative management aimed at reducing sanctions and eliminating
segregation, in practice, psychiatrists still operate within the limits of
the old ideology reaffirming its basic worth and only slightly mitigating
its rigidity (for example, the very limited application of voluntary and
informal admission). (Basaglia, 1980c, p. 24)

Similarly, 20 years before American psychiatry began to tackle the problem
of 'revolving door' or recidivist patients who cycle through repetitive, short-term
hospital stays, Basaglia had predicted this pattern and its effect of keeping the person
tied indefinitely to the overall service system as his or her point of reference. With
the asylum ideology of control following the person into the community, he or she
remains psychologically and culturally confined to a small peer group of people
who similarly congregate in and around mental health service settings. They remain
unable to enter into or engage in the broader community, with the tenuousness
of this existence then continuing to be a factor in their repeated readmissions (cf.
Davidson *et al.*, 1997). Basaglia continues:

> The problem of rehabilitation and chronicity is transformed and
> recycled along the same lines. The practice of confinement for short
> periods and subsequent rapid turnover in the services avoids or at
> least reduces the perpetuation of chronicity in the typical forms the
> asylum presents, such as permanent confinement with no hope of
> ever emerging. Irreversible forms of the disease thus survive in only a
> limited number of patients (the aged and the severely handicapped)
> and chronicity, seen as total dependence on the services is attenuated
> in that it takes the form of regular sessions. Around the services
> themselves, we find the polarization of 'soft' chronicity which keeps up
> contacts with the social fabric by means of an unstable or part-time job
> and the socialization of the patient's own world. Both are controlled
> and supported by resorting to the services where the psychiatrist's
> supervision permits different types of treatment and guarantees the
> homologation of the individual. In other words, a composite area of

> diversified social groups has formed around the services. These groups
> have in common the fact of depending on the institution which is
> resorted to either permanently or periodically . . . As resorting to the
> services is automatically qualified as illness, the status of the sick person
> perilously widens. (Basaglia, 1980c, p. 25)

Over 20 years later, the US President's New Freedom Commission was to
conclude that the community-based mental health service system that had been
developed since the 1970s 'simply manages symptoms and accepts long-term
disability' (Department of Health and Human Services, 2003, p. 1), thereby needing
to be 'transformed' in order to promote recovery and full participation in the
life of the community. What else can be done, then? What kinds of changes was
Basaglia envisioning when he warned against recreating asylums in the community?
While in 1980 he concluded that the new law 'both because of its inherent qualities
and because of the characteristics of the social terrain in which it works, creates
more contradictions than it solves' (Basaglia, 1980c, p. 30), and while he viewed
the challenge of 'how such participation (in community life) can be achieved [as]
a problem for the future' (Basaglia, 1980b, p. 27), he nonetheless offered some
suggestions as to how these contradictions might be resolved. His work, and the
work his colleagues have continued to pursue, in Trieste and elsewhere provide
some insights into what alternative practices focused on facilitating community
participation might entail.

5.9 Social inclusion

> When we began our reform process, in reality we violated society by
> forcing it to accept the 'crazy' person, and this created major problems
> that did not exist before. The important thing, however, was that even
> as we violated society we were there (as new 'technicians') to accept the
> consequences of this violence, and to take responsibility for our actions
> in order to help the community understand what the presence of a
> mentally ill person in society meant . . . The originality of the Trieste
> model perhaps consists precisely in this. Not so much, or not only, in its
> having tried to co-opt the city's population for its project . . . but rather
> in its having proposed a very direct terrain for confrontation, provided
> by the evidence of choices carried out in plain view of everyone. This
> resulted in the staff taking explicit and direct responsibility for every
> single decision taken along the way, regardless of their consequences,
> together with a profound identification of the staff with their patients.
> On the other hand, due to the conflicts that arose, this method offered
> the public possibility of indicating the contents and limits of a special
> form of action, with respect to the discrepancy that existed between
> the abstract adherence to the recognition of the patient's rights and
> the effective possibility of his having a degree of power in the life of
> the city. Verbal consent to the former can be easily obtained; but the
> second will inevitably create contradictions and conflicts which – once

> they have been faced and dealt with in real terms – can constitute the
> terrain for the growth of rights and the enrichment of resources for
> the entire community. (Basaglia, 1979)

This is how Basaglia describes the second major component of his project, and his second major contribution to the recovery movement. As Scheper-Hughes and Lovell had witnessed in visiting Trieste, the first step of closing down the asylum:

> had to be accompanied by the far more radical and difficult task of
> 'opening up' communities, making them more receptive and respon-
> sive, and more than just passively and indifferently 'tolerant' of the
> psychologically different, troubled, or suffering individuals who would
> be returned to their midst. (Scheper-Hughes and Lovell, 1987, p. x)

If individuals with mental illnesses were to be discharged from asylums, or kept out of asylums altogether, communities would have to be prepared to deal with the effects of mental illness among their citizens. As Basaglia (1979) recognized – once again with uncanny foresight – it would be relatively easy for communities to accord people with mental illnesses their full citizenship rights in rhetoric or in principle: 'verbal consent can be easily obtained'. But it would be quite a different matter to respect these rights in practice, especially among individuals who exhibited the signs or symptoms of the illness. It also has proven to be relatively easy, though not entirely so, to honor the rights of those individuals who have progressed far enough in their recoveries to 'pass for normal' (as members of the consumer/survivor/ex-patient movement have described the process of concealing the effects of the illness). It was a new idea in 1980, however, that even individuals who could not conceal the effects of the illness could still 'have a degree of power in the life of the city' (Basaglia, 1979). Making this possible became one of the key responsibilities of the former asylum staff.

According to Scheper-Hughes and Lovell:

> Basaglia did not entertain naïve misconceptions about the readiness
> and willingness of Italian communities to accept the released 'madmen'
> and women. He recognized that his was a deeply cultural as well as
> political task, and that his co-workers had to confront and do battle
> with the Demons of archaic superstitions and negative stereotypes
> about the 'mentally ill'. (Scheper-Hughes and Lovell, 1987, p. x)

Public or community education, as also proposed in the 1963 American legislation creating community mental health centres, would not be enough, however. This could not remain an abstract or merely conceptual acceptance of difference, as it extended to and could conceivably disrupt the everyday lives of ordinary community citizens. Efforts had to take place primarily, therefore, at the level of face-to-face, personal interactions (i.e. those strategies which also have been shown since to be the most effective in addressing stigma). Basaglia and his colleagues channelled these efforts into four related domains.

First, before the asylum was closed and as part of assisting the inmates to become comfortable being around community people as well as vice versa, events were planned to create two-way traffic between the asylum and the community. Patients were taken out on community visits accompanied (rather than supervised) by staff, and community members were invited onto the grounds of the asylum for a range of publicized cultural, recreational and social events. The grounds of the asylum campus were prepared and put to good use for soccer matches, festivals, art exhibits, music concerts, lectures and other public gatherings. Activities that involved children were particularly valued, both for the therapeutic effect that the presence of children had for the patients and for the message this sent to the community in terms of the harmlessness of the patients. In fact, Basaglia and colleagues opened a day care centre for the children of the staff on the grounds of the asylum, much to the alarm and scepticism of the town and his psychiatric colleagues elsewhere. Rather than the anticipated scandal, this turned out to become a valuable asset for the town as a whole.

Like the day care centre, other uninhabited or recently vacated parts of the asylum were put to other uses. This became a second key strategy for community inclusion (as well as a necessary step in honoring the rights of the patients), when Basaglia decided to terminate the patient 'work therapy' programme through which patients cooked meals, did laundry, helped to take care of the physical facilities and performed other menial tasks and were paid only in tokens that they could cash in for cigarettes or other small items. Rejecting the notion of the so-called token economy as indentured servitude or forced labor, Basaglia instituted a system in which patients who were able and interested could do work for the same level of pay they would receive for the same or similar labor in the community. This produced an enormous capacity for employment in a range of industries beyond janitorial and food service, with approximately half of the patient population expressing interest in gainful employment. From this modest beginning, and consistent with the principle that citizens have the right to a decent wage for their labor, the model of social cooperatives was born.

Social cooperatives are industries or service companies that employ a mixture of workers, some with disabilities and some without, that are able to compensate their employees' comparable wages to the rest of the business sector based either on government subsidies used to compensate for reduced productivity or, when possible, on their own self-sustaining productivity. Beginning with their inception within the walls of the Trieste asylum, social cooperatives (or social firms) have since become ubiquitous across the Trieste business sector, at one point numbering 45 different companies or functions. These include catering and cleaning, which were a couple of the original areas, but have expanded to hotels, human services, artisans such as furniture, jewellery, glass-making and a radio station. In fact, it is difficult to spend any time in Trieste and not come into contact with a social cooperative in some form. This social cooperative model has been highly effective in contributing both to the employment rate among individuals with mental illnesses and to the growth and development of the Trieste economy, offering one example of what Basaglia envisioned as 'the enrichment of resources for the entire community' that would come from the community inclusion of people with mental illness. This model has since been replicated in various forms in numerous European countries, Australia and New Zealand, and, more recently, Canada. A 1999 survey found about 2000 social firms in Europe alone employing approximately 47 000 workers, of whom 40–50% were disabled (Leff and Warner, 2006, p. 139).

A third area of focus was in working with groups that represented other marginalized or oppressed peoples within the Trieste community. Given that this work was being done in the early 1970s, that is just after the student revolts of 1968–1969, these groups included the students' movement as well as the labor unions, workers' movement, and the feminist movement, which was particularly active and effective in Italy (e.g. securing rights regarding reproduction, i.e. gaining access to contraception, within a largely Catholic country). We may recall this strategy from Jane Addams' work in the early part of the twentieth century from Chapter 3. In working closely with these movements, there developed once again two-way traffic between different communities: individuals with mental illnesses finding out that they had much in common, and could socialize, with other oppressed people and students, workers and women finding out that people with mental illnesses were in many ways just like them. As was to be demonstrated by the eventual passage of Law 180, considerable political power could be amassed in the collectives formed by sympathetic groups that had similar aims of establishing a just and equitable society for all citizens.

The fourth strategy for promoting social inclusion played out at the individual level and could only be effective one person, one family or one group at a time. Staff worked with each individual to determine the person's interests and needs, and then accompanied the person in his or her efforts to meet those needs and pursue those interests within the broader community. As Basaglia commented, this created entirely new roles and required a new set of skills for the staff, who had viewed their roles as more supervisory than facilitative and who, outside of the asylum, had no more authority or power to achieve results than the patients themselves:

> The approach that underlies this work is in no way an attempt to evade the central point of illness. In this new context, however, the conflicts which had previously been regarded as internal to the patient, or at least to the asylum, are thrown back on the wider society from whence they came ... For the mental health worker, this means an entirely new role: instead of acting as a go-between in the relationship between patient and hospital, he has to enter into conflicts in the real world – the family, the workplace, or the welfare agencies ... Moreover, mental health workers are no longer impartial: they have to face the inequalities of power which engendered these crises, and put themselves whole-heartedly on the side of the weak. Acting outside

> the asylum situation, they of course lack any established expertise
> or authority: thus they have to function without any pre-determined
> responses, on the basis of nothing more nor less than their total
> commitment to the patient. (Basaglia, 1980a, pp. 190–191)

In this case, each person, each issue and each circumstance was unique and
required its own unique response. The staff not only had to be adept at recognizing
and managing effects of the illness but also had to be socially and instrumentally
adept at assisting the person in navigating or negotiating the community terrain,
whether this be securing one's disability pension, resolving conflicts with one's
family or finding the leverage needed to get a neglectful landlord to repair a leaking
sink. It was crucial in all of these circumstances that the staff not take over the
situation and resolve it for the person, as this would be to lapse back into the asylum
role of caretaker. The staff's role was more that of a mediator, who could help
members of the community understand and be responsive to the person with the
mental illness while also helping the person with the mental illness to understand
how the world works and what it requires from him or her. In addition to forming
a core part of the staff's responsibility, this was a function that also could be
performed by community volunteers, of which there were many. Basaglia's energy
and charisma generated large numbers of what came to be referred to affectionately
as 'Basagliani', described by Scheper-Hughes and Lovell as consisting of 'college
students and housewives, artists and artisans, working people and the retired . . .
who rose to the occasion and came out to welcome the ex-mental patients back into
the human community' (Scheper-Hughes and Lovell, 1987, p. xi).

To the degree that all of these strategies were successful, they would help to create
a community which was accepting of differences and in which these differences
would be viewed as secondary in importance to the values that each person's unique
contributions added to the greater good. In other words, by accepting people
with mental illnesses, communities would be moved to lessen their rigid or strict
adherence to the principles of reason and capitalism. As a result, everyone would
stand to benefit from the creation of a world in which people did not have to be
either rational or materially productive in order to have valuable roles to play. In
such a community, members would realize that they did not have a monopoly on
the truth or on one central 'reality', but would appreciate that different people would
have different points of view, each of which could add to, instead of detract from,
the whole. Contemporary readers may recognize this notion of celebrating, rather
than merely tolerating, human diversity as a very timely one that remains difficult
to achieve. It stands as one more testament to the enduring value, and surprising
prescience, of Basaglia's vision.

5.10 Summary of lessons learned

From this review of the work of Goffman and Basaglia, we suggest the following
lessons:

- Institutions can do more harm than good, adding to the burden of disease a sense of demoralization, hopelessness and helplessness.

- Rather than promoting recovery, adopting the identity of a 'mental patient' poses an additional barrier or obstacle to recovery. While some people find it helpful to accept that they have a mental illness, it is important that this not translate into their being absorbed into a mental patient identity within the artificial settings of the mental health system.

- If agency plays a key role in recovery, then the restoration of a person's sovereignty and civil rights needs to precede, rather than follow, recovery. Freedom is a birthright in democratic societies; it cannot be made into something that has to be earned or is bestowed by others as a reward for recovery.

- Many people with mental illnesses want to, and can, work. Innovative structures have been developed to enable people to do so, including social cooperative and social firm models which offer integrated work settings.

- Helping people to exercise their citizenship and helping communities to be more accepting are both appropriate and key roles for mental health practitioners and some volunteers. Playing such roles may require the person to become an advocate and to shed any illusion of being impartial or neutral.

- Two-way streets can be created between the mental health system and the broader community to allow for easier access of people with mental illnesses to community life and to increase the responsiveness of communities to individual needs.

- For people with mental illnesses to be able to live fully as citizens of their communities, communities may have to, and can, change.

  Lessons to avoid repeating:

- Do not recreate asylums or institutions within the community by continuing to view the staff as in charge of or responsible for the person with a mental illness.

- Do not accept stigma and stereotypes as inevitable evils of contemporary society. They can be reduced and perhaps eliminated altogether.

- Do not accept long-term disability and a life confined to artificial mental health settings as the best people can hope for or work towards.

- Do not limit community inclusion activities to educational efforts only. Person-to-person contact is a more effective route to reducing stigma.

6
The Rights and Responsibilities of Citizenship

6.1 Recovery as a civil rights movement

We noted at the outset that this volume was not going to consist of a historical account of the evolution of the recovery movement within psychiatry. At this point in the discussion, however, we do find it necessary to point out one important fact about the recovery movement as a historical phenomenon, and that is that it began in the 1970s – in its contemporary form – primarily as a civil rights movement. Consistent with the aim and overall tone of this book, we will not be concerned in this chapter with the historical events or figures who catalysed and pushed this movement forward. Our concern will rather be in the conceptual realm, exploring the civil rights dimension of recovery and its implications for psychiatric theory, research and practice. What does it mean to say that the recovery movement was, and remains, primarily a civil rights movement? What do civil rights have to do with mental illness or recovery? And how would a psychiatry which explicitly acknowledged the fundamental importance of civil rights look and operate differently?

For guidance in these explorations we again have to look outside of psychiatry or mental health per se, as narrowly defined disciplines, to thinkers who have addressed these issues from a broader point of view. In this case, we propose learning about the nature of civil rights and the conditions for their reclamation from the Reverend Dr Martin Luther King, Jnr. We will see that there continue to be important ways in which the mental health recovery movement parallels earlier stages of the civil rights movement among African Americans in the United States. Following discussion of some of the lessons taught by Dr King, we will then turn to the political thought of the recently deceased French philosopher Gilles Deleuze concerning the rights and challenges associated with community membership, particularly in Western industrial capitalist societies. The notions of Oedipus and desire put forth

The Roots of the Recovery Movement in Psychiatry   Larry Davidson, Jaak Rakfeldt, John Strauss
© 2010 John Wiley & Sons, Ltd

by Deleuze, in conjunction with his psychiatrist collaborator Felix Guattari (1982), push King's insights to a deeper level of analysis. They bring out the basic tensions involved in according civil rights to citizens whose behaviors threaten to undermine, rather than confirm or support, a society's vision of the good life. Having resolved this tension in the present chapter, we will then be able to move on in the chapter which follows to explore in a more positive fashion what such a sense of citizenship might entail.

6.2 The incomplete world of Martin Luther King, Jnr

> Today, psychologists have a favorite word, and that word is malad-
> justed. I tell you today that there are some things in our social system to
> which I am proud to be maladjusted. I shall never be adjusted to lynch
> mobs, segregation, economic inequalities, 'the madness of militarism,'
> and self-defeating physical violence. The salvation of the world lies in
> the maladjusted. (King, 1981, p. 23)

What does it take for a person to lead a civil rights movement? At the risk of seeming to dwell on the obvious, that person must first and foremost be able to envision a world that is significantly different from the one that currently exists. For Dr King, this was a world in which children would be judged 'by the content of their character rather than by the color of their skin'. King had to believe that such a world was possible, even if it was not a world that he or anyone else he knew had yet experienced. Franco Basaglia felt that he had to take just such a leap of faith as well, suggesting shortly before his untimely death that he and his colleagues had been successful in 'showing that the impossible could be possible' (Basaglia, 1979). In this case, it had been possible for people with serious mental illnesses to live outside of asylums. This language was more recently borrowed by the *Federal Action Agenda*, in which we read that the 'transformation' of mental health care to recovery will entail 'creating something possible from the perceived impossible' (Department of Health and Human Services, 2005, p. 1). Before turning to what it is precisely that we need to create through the process of transformation that is currently perceived to be impossible, it is worth exploring first this notion of the world as incomplete. It is at the foundation of any battle for civil or human rights, or, for that matter, of any transformation.

Though it may seem obvious to suggest that some things that are currently considered impossible may become possible over time, we ordinarily think of this principle as applying to science fiction and to inventions or technological breakthroughs such as Edison's invention of the light bulb, Marconi's invention of the radio or the Wright brothers' invention of the aeroplane. Having electric lights and radios, and being able to fly, certainly have changed the world in fundamental ways, and each was of course considered impossible before being demonstrated to be possible. But these breakthroughs took place at the level of the concrete and particular; they added to the existing world a new component or capacity.

Underlying each of these inventions was also a more basic insight into the nature of the world as it was already. Inventing the light bulb required an understanding of the nature of electricity, the radio involved using air as a medium for communication and the aeroplane resulted from the study of aerodynamics. In each case, it was human understanding as well as the world itself which had been incomplete. In each case, what had seemed impossible became possible when a previous human understanding was shown to be incomplete or incorrect. While no one now needs to understand the nature of electricity in order to turn on a light, it was necessary initially for someone to do so in order for there to be electric lights.

What relevance does this have for civil rights in the short term or for mental illness and recovery in the long term? Its relevance lies in the fact that to bring about a new world one must first recognize the incompleteness of the existing world. In the case of civil rights for people of African origin in the United States, Martin Luther King, Jnr and his contemporaries grew up in an era and in a place (i.e. in a world) in which people of color were viewed and treated as less than human. Assumed inferior to whites as a matter of biological, theological and/or moral fact, they were denied access to the lunch counters, bus seats, bathrooms and drinking fountains used by whites, not to mention denied equal rights and access to the marketplaces, schools, job sites or voting booths of mainstream America. This was the world that was inherited by the founders of the civil rights movement and their white detractors alike. What is a person, or a people, to do in the face of such a world?

Were the world predetermined and complete, people would have little choice but to find a way to accept and adapt to such a state of affairs. And many people, of course, tried to do just that. But we know now that that was not the only possibility. King's derision of the concept of 'adjustment' in the passage with which we opened this section speaks to what he thought of the false necessity of adjusting to the world into which one happened to be born. The world of racial inequality was neither necessary nor complete. It was a world to which one could and should refuse to adjust. In these, and similar, circumstances, 'the salvation of the world' resides in those who can see beyond the world as it is and who choose instead to create a world as it should be. Once we recognize the possibility of doing so – of not accepting the ways things are and choosing to change them – we come to realize that even accepting and adjusting to the world the way it is requires active choice and participation on the part of each person. It may seem to be the path of least resistance, it may even seem to require no effort on the person's part at all, but each person each moment is either working towards the creation of a new world and/or endorsing an existing one.

The existentialist philosopher Jean-Paul Sartre pointed this out in describing the dilemma of the French living under German occupation during World War II, insisting that all citizens were faced with the choice of joining the resistance or being complicit with the Nazis. King framed this similar dilemma in terms of 'adjustment': you either refuse to adjust to lynch mobs, segregation and inequality or, by not refusing, you become complicit with and contribute to their perpetuation. People of conscience in an earlier century were faced with the same issue regarding slavery. It was not only a question of who would join the abolitionists, but who, by virtue of their own actions, would continue the enslavement of another human being or instead would view and treat this person as a free and sovereign agent (who had been enslaved by others in the past). In these and other ways, people are always engaged in creating a world, even if their actions serve only to perpetuate a world that existed previously.

With these examples of slavery, occupation and discrimination we have arrived at one issue we consider key to the transformation required of psychiatry and mental health care for people with serious mental illnesses to reclaim their civil rights as citizens of their communities. A basic driver of the recovery movement has been the perception that adults with serious mental illnesses have themselves been a population subjected to slavery, occupation and, most recently, discrimination. The challenge posed by transformation therefore is whether we choose to continue to confine adults with serious mental illnesses to the second-class status of 'mental patient' or we instead find new ways of viewing and treating them as full, contributing citizens, capable of self-determination and worthy of being included fully in community life. As has been true with racism, the institutions, social structures and mechanisms of slavery, occupation and discrimination may no longer be as blatant or obvious as they once were. Just as people of African origin are no longer slaves on Southern plantations, people with serious mental illnesses are no longer made to work without pay to tend the farms and take care of the hospitals in which they live. And just as lunch counters and bathrooms are no longer segregated, people with mental illnesses can no longer be confined against their will arbitrarily and for extended periods by others under the guise of acting in their best interests. Though things have improved significantly, and people with mental illnesses spend less and less time in confined settings, segregation and discrimination remain fundamental realities in their everyday lives. Dr King understood these more subtle forms of oppression as well, as we will see next.

6.3 Can rights be given?

During a grand rounds presentation one of us recently gave at a medical centre in which the issue of civil rights was being discussed, a psychiatry resident stood up and asked whether the presenter could specify precisely which civil rights were being denied to adults with serious mental illnesses at the current time. No longer confined to state mental hospitals for extended periods, it was not obvious to this well-meaning and compassionate young doctor in what ways her current patients were being discriminated against because of their mental illness. Before responding, the presenter asked other members of the audience if they would like to reply to this important question, and a couple of audience members who were themselves in recovery gave a few examples of losing a job and a girlfriend because of people finding out about their illness, as well as not being accorded respect and having others not take them seriously because of their status as a recipient of mental health services. Though poignant, these offences did not seem to be of the magnitude other participants associated with the weighty issue of civil rights. The presenter then asked the young doctor what she thought she was doing herself to respect the rights of her patients. If these rights were not being denied, how was she in fact honoring them in practice? Her response was that she and her treatment team allowed, even encouraged, their patients to make as many of their own decisions as they could. When asked how she determined their capability, she replied that it was a matter of clinical judgement. It was part of the staff's job, and her societal obligation, she assumed, to determine which of, when and under what circumstances her patients were capable of making their own decisions.

This vignette is as complicated as it is true, real life typically being complicated. By using this example, we do not mean to raise questions about this particular professional's care, compassion or competence. We draw no conclusions regarding her ethical standards or integrity. We do not accuse her of being personally prejudiced or discriminatory. In fact, we thanked and congratulated her for her courage and willingness to address the substantive issues involved in re-orienting care to the promotion of recovery, for going beyond the simplistic rhetoric to the real-life issues encountered in everyday practice. In doing so, she drew our attention to the heart of the matter: who decides, based on what criteria, which of, when and under what circumstances a select population of people are entitled to make their own decisions? Rather than being a matter of clinical judgement, these are the questions that cut right to the heart of matters of civil rights. The fact that such questions are taken as a matter of course to be under the purview of psychiatry suggests the degree to which certain prejudices have become entrenched within the profession itself. Like institutional racism, discrimination against individuals with serious mental illnesses has been institutionalized. It is simply how services are provided. As mental health practitioners, we have become much more acutely aware of our societal obligation to protect people and the community from the ravages of mental illness (which are themselves very real) than of our equal societal obligation to honor and respect the rights of the people we serve. According to current laws and previous judicial interpretations, individuals with serious mental illnesses retain their fundamental rights to personal sovereignty and self-determination unless, until, and then only for as long as, they pose serious imminent risks to self or others or have been determined to be incapacitated and/or require conservatorship by a judge. In all other cases and circumstances, we have no legal authority to determine when and under what circumstances another person is entitled to make his or her own decisions. Even though it may not be enacted until adulthood, the right to make one's own decisions is the birthright of every citizen of a democratic society. This includes citizens who happen to have serious mental illnesses. In practice, however, this right is often made contingent on the person's recovery. It is as if the mental illness has robbed the person of his or her birthright and this right can only be restored to the person once he or she proves that the illness has abated or is cured. You can make your own decisions as long as (i) I agree with the decision and/or (ii) you have proven yourself capable of making good decisions– 'good' unfortunately being defined de facto as decisions I would agree with or condone. In reality, however, it has been as much the mental health system that has robbed people of their birthright of self-determination as it has been the illness itself.

It may help in gaining some distance from prevailing assumptions about the capacity of individuals with serious mental illnesses to turn back to the example of the civil rights movement and Dr King. An analogous situation was faced in the civil rights movement when some white community leaders in the South, in particular members of the clergy, became simultaneously outspoken critics both of segregation and of the civil rights movement's strategies for fostering integration. Like the psychiatrist mentioned above, they saw themselves as being in the position of deciding what rights could be accorded to which citizens on the basis of what circumstances and, in this case, according to what timeline. In his now classic 'Letter from Birmingham Jail' (King, 1981), King challenged this position, concerned that the goodwill, best intentions and eventual impact of what we had come to call the 'white moderates' in the Southern clergy would pose more of an obstacle to true progress in ending racism than the more blatant and violent attacks of the Ku Klux Klan. The letter was written specifically to a group of white clergy in Birmingham who had admonished the civil rights activists for what they considered their ill-timed and unreasonable demonstrations. They urged King to replace his demands for redress with patience, to allow the white community leaders the time to institute incremental and presumably less controversial steps towards social change. To this plea, King made the following response:

> We know through painful experience that freedom is never voluntarily given by the oppressor; it must be demanded by the oppressed. Frankly, I have yet to engage in a direct action campaign that was 'well-timed' in view of those who have not suffered unduly from the disease of segregation. For years now I have heard the word 'Wait!' It rings in the ear of every Negro with piercing familiarity. This 'Wait!' has almost always meant 'Never'. We must come to see, with one of our distinguished jurists, that justice too long delayed is justice denied. (King, 1981, p. 278)

6.4 Recovery delayed is recovery denied

We saw in Chapter 4 how Franco Basaglia and his colleagues had come to a similar conclusion regarding the role of freedom. If freedom were made contingent on cure or recovery, then inmates of the asylum would never be free. Having one's freedom restored was rather one of the first preconditions *for* recovery. Freedom, we recall, was considered 'therapeutic' and one could only gain mastery over one's illness and manage one's life outside of the asylum by first being accorded one's freedom. King's point here is similar. Justice for one party cannot be made contingent on or left up to the whims of another party, as in that case it will inevitably be delayed indefinitely and, as a result, denied. The time would never be quite right for people of African origin to be afforded full citizenship as long as this concession were viewed as threatening to, or taking something away from, white Americans. But justice cannot be made a matter of charity.

We suggest that the same is true for recovery in serious mental illness. While it may seem a stretch to those of us who have never experienced serious mental illnesses personally, the word 'wait', unfortunately, seems to ring with an almost equally piercing familiarity in the ears of many people who have. In their case, they have been told to wait for over a half-century before they will be allowed to live in their own homes, work in meaningful jobs, make friends or become lovers with the people they choose, have sex, attend church or pursue their other dreams (Davidson et al., 2001). Regardless of whether it is due to the interference of symptoms, the presumption of skill deficits, the lack of supports, the inadequacy of entitlements or the insufficiency of funding for care, people with mental illnesses have been told repeatedly that they are not yet ready or able to participate in the lives of their communities. And when informed that the vision of the President's New Freedom Commission on Mental Health was 'a life in the community' for everyone (Department of Health and Human Services, 2003, p. 1), well-meaning practitioners often agree in principle with this goal, but suggest that it is not yet the right time, or that we do not yet have the requisite means, to achieve it. Their patients are too sick or disabled to recover; there is not yet an adequate evidence base to support recovery (despite 30 years of rigorous longitudinal research; Davidson, Harding and Spaniol, 2005) or the systems in which they work lack either the resources or the political will to honor the *Olmstead* decision by no longer viewing institutions as acceptable places for people to live.

At the same time, these are the same practitioners who suggest that the current system of care is not yet so broken as to require fixing. In their estimation, the fact that tens of thousands of people with serious mental illnesses continue to live in hospitals, that the unemployment rate among people with mental illnesses remains at 85% and that people continue to have their hopes, aspirations and passions squelched on a daily basis by 'outdated science, outmoded financing and unspoken discrimination' (Department of Health and Human Services, 2003) appear not to be sufficient to justify more drastic measures. 'Perhaps it is easy', as King suggests, 'for those who have never felt the stinging darts of segregation to say "Wait"' (King, 1981, p. 278). But for people with serious mental illnesses and their families, 'Wait' can no longer be considered a reasonable, adequate or acceptable response.

In King's letter, he goes on to poignantly list the abuses, violations, discriminations, horrors and indecencies that people of African origin had been subjected to for the preceding 350 years, which made them legitimately and unavoidably impatient. These travesties ranged from slavery, lynching and police brutality to having to explain to his six-year-old daughter why she would not be allowed to visit the amusement park she had just seen advertised on television because it was for whites only.

For people with serious mental illnesses, societal abuses and discrimination similarly did not end with the depopulation of over-crowded and under-staffed custodial institutions. To this day, people with serious mental illnesses continue to be suspected to be serial killers, continue to be told that they cannot return to school or that they will never work again, to be discouraged from having children because they are told they cannot even take care of themselves and to be discouraged from talking about their spiritual beliefs or sexual desires because they reflect their illness. To this day, their families continue to be told to grieve for their loss as if the person had died. To this day, people in recovery are allowed, and even encouraged, to make their own decisions only when staff have decided they are capable of doing so. And to this day, even people in recovery who take on roles within the mental health system in order to give back and to help others are told that their job description is to do all of those 'messy' things (i.e. help people get food, shelter, clothing and their other basic needs addressed) that 'real' staff are too busy to attend to, are told that they can only provide 'support' (which is never defined) since they are not trained or qualified to do anything else or find their insights about a person's assets or interests dismissed because they are considered relevant only to recovery and not to treatment – as if treatment can be divorced from, or made superordinate to, recovery. Perhaps it is only when you are yourself in such a position, as King suggests, that 'then you will understand why we find it difficult to wait' (King, 1981, p. 278).

We suggest that mental health care will continue to be limited in its effectiveness as long as people with serious mental illnesses continue to be made to wait to reclaim their lives in the community. It is not surprising, therefore, that many of those people in recovery who fought long and hard for their rights to self-determination and social inclusion distrust the current rhetoric of recovery and transformation. Their distrust, dissatisfaction and demands must be understood as analogous to the position King was eventually forced to take with respect to those white clergy who were forever delaying ending segregation to some mythical point in time, always 'later', when all of the stars would be aligned. Consistent with his message above, we suggest that recovery too long delayed is also recovery denied. As King sadly concludes:

> I must confess that over the past few years I have been gravely disappointed with the White moderate. I have almost reached the regrettable conclusion that the Negro's great stumbling block in his stride toward freedom is not . . . the Ku Klux Klanner, but the White moderate, who is more devoted to 'order' than to justice; who . . . paternalistically believes he can set the timetable for another's freedom . . . Shallow understanding from people of good will is more frustrating than absolute misunderstanding from people of ill will. Lukewarm acceptance is much more bewildering than outright rejection (King, 1981, p. 280)

While it may seem unreasonable to some to suggest that well-meaning mental health practitioners are at times 'more devoted' to symptom reduction and skill acquisition than to the person's day-to-day life, and that they at times 'paternalistically believe' that they can set the conditions for their patients' self-determination or participation in the life of their communities, we suggest that these examples capture some of the more concerning elements that appear to be emerging in the field under the rubric of recovery. In a variety of venues, the term 'recovery' has come to be used to refer to what happens after care or cure, to repackaged models of treatment or rehabilitation or to the adding on of new services to existing systems of care. But as several leading recovery advocates have suggested, recovery refers primarily to the fundamental personhood of people with serious mental illnesses (Deegan, 1988; Anthony, 2004; Davidson, 2006). A similar point was made by former president Bill Clinton when he took the podium to eulogize Coretta Scott King, Martin Luther King, Jnr's wife and one of the few remaining towering figures of the civil rights movement. Coming after lofty tributes that praised Mrs King as embodying various virtues and noble principles, Clinton pointed to her casket and began his comments with: 'Now, I want to remind you all that there is a woman in there. That's no symbol in there, but a flesh-and-blood woman.' This admonition returns us to the original civil rights dimension of the recovery movement: people with mental illnesses are first and foremost people who belong here, in the community, participating alongside other citizens in the naturally occurring community activities of their choice regardless of their disability status.

What is it precisely that has led us to view people with mental illnesses as less than, as inferior to, those who presumably are without mental illness? What leads us to believe that we, acting as mental health professionals, are in the position of determining who, when and under what circumstances another person is to be allowed to make his or her own decisions? If it were merely a matter of risk aversion, such intrusions into another person's sovereignty would not extend to and pervade the entirety of the person's life, as it often continues to to this day. What makes me think, for example, that a person who is hearing voices can no longer decide what he or she would like to eat for lunch? Why would someone with a mental illness need to be told when he or she can take a shower or be made to take one at a certain hour? What puts me in a better position than the person him- or herself to decide where, or with whom, the person should live or what kind of job he or she should have? Why do we require people with mental illnesses to attend educational or therapeutic groups in order to have safe and affordable housing, in order to access other needed resources, in order to remain out of jail or in order to apply for a job? King's efforts established that no one could be judged to be 'too black' to sit at a lunch counter, to use a bathroom or to sit in the front of a bus. In a similar vein, Bill Anthony, one of the founders of psychiatric rehabilitation, has reminded us that no one can be determined to be 'too blind' to learn Braille. Why do we continue to think that a person can be 'too mentally ill' to benefit from rehabilitation, to learn compensatory strategies and to exercise autonomy in making his or her own decisions on a day-to-day basis?

In order to understand fully the basis for these discriminatory beliefs, we must first understand better the world to which they belong. King inherited a world in which people of color were considered inferior to and less than whites. His efforts, and those of many other courageous and visionary people, have helped to create a world in which a person of color can now be elected president of the United States. We likewise have inherited a world in which people with serious mental illnesses are considered inferior to and less than people who do not have a serious mental illness. We have inherited a world in which people are expected to recover fully from a mental illness first – despite the fact that we do not yet have cures for these illnesses – before they will be allowed to make their own decisions, pursue their own hopes, dreams and aspirations and otherwise participate fully in the life of their communities. It will be helpful in establishing the incompleteness of this world, and in beginning to envision a new world in which these assumptions will no longer be held, to understand where these beliefs came from and what societal purposes they might have played, and continue to play, in perpetuating an old world order, that is the world as it currently exists. For this task, we turn from the example of King to the thinking of the contemporary French philosopher Gilles Deleuze.

6.5 Color blindness and capitalism

Before turning to the challenging and world-shifting thought of Deleuze, it may help to ease us into this complex territory to revisit first a seminal article about serious mental illness by a leading figure in the American psychiatry of a generation or so ago. In his theoretical essay entitled 'Schizotaxia, schizotypy, schizophrenia', Meehl (1973) explores the possibility that the genetic dimension of psychosis may be responsible for a common or underlying trait, or combination of traits, possessed by people who display a variety of conditions differing both in level of severity and in degree of associated disability. All of these individuals may share an underlying schizotaxic proclivity, but some may only manifest this in mild or unobtrusive ways, in what Meehl refers to as 'schizotypy'. It is even possible that in some of these individuals this condition of schizotypy may put them at an advantage for certain kinds of creative pursuits, for example pursuits in which thinking outside of the box, so to speak, is an asset rather than a liability. In other individuals, however, this condition may be more severe or may generate a certain degree of disability, such as that condition that has traditionally been referred to as 'schizophrenia'. What is most useful to us about Meehl's rather sophisticated argument – which in fact anticipates developments in genetics and evolutionary biology that are just now coming to maturity – is that it is not only the genetic inheritance itself but also the environment that can determine which of these conditions result. It is not only a matter of individual 'vulnerability' that determines how this genetic inheritance will influence the person's character and life, but the very fact of whether this genetic inheritance will be understood *as* a vulnerability may also be determined by the social context into which the person is born.

To illustrate this point, Meehl suggests the analogy of color blindness. Color blindness may itself be an inherited trait. This alone, however, will not determine the degree or nature of the influence this inheritance has on the person and his or her life. Within our current context, the vast majority of individuals with color blindness function perfectly well in society. If you do not know someone well, or if they choose not to disclose this fact to you, you would have little ability (outside of a vision test) to detect that someone cannot in fact see certain colors. Most likely, such individuals would not choose to pursue activities or careers in which keen color vision is required, such as painters, interior decorators, graphic artists and so on. At the same time, such individuals may find that their color blindness prepares them especially well for other kinds of pursuits, such as taking black and white photographs. Otherwise, though, the influence of this particular genetic inheritance would be rather mild and unobtrusive.

Imagine for a moment, however, suggests Meehl, that there is 'a society entirely oriented around the making of fine color discriminations' (Meehl, 1973, p. 139). Within the context of such a society, being born with color blindness, with a biological inability to discriminate colors, would place a person at a distinct disadvantage. Such a person may even be considered to have a 'vulnerability' to what Meehl describes as a 'color psychosis'. Such a person would have the misfortune of being born with a biologically determined inability to perform precisely those functions most required, and therefore most valued, by his or her community. He or she may in fact have considerable gifts and talents in other domains; the person may be a virtuoso violinist or sculptor, or even an exceptional visual artist of black and white photography. Still, he or she would still be at a grave disadvantage in terms of membership in this particular society, in terms of navigating and negotiating his or her ordinary life in a society in which the making of fine color discriminations is involved in the simplest of everyday tasks. The more these kinds of discriminations are required, and the more life domains in which they are required, the more likely will such a person be diagnosed with an illness and/or disability. Should the blindness be severe and the need to make color discriminations frequent, it is even conceivable that the other domains in which the person is gifted or talented would be affected and his or her functioning in these domains be compromised. In this case, it is quite possible that we would never come to learn that this person could play the violin or take black and white photographs at all. He or she may be defined entirely in terms of his or her color blindness, and his or her own sense of identity may be subsumed or engrossed by the disability. If I cannot discriminate colors, then I must be less of a person than those, who comprise the vast majority of people, who can.

For this analogy to be useful for our purposes, we would need to identify what it is precisely that our current context requires of people, and therefore values in people, for which individuals with serious mental illnesses are at a distinct disadvantage. What is the equivalent in our culture of the making of fine color discriminations in Meehl's imagined world? What core assumption of our current world, what fundamental requirement of everyday life, is challenged by the particular socio-cognitive, emotional, attitudinal and/or behavioral proclivities of people experiencing a serious mental illness? According first to Michel Foucault, and then confirmed and expanded upon by his close friend and colleague Gilles Deleuze, the assumptions and daily requirements in question appear to be those associated with – both produced by and necessary for – the emergence and maintenance of capitalism in Western industrial societies.

At the same time that Western societies were first beginning to grapple seriously with the depopulation of mental hospitals and institutions, Michel Foucault was looking instead into what had happened that so many generations of people had had to live inside of them in the first place. Much of the rhetoric of de-institutionalization, as we have seen (see Chapter 5), focused on the challenges of supporting people with serious mental illnesses outside of hospital settings. The assumption that people with serious mental illnesses required and therefore needed to be placed in such confined settings was so entrenched and unquestioned by the 1960s that the Basaglias' major challenge was to prove otherwise. As we noted in the previous chapter, the 'impossible' that Franco Basaglia had thought he had shown to be possible was precisely that people with serious mental illnesses could, in fact, live outside of the asylum. But where did people think individuals with serious mental illnesses had lived before there were asylums? If, as Basaglia was able to show, they could live outside of hospitals, why had they been sent there to begin with? Foucault's research extended further back than Dorothea Dix and her advocacy to secure treatment for all in need to the more basic question of why was *this* population determined to need *that* kind of treatment (i.e. in confined settings). What problem was 'moral treatment' a response to? What societal function did confinement serve?

The answers to these questions, Foucault (1965) suggests, are to be found in the origins and history of the Industrial Revolution and the 'imperative of labor' that it introduced. The story, however, begins in the fifteenth century, when 'madness' came to replace leprosy as a main object of societal concern and censure. With the diminution of leprosy, leper colonies began to be emptied out, leaving large institutions increasingly vacant and unused. Shortly thereafter, European societies became increasingly concerned with those of its citizens who could not, for a variety of reasons, provide for themselves. By the beginning of the seventeenth century, according to Foucault, these vacated institutions had become 'homeland to the poor, to the unemployed, to prisoners, and to the insane' (Foucault, 1965, p. 39). Viewed through the lens of the Enlightenment as a moral imperative, the state took on the responsibility of caring for those who apparently could not care for themselves. As this was determined primarily through whether the person was able to support him- or herself financially, leprosy became replaced with the lack of labor as the cause for confinement. This was what the populations listed above had in common. Writes Foucault:

> Before having the medical meaning we give to it, or that at least we like to suppose it has, confinement was required by something quite different from any concern with curing the sick. What made it necessary was an imperative of labor. Our philanthropy prefers to recognize the signs of a benevolence toward sickness where there is only a condemnation of idleness. (Foucault, 1965, p. 46)

'From the beginning, the institution set itself the task' continues Foucault, and here he quotes from a royal edict of 1656 that led to the creation of an early mental hospital: 'of preventing "mendicancy and idleness as the source of all disorders"' (Foucault, 1965, p. 47).

In this respect, people with serious mental illnesses were confined together with any other person who could not, or chose not to, work for a living, unless, of course, that person was supported by his or her family. Once inside the walls of the institution, however, those inmates with mental illnesses did not remain inconspicuously interspersed among prisoners, the poor and the unemployed. Rather, they differed from their similarly impoverished fellow inmates by virtue of their inability or refusal to work even under these supervised circumstances. Unless physically unable to do so, everyone who was confined was subjected to forced labor, both to lessen the burden they imposed on the state and as part of their own rehabilitation. Since the previous state of impoverishment that brought them to the institution was viewed as due neither to 'scarcity of commodities nor unemployment' but to 'the weakening of discipline and the relaxation of morals', all inmates were closely scrutinized and supervised in the process of being restored to a moral, productive life. In this setting of what he describes as a 'forced labor camp', people with serious mental illnesses 'distinguished themselves', writes Foucault, 'by their inability to work and to follow the rhythms of collective life' (Foucault, 1965, pp. 58–59). Even when supervised and under the pressure of coercion, people with serious mental illnesses could not be made to contribute to the community. People who were simply poor or unemployed, and those who had committed crimes, appeared to be easier to rehabilitate than those with mental illnesses were, whose conditions proved to be refractory to any attempts at change, including those attempts using physical force and violence. It was with this recognition, according to Foucault, when madness was 'perceived on the social horizon of poverty, of incapacity for work, of inability to integrate with the group', that the asylum was born as a speciality institution for the insane (Foucault, 1965, p. 64).

Returning to Meehl's analogy of color blindness, this step would be equivalent to placing everyone in a community who could not make fine-color discriminations into an institution whose main aim was to restore their color vision. Once their condition was found to be refractory to intervention, once their vision could not be restored (when, in fact, they had never had the ability to discriminate colors to begin with), then their condition would come to be recognized as an illness or disability, and then, as a result, would come 'to rank among the problems of the city' (Meehl, 1973, p. 64). This was the problem that the asylum, and eventually moral treatment, was meant to address: what to do with people who could not be made to work? But how had work come to be such an important and essential activity? What was happening that had generated this 'imperative of labor'? People had survived for millennia without 'working' in the sense that this concept took on in the seventeenth century and beyond. What had made labor such a defining trait of humanity and citizenship that its transgression was accorded the status of an illness, a disability? For answers to these questions, we turn to Deleuze.

6.6 The complete subject of Gilles Deleuze

How is labor understood within an industrial capitalist economic system, and how may it be understood differently? When we wrote above that people had survived for millennia without 'working', this provided an initial clue. Hunting and gathering were not understood to be labor or work in the sense that emerged with the Industrial Revolution, neither, for that matter, were child rearing or house keeping. These were necessary activities of daily life, but they were tied directly and immediately to both their purposes and results. One hunted or gathered so that one could eat, because one was hungry and one cared for one's environment and one's offspring so that one, and one's family, could survive. Gathering food or building one's house would in this way no more be considered work in the current sense of the term than running to escape a tiger or picking up a sword to defend oneself. All of these are tactics of survival.

If one were to attempt to make the same case for delivering mail, greeting customers at Wal-Mart or teaching neuroscience, the argument would inevitably have to pass through the mediation of money – similarly to when our children ask us why we have to go to work in the morning and we respond: 'So that we can pay our bills.' When the inmates of the poor houses and prisons who had mental illnesses were described as being unable to fend for themselves, it was because they refused to do, or were incapable of doing, tasks or to take on responsibilities for which they would have received the money needed to pay their own bills. For the most part, they ate when hungry, slept when tired and performed the other bodily functions necessary for their survival. What they did not or could not do was 'make a living'.

When did human beings start making a living instead of simply surviving? Although there certainly were precursors to the conversion of capital, the Industrial Revolution and its aftermath seem to have marked a period of dramatic transition in this regard. Currency was initially introduced as a means of barter, the way in which Native Americans used beads, for example. With the Industrial Revolution and capitalism, however, currency came to reflect, represent and require a very different relationship between human activity and its purposes. As Marx was to demonstrate, at the very heart of capitalism is the transformation of capital from being that which is produced by labor to that which comes to be viewed as its source. It is the process of human engagement and activity in the world which produces goods which then have a value. Activity is originally and primarily a productive function: it creates goods and services; it makes things happen. With the disconnection of activity from its survival function, and the disconnection of capital from that activity which produced it, it became possible for products to be elevated above process and for currency or capital to be elevated above labor. Labor, or so it seems, can be purchased with capital. And activity, or so it seems, can be re-oriented to become a form of labor that is used to acquire further capital. Rather than desiring their own survival, including their engagement in life-affirming activities, human beings can come to desire capital as that which appears to give life in the first place. Even though, in reality, capital is always produced by and dependent upon human activity.

Deleuze and Guattari consider this classically Marxist position to have implications not only for the political economic system in which we work and live but also for our sense of identity as well (Deleuze and Guattari, 1982). If human activity is transformed from being productive in nature (from doing) to being acquisitive in nature (to wanting), what does this do to our sense of ourselves as active agents? For Deleuze and Guattari, this tension between production and acquisition goes back much further than the Industrial Revolution to antiquity, but its fundamental repercussions for understanding human activity and identity could not be more current. They write:

> The traditional logic of desire is all wrong from the very outset: from the very first step that the Platonic logic of desire forces us to take, making us choose between *production* and *acquisition*. From the moment that we place desire on the side of acquisition, we make desire an idealistic (dialectical, nihilistic) conception, which causes us to look upon it as primarily a lack. (Deleuze and Guattari, 1982, p. 25; italics in the original)

Does desire arouse out of a perceived lack of something? Or is desire experienced rather as an abundance, an overflowing, of something? Is human activity necessarily oriented to filling the coffers, whether for oneself or for one's company and share holders? Or is human activity what Deleuze and Guattari (1982) propose to describe as 'desiring-production'? Given that it is human activity which produces capital, what sense does it make to view human activity as lacking or needing to acquire capital? It is only through the conversion of capital that human beings come to view themselves as being fundamentally deficient, as fated forever to be in search of a part of themselves that is missing. Only in this way do they become like the protagonist in a Shel Silverstein children's book, who cannot rest until he or she finds his or her 'missing piece' (Silverstein, 1976).

As a result of this conversion, Deleuze (1983) suggests, there arises an image of humanity that is fundamentally fictional and illusory. People are no longer complete in and of themselves, they no longer understand themselves to be 'desiring machines' who create a world in their own image, but rather they consider themselves lacks, deficits or gaps to be filled in by others and by any number of diverse things (e.g. food, money, status, prestige, etc.). Subsuming all of these various attempts at gap-filling as ways of paying homage to Freud's icon of Oedipus, Deleuze and Guattari's enigmatic title for the first volume of their series on capitalism and schizophrenia, *Anti-Oedipus* (Deleuze and Guattari, 1982), is meant to call into question, and eventually raze, the foundations of this approach. Rather than being an ideal to which humans should aspire, Oedipus – which they take to represent Freud's notion of a 'mature ego' – is an illusion which seduces human beings away from an appreciation and, even more importantly, an affirmation of their own nature as desiring machines. Oedipus embodies the culmination of the contemporary search for the Holy Grail that will make one whole, a transformation of the activity of desire into an immovable object. In Oedipus, we seek the complete satiety of our needs that results in our coming to, and remaining, at rest in an undisturbed state of quiescence. Drawing from Nietzsche, Deleuze suggests that this version of maturity or 'normality' 'appears essentially as a narcotic drug, rest, peace, "sabbath", slackening of tension and relaxing of limbs, in short passively'. This version of Oedipus 'does not know how to and does not want to love, but wants to be loved. He wants to be loved, fed, watered, caressed, and put to sleep' (Deleuze, 1983, pp. 117–118). But we are not, and cannot become, sated in this way. As Freud had himself recognized, the only time human beings ever reach such an undisturbed state of quiescence is in their eventual death (i.e. his thanatos or 'death instinct').

While with Martin Luther King, Jnr, we learned that the world is, and remains, basically incomplete (as a function of human understanding), with Deleuze we learn that the self, on the contrary, is always and already complete. The subject, as a desiring machine, does not lack anything. It is always already in motion, creating a world that it will never completely know or understand. In this case, Deleuze and Guattari (1982) ask, why bother trying to become Oedipus when all of us are always and already Laius? Why bother plotting to overthrow the father when we are all already the kings or queens of our respective domains? Presumably because the father has something we want which, if we succeed in obtaining it, will somehow make our lives better. It never does, of course, but not because it is the wrong thing or because there isn't yet quite enough of it (assumptions which form the basis for marketing in a capitalist and consumerist world), but because human nature is fundamentally other. No matter how many things we acquire, no matter how full we become, we will never be turned to stone. Not until we die will we reach such a permanent state of quiescence. Desire, for Deleuze and Guattari, is not the wish to return to the womb, but rather refers to the fundamentally active nature of the subject. Rather than being the search for our missing piece, desire creates hunger in the same way that it creates other human functions and passions. We are our desires, not their objects. In this sense, the father does not possess anything that we do not also already have ourselves.

For our present purposes, it is important to recall that Oedipus, as a symbol of insatiable acquisitiveness, is the product of a socio-political process. Specifically, as the title of their series suggests, the ascendancy of Oedipus is associated with the rise of industrial capitalism. From what other source would acquisitiveness per se take on such prominence and be accorded such a foundational role in the constitution of human agency? The argument of *Anti-Oedipus* identifies the same transformation that Marx identified as having taken place between labor and capital as also having taken place with respect to the relation of desire to the self. Oedipus, or the ego, which is originally produced by desire, comes to be seen as its source. Desire becomes a function of the ego, an acquisitive pursuit of those objects and entities that the ego needs in order to be whole. The ego, in turn, comes to be seen as that which makes desire possible, as that which creates desire as a means to achieving wholeness. But what if the person, as a so-called desiring machine, is always already whole?

6.7 Oedipus and anti-Oedipus

In more prosaic terms, this is the fundamental philosophical presumption of the positive alternative to Oedipus proposed by Deleuze and Guattari (1982). Human agency, like human labor, is an active and creative process of desire *as production* (thus 'desiring-production'). Among the many objects created by human agency is the edifice of Oedipus. When mistaken as the source, rather than as an object, of human agency, Oedipus, like capital, becomes a problematic, yet seductive, illusion (reminiscent of Sartre's 1956 notion of the seduction of 'being-in-itself' for consciousness). Like capital (of which there can never be quite enough), Oedipus can never be quite big or strong or full enough (of whatever) to be complete; it is, by definition, forever in a state of deficit. But human agency, desire and subjectivity are neither gaps to be filled in by commodities nor commodities themselves. The act of production is just that: an act.

What does this have to do with mental health and recovery? Why did Deleuze and Guattari (1982) tie their critique of industrial capitalism to schizophrenia? Because for them the very possibility of schizophrenia as a human condition calls into question the necessity of Oedipus. By being unwilling or unable to work for a living, people with serious mental illnesses – by default as much as by design – fail to subordinate their labor to the acquisition, control and never-ending growth of capital. By being unwilling or unable to inhabit the valued social role of worker – again by default as much as by design – people with serious mental illnesses fail to subordinate their desire, agency or activity to the creation, preservation and polishing of their own personal replica of Oedipus. They stubbornly resist becoming a cog in the industrial capitalist economic machine. And yet they remain human beings, they continue to desire, to act and to produce, even if what they produce is not considered of much value. But here, for Deleuze, lies the rub. What determines value? How are the various products of human labor to be valued? Who makes those determinations and on what basis?

Within the context of a capitalist economic system, value is primarily determined in relation to capital. What has the most value is capital (i.e. money) because it truly 'makes the world go "round"', it is required at every turn for anyone to be enabled to do just about anything. Other products are valued in terms of how much they contribute to capital and its growth. In some circles, and for some individuals, the same is true of people as well. A person may be valued in terms of his or her material wealth and how much he or she controls capital. This is, of course, not true for everyone, nor is it true of everything. It is not true, for example, in the arts, where it would be hard to justify paying tens, if not hundreds, of millions of dollars for a painting by Van Gogh when there is no conceivable relationship between owning such a painting and being materially productive. But, again, that is consistent with Deleuze's (1983) point. Capitalism is neither necessary nor all-encompassing. No one is, or can ever be, solely Oedipus. There is much more to life, and to human nature, than there is to capitalism, and the possibility of having a serious mental illness proves this point.

It is important at this point not to mistake Deleuze's (1983) perspective on schizophrenia for a romantic idealization of mental illness. The provocative title of *Anti-Oedipus* should not be taken to suggest that Deleuze and Guattari (1982) encourage people to become or remain psychotic as a way of rebelling against the capitalist monolith at the centre of contemporary Western culture. They do not valorize individuals with schizophrenia for having the condition as if that alone were a heroic act, nor do they minimize the suffering and impoverishment that currently is associated with having a serious mental illness for many people unfortunate enough to be afflicted with one. They suggest, though, that some of the suffering and impoverishment associated with mental illness is due to the nature of the society in which people live rather than to the illness itself.

We remember Meehl's analogy of color blindness. For Deleuze (1983), people with serious mental illnesses unfortunately may lack some of those very capacities that are most required, and therefore most valued, by the particular society in which they happen to live. As with color blindness, however, we can imagine societies in which this were not true. More importantly, we understand that this does not make a person with a serious mental illness any less of a person than anyone else. Those particular capacities are no more central or essential to human nature than the ability to make fine-color discrimination or any of the other various capacities human beings have. And it is possible that outside of the context of a capitalist economic system those particular capacities also would not be viewed as having any more value than any others have as well.

In this way, Deleuze does not romanticize schizophrenia as much as insist that it involves a process to which all of us are vulnerable and which makes none of us any less human. He can only be described as romanticizing psychosis if by this we understand him to be insisting that people with psychosis remain just as human as everyone else, a position that we may recall is at the heart of the recovery movement. As we noted in our first chapter, for example, Pat Deegan suggests that: 'The concept of recovery is rooted in the simple yet profound realization that people who have been diagnosed with a mental illness are human beings' (Deegan, 1993). Although he never addressed the issue of recovery per se, this statement can be taken to be consistent with Deleuze's (1983) position as well. One of the central things that are required of people living within a capitalist economic system is that they subordinate their own processes, their desire and activity, to the creation, preservation and growth of capital. To the degree that one does not do this, for whatever reason, one may be considered a bad capitalist, an under-performing employee or even a dissident citizen, but one is no less of a human being.

We dwell on this point at length for two reasons. One, as Deegan (1993) suggests, it is perhaps the most core belief and principle of the recovery movement, from which most other beliefs and principles follow. Two, the implications of this point for mental health are challenging yet crucial. If the capacities required by capitalism were also required by human nature, then people with serious mental illnesses would have to develop these capacities in order to be considered fully human. More practically speaking, they would have to develop these capacities – that is be cured of their illnesses and have no remaining disability – before rejoining community life, before reclaiming their citizenship. Prior to that, or in the case that skill acquisition and cure are delayed indefinitely, they will remain marginal to society at best, if not enslaved, oppressed or otherwise destroyed. It is for this reason that we spent the first half of this chapter on Martin Luther King, Jnr. It is from just such a position of marginalization, enslavement and oppression that people with serious mental illnesses are struggling to reclaim their rights to full citizenship.

What difference does it make to suggest that the capacities required by capitalism are no more essential to human nature than those required by 'a society entirely oriented around the making of fine color discriminations'? A first implication is that these capacities are developed in part as a response to the socio-political environment. There are other processes underlying these capacities that are necessary to their development but which may be channelled differently under different circumstances. Deleuze (1983) uses the example of speech. All speech involves certain underlying processes, both physical and mental in nature. All speech is itself a process, but one that can be put to different uses. Some speech, for example, is particularly useful in enabling business to be carried out, in greasing the wheels of the capitalist machine, while other speech does not serve this particular purpose. Speech can serve other purposes, such as those involved in poetry, song or humor, or those involved in expressing love and affection. Those uses of speech which may be most prominent or valued in a capitalist system are no more intrinsically valuable than the others; their value is determined instead by their context. Thus, Deleuze and Guattari write that:

> The language of a banker, a general, an industrialist, a middle or high-level manager, or a government minister is a perfectly schizophrenic language, but that functions only statistically within the flattening axiomatic of connections that puts it in the service of the capitalist order. (Deleuze and Guattari, 1982, p. 246)

6.8 Schizophrenic speech and Watergate

But why do Deleuze and Guattari describe this language as 'schizophrenic'? Guattari, at least, was a psychiatrist. Didn't he know that people with schizophrenia use language differently from others? Aren't there typical ways in which speech is disorganized, derailed, disordered or otherwise deficient in people with this condition? Doesn't the *DSM-IV-TR*, the current diagnostic manual of the American Psychiatric Association (2000), for example, suggest that impairment of speech is a core characteristic, and therefore a core diagnostic indicator, of schizophrenia?

In answering these questions we run up against a fundamental problem with both psychiatry broadly and psychopathology more specifically. The problem is that neither of these sciences has given much consideration to what constitutes 'normal' or 'healthy' functioning as the foil against which they define 'psychopathology'. It is easier to describe the purported speech patterns of individuals diagnosed with schizophrenia as being disorganized, derailed, disordered or otherwise deficient than it is to characterize normal speech. But as Claude Bernard, the noted father of physiology and experimental medicine, pointed out: in order to understand pathology one must first understand normality. What constitutes 'normal' or 'healthy' speech? If one takes the rules of grammar and syntax to represent normal or healthy speech in a formalistic way, then most people do not use normal or healthy speech. Most people's speech would be considered deficient in some ways. What does this suggest about the speech of people with schizophrenia?

A cursory glance at the empirical evidence for speech pathology in schizophrenia is revealing and suggestive. Very few studies compare the speech of people diagnosed with schizophrenia with the speech of people who have not been diagnosed with a mental illness. One line of investigation has done so, however, and it confirms Deleuze's position, which we will describe below. First, however, let us consider these elegant, if overlooked, studies which were conducted in the 1970s by Tucker, Rosenberg and Harrow.

Struck by just how little empirical verification could be found for 'even the most generally accepted truisms about the structural properties of the speech' of people diagnosed with schizophrenia, Rosenberg and Tucker (1979) explored the formal and semantic characteristics of the speech of both people who had been diagnosed with and those who had not been diagnosed with schizophrenia. Through their review of the existing empirical studies on 'thought disorder' (the technical psychiatric term for disordered speech), it became 'increasingly clear' to them that the speech of individuals diagnosed with schizophrenia did not 'represent a characterizable linguistic entity in terms of shared formal properties' (Rosenberg and Tucker, 1979, p. 1331). Rather, they found that the degree of disorganization supposedly found in the speech of individuals diagnosed with schizophrenia could be equally well found in the free speech of presumably 'normal' people, especially when such people were in a 'highly anxious or agitated state' (such as the state in which many individuals diagnosed with schizophrenia had been studied, i.e. in the hospital). They drew this conclusion from their review of the Watergate hearing transcripts, in which we find the free speech of presumably competent and 'normal' people, but in which they also found marked levels of disorganization, levels high enough to be considered evidence of a 'thought disorder' if discovered in the speech of people diagnosed with schizophrenia.

In an earlier analysis of these transcripts, Tucker and his colleagues (Reilly, Harrow and Tucker, 1975) had found only a slightly more frequent occurrence of specific formal defects in the speech of individuals diagnosed with schizophrenia than in the speech of these 'government ministers' (to borrow Deleuze and Guattari's (1982) term). The formal disorders of speech thought to be signs of schizophrenia could be found in all spontaneous speech; it is only that they may be a bit more frequent or more severe in the speech of people diagnosed with having schizophrenia, especially when they are in an acute, anxious or agitated state (Harrow and Quinlan, 1977). We apparently are all disorganized in our speech; it is just that some of us have managed to become less disorganized than others. As Deleuze (1983) suggested above, we all use 'schizophrenic' language, it is just that sometimes we learn how to place this language in the service of other aims.

Why, then, do the fields of psychiatry and psychopathology continue to think that people with schizophrenia have disordered speech? Why do we notice the presence of these formal defects in the speech of individuals diagnosed with schizophrenia but appear not to be aware of them in our own speech? What draws our clinical/scientific attention to them as evidence of an underlying illness? Rosenberg and Tucker (1979) found that while the speech of individuals diagnosed with schizophrenia did not differ markedly from the speech of presumably 'normal' people on the formal, structural level it did differ on the semantic level. The speech of (some) individuals diagnosed with schizophrenia differed in terms of its content, in terms of the 'thematic concerns' that were being addressed. And it is this 'deviation from expected thematic concerns, which are linked both to general and sex-specific social role expectations', suggest Rosenberg and Tucker, 'that is associated with the diagnosis of schizophrenia' (Rosenberg and Tucker, 1979, p. 1334).

The speech of (some) individuals diagnosed with schizophrenia draws attention to itself by deviating from the socially determined expectations of what it should be about. Once such a transgression is noticed, formal elements of speech which might otherwise have remained unremarkable become a focus of clinical and scientific scrutiny. 'Linguists and anthropologists', point out Rosenberg and Tucker, 'observe that there are implicit semantic baselines in each culture that create norms for speakers of each sex, age, social class and so on' (Rosenberg and Tucker, 1979, p. 1336). A person demonstrating what comes to be considered a sign of schizophrenia, they suggest, 'creates a sense of disorder in the listener by subtly deviating from these expectations. The listener may then perceive the deviation as being on a structural or syntactic' – as opposed to semantic – level (p. 1336). In their own research, they found the majority of the semantic content of their conversations with people diagnosed with schizophrenia to revolve around two major themes: being unable to work and having difficulty following 'the rhythms of collective life'. We recognize these two themes from our discussion of Foucault's work at the beginning of this chapter, of course. Rosenberg and Tucker observed the same difficulties being described by their participants in the 1970s that Foucault had suggested characterized this particular subgroup of inmates of the poorhouses, almshouses and jails of the 1790s.

So doesn't this suggest that people with schizophrenia *are* disordered and deficient? No, it suggests that many people with serious mental illnesses have difficulties working and relating to others, they do not readily 'fit in' at the work site or among groups of their peers. We have already established that this makes them no less human, even if it leaves them impoverished and isolated within the context of a capitalist system. But how are we to understand their difficulties? Just as they did in the case of speech, Deleuze and Guattari (1982) suggest that all of us are vulnerable to and can identify with these kinds of experiences. Who of us, they might ask, has not fantasized at times about not having to work for a living? Who of us has not shut off the alarm clock and wished to remain in bed? Who of us has not decided at times not to cooperate with the expectations or requirements of others – or at least wished that we could do so? What person, Deleuze and Guattari ask, 'is not leaning against the rock of schizophrenia, a rock in this case mobile, aerolitic' (Deleuze and Guattari, 1982, p. 67)? From such a position, the question is not so much one of 'How does one develop schizophrenia?' but rather 'How do so many people avoid schizophrenia?' Or, in the terms we used above, 'How and why do most people in this culture agree to place their desire, their lives, in the service of capital?' A similar point was made by Gregory Bateson, a leading social scientist and central figure in schizophrenia research between the 1950s and 1970s, when he argued that it was not so surprising that some people developed schizophrenia. Rather, he quipped: 'The surprising thing is that some of us are less schizophrenic than others – but we have trouble deciding how that came about' (cited in Berger, 1978, p. 82).

Does this kind of turning on its head of our conventional view actually make a difference in how we understand and respond to individuals with serious mental illnesses, or have we taken instead a temporary excursion through Alice's Wonderland and merely play with words? To us, and we suggest to Deleuze, it is a difference that can make all the difference in the world.

6.9 Community inclusion vs community integration

In the first place, if all of us are vulnerable to serious mental illnesses, and if all of us can identify with the core experiences associated with serious mental illnesses, then that makes them less foreign or alien to us and more likely that serious mental illnesses are conditions from which people can also return. Given what we have most recently said about schizophrenia in particular representing a failure to subordinate our lives and desire to capital, we will need to return eventually to the question of whether these are conditions from which people will or should want to return. But for the moment, let us assume that having a serious mental illness is worse than being a functioning part of the capitalist machine and that these are conditions from which people desire to return. In that case, the boundaries between a universal vulnerability to psychosis, an active state of psychosis and a return to a state of 'normal' vulnerability should be more permeable in non-capitalist societies. People whose capacities for gainful employment and following 'the rhythms of collective life' are not as well developed would be less conspicuous and less disabled in a non-capitalist system than they currently are in the industrial West. If the incapacity were considered permanent but not terribly relevant to cultural values (as with color blindness), then perhaps people with such incapacities would not be identified as such at all. If, on the other hand, the incapacity were a state into which people fell and from which they could return, then these processes would appear more fluid when divorced from the 'imperative of labor' essential to industrial capitalism (newer forms of capitalism may not pose the same challenges).

What empirical evidence exists to date suggests that the latter situation is more common. These data can be found in a number of cross-cultural studies of the course and outcome of schizophrenia, including and beginning with the International Pilot Study of Schizophrenia launched by the World Health Organization (WHO) in the late 1960s. Owing to their unexpected and even provocative findings, these data have been examined, re-examined and reviewed by numerous investigators since then, but almost unanimously drawing the same conclusions. Although the incidence and prevalence of acute schizophrenic-like episodes appear to be the same across cultures, there has been a consistent disparity in the course and outcomes of these episodes. According to one of the leading authorities on this issue, cross-cultural anthropologist and psychiatrist Richard Warner: 'Patients in the developing world showed outstandingly better results' (Warner, 1983, p. 201). Explains Warner:

> The general conclusion is unavoidable. Schizophrenia in the Third World has a course and prognosis quite unlike the condition as we recognize it in the West. The progressive deterioration which Kraepelin considered central to his definition of the disease is rare in non-industrial societies, except perhaps under the dehumanizing restrictions of a traditional asylum. The majority of the Third World schizophrenics achieve a favorable outcome. The more urbanized and industrialized the setting, the more malignant becomes the illness. (Warner, 1983, p. 203)

While much has changed since the early 1980s – we no longer refer to the developing world as 'the Third World', we no longer refer to people with serious mental illnesses as 'schizophrenics' and we no longer believe in the necessity of the Kraepelinian prognosis of progressive deterioration in schizophrenia, even in the industrial capitalist West – these findings, however, have not. Despite the fact that we now know that outcomes for psychotic disorders in the West are much better than we had expected before we undertook these long-term longitudinal studies (cf. Davidson, Harding and Spaniol, 2005), outcomes in the developing world remain superior to those in industrialized, capitalist countries. As summarized by another leading authority on the cross-cultural studies:

> All findings point to the conclusion that persons suffering from schizophrenia in non-industrial societies have a greater chance for complete remission of symptoms and normal social adjustment than do similar persons living in modern industrial societies. (Waxler, 1979, p. 156)

Such a finding is surprising not only due to what may be described as an unfortunate, if persistent, arrogance of the West towards the rest of the world but also because schizophrenia and other serious mental illnesses have been declared for the last 30 or so years to be 'brain diseases' (Andreasen, 1982; Torrey, 1983). Given the exponentially higher amount of funding devoted to medical care and research, and the significantly more developed systems of health care delivery, in the West, how could people with brain diseases fare better in countries where health care is less accessible and presumably of a lower quality? The only credible answer to this question that has been suggested thus far was stated succinctly by Harding, Zubin and Strauss – three of the world's leading investigators into the course and outcome of schizophrenia from the 1970s to the present – as follows:

> The possible causes of chronicity may be viewed as having less to do with any inherent natural outcome of the disorder and more to do with a myriad of environmental and other psychosocial factors interacting with the person and the illness. (Harding, Zubin and Strauss, 1987, p. 483)

As we now know, Foucault, Deleuze and cross-cultural studies suggest that these factors are somehow related to the introduction, growth and requirements of industrial capitalism. Cooper and Sartorius, two of the original investigators in the WHO-initiated study that involved visiting and collecting data from 11 countries across the globe, agreed, concluding that: 'Industrialization introduces new social effects which increase the likelihood of a poor outcome in patients with schizophrenia' (Cooper and Sartorius, 1977, p. 50). Perhaps the most important of these effects is the 'specialization of work roles and social functions'. They explain:

> In modern industrial cultures there is usually an overt pressure or expectation for individual education and specialization aimed directly at a rise in highly correlated financial and social status. The more tightly the social and work roles are defined, the more likely and more severe will be the punishments and stigmata resulting from deviations from these roles, and the more difficult will be the re-integration of the individual recovering from the illness. (Cooper and Sartorius, 1977, p. 52)

Warner makes this same point in more concrete and practical terms. He writes:

> The return of a psychotic to a productive role in a non-industrial setting is not contingent upon his actively seeking a job, impressing an employer with his worth, or functioning at a consistently adequate level. In a non-wage, subsistence economy, psychotics may perform any of those available tasks which match their level of functioning at a given time. Whatever constructive contributions they can make are likely to be valued by their community, and their level of disability will not be considered absolute . . . The more flexible use of labor in pre-industrial societies may encourage high rates of recovery from psychosis . . . High productivity requirements and competitive performance ratings may be particularly unsuitable for a rehabilitating schizophrenic. (Warner, 1983, p. 203)

Re-integration into the community is thus more difficult for people with schizophrenia when they happen to live in the industrial West. Re-integration involves taking on the roles and responsibilities of an aspiring capitalist. Re-integration may nonetheless be desired by people with serious mental illnesses who wish to 'fit in' to the community into which they were born, and who for the most part are unaware of the social and economic forces which determine or shape what it means for them to 'fit in'. As long as these individuals do not believe that they *have* to 'fit in' to this particular social, political and economic order in order to feel and be considered worthwhile human beings, then we accept this as a personal choice and do our best to support them in their efforts to do so. The psychiatric rehabilitation strategies of supported housing, supported employment, supported education and supported socialization are perhaps the best interventions we have to offer them at this time, and we can hope along with them that they can regain, or perhaps learn for the first time, the skills they need to be successful in the world in which they currently live. We do not think it reasonable to expect or demand of people with serious mental illnesses more than we expect or demand from anyone else, and we accept that it is perfectly reasonable for people with serious mental illnesses to want to be just like everyone else. While a line of anthropological research by Corin and Lauzon suggests that those who do try to 'fit in' to contemporary Western culture have a harder time than those who assume a stance of what they call 'positive withdrawal' (Corin and Lauzon, 1992), we do not begrudge the desires of those who wish to 'fit in' more comfortably and effectively into the world as it is. We do not accept, however, that the world as it currently is represents the only way that the world can be.

If we return to our discussion of the civil rights movement, we readily acknowledge that in the 1950s many people of color, perhaps the majority, did their best to 'fit in' to the roles offered to them by the segregated American society of the day. They did their best to survive, and in some ways even thrive, within the limitations imposed by the continued oppression and discrimination enforced by the white majority. It took people of uncommon vision, courage and uncountable other skills to question this world and then to take up the fight for a better one. We return to where this chapter began, with what it took for Martin Luther King, Jnr to envision a world different from the one he inherited. We suggest here that restoring civil and human rights to individuals with serious mental illnesses requires a similar questioning of the necessity of the world we have inherited and an envisioning of one in which these people will not be limited to such a marginalized status or required to shed the vestiges of their illness in order to return to the mainstream. We suggest, in other words, that there should be an alternative for people with serious mental illnesses to having to 'fit in' in order to have a safe, dignified and meaningful life. Without having to relocate individuals with serious mental illnesses to developing countries where their 'constructive contributions . . . are [more] likely to be valued by their community', there should be a way to change the community itself.

As we recall, this was precisely the task that Franco Basaglia saw as the next step in helping people with serious mental illnesses to establish and lead gratifying lives outside of the asylum. He unfortunately died a premature death before he could take any more significant steps in this direction. At the same time, the linguistic and cross-cultural studies we have been citing in this chapter have received little attention in the 35 or so years since they first appeared. The work of changing the community to offer alternatives to 'fitting in' to the mould created and required by industrial capitalism thus remains, for the most part, still to be achieved. There have been steps taken, certainly, such as the passage of the Americans with Disabilities Act in 1990 and the Supreme Court's *Olmstead* decision of 1999 which reaffirmed that a life in the community is a fundamental right of American citizens regardless of their disability status. These were steps taken in response to assertive, persistent advocacy on the part of people with serious mental illnesses and other disabilities, and with the support of those who care about them. But there remains much work to be done.

The following chapter will begin to lay out some of the elements of what can be accomplished in a more accepting and accommodating world. In closing this chapter, though, we wish to reassure our sceptics (and we are sure that we have some) that this challenge is not as daunting or even impossible as it may seem. What we are referring to here can be reframed as the tension between what social scientists have referred to, and we named this section, as 'community inclusion vs community integration'. In simple terms, 'community integration' refers to ways to assist people on the margins of a community to assume the normative roles that they wish to occupy, such as student, worker, car-owner, parishioner and so on. For the most part, community integration requires the person to change, or be changed, in order to fit into these roles as they currently exist. For a person with a serious mental illness, this would mean overcoming or recovering from the illness first, or at least learning how to manage and hide the illness well enough to 'pass for normal' (Flanagan, Miller and Davidson, 2009), before rejoining community life. In racial terms, this would mean that people of color would need to pass for white in order to enjoy fully the opportunities and resources of community membership.

While perhaps it is easier for some people with serious mental illnesses to 'pass for normal' than it was for Americans of African origin to pass for white, we argue that this remains nonetheless an unreasonable requirement. Unfortunately, the majority of the mental health system continues to insist precisely on this vision of integration, requiring people to have fewer symptoms, to acquire more skills, to have better insight into their condition, to adhere more strictly to their medication regimen, to be compliant and cooperative patients, before they can get their lives back. As we suggested above, this misses the basic point of the civil rights argument. King established in principle that people of color did not need to become or pass for white in order to reclaim their full citizenship in American society. Deleuze can be taken to be arguing similarly that people with serious mental illnesses do not need to become or pass for replicas of Oedipus in order to reclaim their full citizenship in society. The Americans with Disabilities Act insists that people with disabilities have the right to community access and social inclusion *while* they are disabled, not once they overcome their disability. Otherwise, no law would be required. The same is true for application of the Americans with Disabilities Act to people with serious mental illnesses. They have the right to community access and social inclusion, to 'a life in the community' in the words of the New Freedom Commission, while they continue to suffer from the effects of a mental illness.

Such a vision of a fundamental right to community access and social inclusion is a more recent development in social policy than community integration, and we refer to it under the rubric of 'community inclusion'. Although the difference between integration and inclusion might strike some readers as picky or merely semantic, we have tried to show in this chapter how it is a difference that truly makes a difference for a person with an enduring mental illness. For this person it can mean the difference between his or her recovery being indefinitely delayed (and therefore, we recall, being ultimately denied) and his or her recovery occurring today and every day on an ongoing basis.

In contrast to community integration, community inclusion requires change on the part of the community as well as, and at times even more than, the person him- or herself. Strategies for the community inclusion of people with physical disabilities include such things as wheelchair ramps, the posting of signs in Braille, the use of perceptual alarms or notifications for people with auditory impairments, and the use of assistive technology (e.g. touch tone dialling devices) and animal companions. Some similar accommodations have been identified and developed for people with serious mental illnesses, such as flex time, ready access to support on-site and various cognitive adaptations. In addition to these strategies, though, we suggest that accommodations may need to be made in affording people opportunities to lead meaningful and gratifying lives that do not conform to the moulds of acquisition and material production inherent to industrial capitalism. Many people would benefit from the opportunity to make meaningful and valued contributions to their communities that do not necessarily promote the further acquisition and production of capital or material wealth. Many people would benefit from exploring and occupying alternatives to becoming a cog in the capitalist machine, from finding other ways to be a respected and valued member of society without necessarily being gainfully employed or fitting in to existing social spheres or structures. What appears at the beginning of 2009 to be the beginning of the end of American capitalism and the exploration of alternative economic theories suggests that the community inclusion of people with enduring mental illnesses may not be as far off as some imagine. The following chapter begins to explore some of the ways this may be pursued.

6.10 Summary of lessons learned

From this review of the work of King and Deleuze, we suggest the following lessons:

- We do not have to accept the world as it currently is, as this is not the only way it can be.

- It is within our power to make changes in the way the world works, especially as they relate to how people who are marked as different are viewed and treated by society.

- The world as it currently is, especially in Western industrial capitalist economic systems, is not particularly conducive to recovery and is not very accommodating of people with enduring mental illnesses. People appear to have better outcomes when there are more alternative ways for them to make valued contributions to the life of the community.

- We should not equate recovery from a mental illness with fitting in to the mould of what has been created by, and is required by, our current preoccupation with the production and acquisition of material wealth.

- People are no less people just because they happen to have a mental illness. Having a mental illness does not rob a person of his or her humanity and worth as a human being.

- People have the right to be included fully in the life of the community despite being disabled by a mental illness, but enforcing this right may require changes on the part of the community as well as the person.

- People can be valued for many things and in many ways. We can do better in creating and expanding ways of contributing that are not tied to gainful employment and/or fitting in with existing social spheres or structures. The downfall of American capitalism (and the continued growth of the Internet), among other things, may make this much more possible.

Lessons to avoid repeating:

- Do not make assumptions about psychopathology in the absence of a clear, consensual and empirically grounded view of what is 'normal' or 'healthy' functioning.

- Do not make fundamental human and civil rights contingent upon a person's willingness to promote certain social norms or values (especially when they do not endanger others).

- Do not insist that people recover from a mental illness first before rejoining community life, as community life provides a foundation for recovery.

- Do not confuse leading a meaningful and gratifying life with capitulating to someone else's ideals of how life should be. Mental health practitioners need to adopt much more humility about how little they know before presuming to define the 'good life' for another person.

7
Agency as the Basis for Transformation

7.1 The need for a new conceptual framework

> Mere reforms to the existing mental health system are insufficient ...
> Applied to the task at hand, transformation represents a bold vision
> to change the very form and function of the mental health service
> delivery system ... It implies profound change – not at the margins of
> a system, but at its very core. (*Federal Action Agenda*, US Department
> of Health and Human Services, 2005, pp. 5, 18)
>
> The Commission should be ready to recommend radical recon-
> struction of the present system. (*Action for Mental Health*, Joint
> Commission on Mental Illness and Health, 1961, pp. xxx–xxxi)

The first passage above was taken from the *Federal Action Agenda* released in 2005, which we discussed in the Introduction to this book. As we noted earlier, the reform that mental health services are to undergo in order to become recovery-oriented will be profound, substantive and long term, characteristics captured by the federal government in describing the magnitude of this reform as 'a transformation' of the nature of care 'at its very core'. The second passage harks back to the last time such a radical reform of mental health care was attempted in the United States, quoting from the *Action for Mental Health* report issued by the Joint Commission on Mental Illness and Health convened by the Eisenhower administration that provided an initial blueprint for the de-institutionalization efforts which had begun in 1954. One of the questions with which this chapter will be concerned is how current and future efforts need to differ from these previous efforts in order to be more successful.

According to the Eisenhower commission, it was already 'the objective of modern treatment of persons with major mental illness [in the early 1960s] to enable the patient to maintain himself in the community in a normal manner' (Joint Commission on Mental Illness and Health, 1961, p. xvii). This objective of a normal

The Roots of the Recovery Movement in Psychiatry   Larry Davidson, Jaak Rakfeldt, John Strauss
© 2010 John Wiley & Sons, Ltd

life in the community is the same 'promise' to which the title of the 2003 New Freedom Commission on Mental Health Report refers (i.e. *Achieving the Promise: Transforming Mental Health Care in America*). As this recent report makes clear, it is widely accepted that the promise made to people with mental illnesses, their families and society at large in passing the de-institutionalization legislation has not been kept (Department of Health and Human Services, 2003). A similar sentiment is now becoming apparent in Canada, where the Senate issued its own commission report entitled: *Out of the Shadows at Last: Transforming Mental Health, Mental Illness, and Addiction Services in Canada* (Standing Senate Committee on Social Affairs, Science, and Technology, 2006). As their titles imply, both reports emphasize that it is now time, finally ('at last'), to make good on ('achieve') these promises. But how? How can we ensure that we get it right this time round, rather than merely repeat the mistakes of the past?

In prior publications, including the previous chapter, we have argued that one dimension that was missing from previous efforts to transform mental health care, and to which we must give priority in current efforts if we are not simply to repeat past mistakes, is that of restoring the civil rights of people with serious mental illnesses (Davidson, 2006; Davidson *et al.*, 2006). This position is affirmed in the *Federal Action Agenda*, where we read that: 'A keystone of the transformation process will be the protection and respect of the rights of adults with serious mental illnesses' (Department of Health and Human Services, 2005, p. 3). While certainly not sufficient to overcome the range of formidable political and economic barriers that undermined previous efforts, we believe that it is nonetheless crucial to offer a new conceptual framework to inform and guide the work of transformation, a framework that, following Addams, Meyer and Basaglia, is based on the fundamental role of freedom and agency in enabling individuals with serious mental illnesses to exercise their rights of citizenship and to live fully human lives.

Previous reform efforts focused almost exclusively on what mental health practitioners needed to do to treat and ameliorate illness and dysfunction, and where people needed to be in order to receive such treatment (e.g. community vs hospital). We suggest that for our current transformation efforts to be successful, equal, if not more attention, needs to be paid to what people with mental illnesses need to do for themselves. In this chapter, we develop this line of argument further to propose the adoption of a 'capabilities approach', grounded in the political and economic theory of Amartya Sen, and an action theory perspective, as envisioned by the Russian psychologist Lev Vygotsky, as offering a new conceptual framework for incorporating a rights perspective into the work of transformation. Our proposal is based on our assessment that the conceptual framework offered a half-century ago by the leaders of de-institutionalization is no longer adequate to the task in hand, and that a new conceptual framework is needed for the 'post-institutional' era (Minkoff, 1987), an era which we view as being guided by the emerging recovery vision. We begin by highlighting some of the limitations of the current approach, and then move on to describe and begin to apply the capabilities approach and action theory as offering promising foundations for the current 'revolution' in mental health care.

7.2 Beyond de-institutionalization and community tenure

Veterans of mental health policy reform will undoubtedly and legitimately point out that many of the seeds for the current revolution were present in the thinking of the early 1960s. As we suggested above, the objective described in 1961 of enabling people to 'maintain' themselves in the community in a 'normal manner' is not that different from the vision of the 2003 New Freedom Commission on Mental Health of 'a life in the community for everyone' (Department of Health and Human Services, 2003, p. 1). What may be different, however, is how that life, and what is entailed in affording people with mental illnesses such a life, is conceptualized, and the implications this conceptual framework has for the provision of services and supports.

In reading through materials from the early days of de-institutionalization, and in reflecting on the basic mechanisms developed to effect the depopulation of state hospitals (e.g. community mental health centres, entitlement programmes), one gets the impression that the sole function of mental health services was to treat and minimize, if not eradicate, the illness. The fact that this statement may appear to be a statement of the obvious is confirmation of its central, if implicit, role as an underlying core assumption of the overall approach. But what other functions could mental health services serve? Is not the primary focus of mental health treating mental illness? It is true that several functions were proposed for the developing community mental health centres, including prevention and community education and consultation (Snow and Swift, 1985). As primarily a treatment facility (Snow and Newton, 1976), though, the model of service delivery initially was one of acute care involving office-based psychotherapy and the administration of psychiatric medication. The assumption of this approach was that people with psychiatric disorders would be able to benefit from these available treatments to resolve their episodes of illness so that they would then be able to live in the community in a 'normal manner'. Treatment would ameliorate or reduce the illness to a point at which normal life could be resumed, with minimal, if any, residual symptoms or signs of the illness. People would be cured of the illness first and then return to a normal life afterwards.

Paradoxically, perhaps, this policy direction evolved during a time when the illnesses for which people were being treated were considered largely incurable. Even if not incurable, the field quickly learned that a combination of chlorpromazine and therapy was inadequate to engage people with mental illnesses in care, not to mention to eliminate the barriers to their returning to a normal life. By the 1970s, when it had become clear that this model was not adequate to meet the many complex needs of people with serious mental illnesses – who were increasingly being seen on city streets around the country 'shuffling off to oblivion' (Johnson, 1990) – the Carter administration launched the community support movement (Turner and TenHoor, 1978; Parrish, 1989). An idealistic effort from which the recovery movement derives many of its core ideas and approaches, the community support movement has played a key transitional role in bringing the field to where it is today through the introduction of such advances as assertive community treatment; supported housing, education and employment; and self-help, peer support and family support approaches. With recognition that many people with serious mental illnesses were not being served adequately or effectively by office-based practice and medication, an array of intensive community-based services and supports were developed to close the gap in care people faced upon discharge from the hospital.

We view the community support movement as transitional for several interrelated reasons. First, with the inauguration of Ronald Reagan in 1981, this movement never received the level of support – financial, practical or conceptual – that was needed for it to take firm hold within the broader field. While the recovery movement which has emerged this century can be viewed as a continuation of the work begun with the community support movement in the 1970s, the fiscal policies of the 1980s and introduction of privatization and managed care in the 1990s effectively disrupted its maturation (Hoge et al., 1998).

Second, and possibly as a result of these factors, the community support movement did not bring about a fundamental rethinking of the original conceptual model of 'recover first and get your life back later'. The community support movement made initial forays away from acute care towards a disability model, but was not able (or afforded the opportunity) to achieve this 'transformation'. This is one of the reasons why current systems are faced with the contradictory mandates of providing community supports to people with enduring disabilities but then having to terminate those same supports (e.g. job coaches) after an initial three- to six-month period when the person fails to show adequate improvement. When viewed from the perspective of a disability model, this would be equivalent to retracting a person's wheelchair after a year or so because he or she had not relearned how to walk or, for those of us who wear glasses, having our insurers deny funding for new glasses because the old ones had failed to restore our vision.

The third and final reason for viewing the community support movement as transitional is that, like the de-institutionalization movement which preceded it, it continued to focus almost exclusively on what mental health practitioners needed to do, or to provide, in order to treat the illness. The idea that recovery is actually the responsibility of the person with the illness, and that it is primarily up to him or her to pursue, establish and enhance his or her own recovery – as opposed to recovery-oriented care, which it is the responsibility of practitioners to offer – is a fairly recent development (Davidson et al., 2006; Davidson and White, 2007). We view this fact as a further by-product of the acute care model we described above, in which the person's only role while he or she was ill was to receive, or at best to participate in, treatment. Is it merely a semantic difference, or does it lead to a substantive difference in practice to shift from viewing people with mental illnesses as passive recipients of the actions of others to viewing them as active agents in their own recovery?

It is our hypothesis that such a shift does lead to a substantive difference in practice and, moreover, that it requires a change in the conceptual framework. It is perhaps easiest to see the implications of this framework in how we currently assess the 'outcomes' of care. How is it, in other words, that we currently conceptualize the 'life in the community' that we are striving to make available to everyone? How can we tell when we are being successful in our efforts?

Historically, one way we have assessed outcome is by counting the days a person spends outside of the hospital and, more recently, outside of other institutional settings such as jails, a concept we might term 'time *in* the community' or 'community tenure'. From the prominence of this outcome indicator, one could surmise that the objective of de-institutionalization was not so much to enable people to have a life in the community as it was to get and keep people out of the hospital. At its inception, for instance, assertive community treatment was conceptualized as an alternative to the hospital, a 'hospital without walls' (Stein and Test, 1978, 1980). And this approach made sense earlier in the process of closing mental hospitals, when it still seemed like a formidable challenge to find ways to support people outside of hospital settings. But now we are faced with entire generations of individuals with serious mental illnesses who have never lived in hospitals in the first place, and whose use of hospitals, if any, is limited to acute stays of days or perhaps weeks. The goal of getting and keeping people out of hospitals is clearly not equivalent to the goal of affording them a 'life in the community' to be maintained in a 'normal manner'. *Time* in the community is not the same as *a life* in the community.

What is missing in this approach? One thing that appears to be missing is any positive conceptualization of what such a life may entail beyond the desideratum of staying outside of a hospital or jail. This is not because we do not believe that people with mental illnesses have lives outside of the hospital, but because we have not seen that as within the purview of our field. Our role has been to eradicate the illness; it has been the person's responsibility to pursue his or her life once the illness has been contained. Such a division of labor may not only be simplistic but also overlooks the active role people have to play in learning how to contain, or how to deal with the enduring presence of, the illness. Now that we are in a post-institutional era, it is important to recognize that both of these tasks take place within the context of the person's ongoing life *in* the community (Davidson and Strauss, 1995). People can no longer be viewed as resuming their lives at some point later (i.e. when the illness becomes more manageable) when they are always already engaged in the process of having to live their lives now (Davidson, Tondora and O'Connell, 2006).

The fact that people are always already having to live their lives in the community in the presence of mental illness is a fact that previous models did not have to grapple with directly. It is a fact that has been introduced with moving the goal posts of care from hospital discharge, to community tenure, to emerging visions of recovery, visions which hold out the expectation that people with serious mental illnesses will be supported in their efforts to 'live, work, learn, and participate fully in their communities' (Department of Health and Human Services, 2005, p. 3). It is in order to embrace this fact of the active role people play in their own recovery, and to explore its various implications for practice, that we suggest a capabilities approach and action theory are needed. Before taking up this framework, though, we need to turn to one additional perspective on this argument that provides an essential context for transformation: the perspective of rights.

7.3 Rights and recovery

With the benefit of hindsight, we can see that the 1961 *Action for Mental Health* agenda is striking in terms of one of its major differences from current policy discussions. Even at the time of this report, the commissioners were already concerned with why previous reform efforts had failed and how they could pursue their current efforts in ways which would not repeat mistakes of the past. In this case, however, the commissioners determined that a root cause of previous failures was the fact that people with serious mental illnesses 'lack appeal' and, instead, pose a 'nuisance' to others (Joint Commission on Mental Illness and Health, 1961, p. 58). For this reason, they argued, people with serious mental illnesses did not invoke much in the way of sympathy, and did not elicit the kind of compassion that was aroused by other groups of people with other serious illnesses (e.g. polio) or disabilities (e.g. Down syndrome). Their strategy to address this basic problem was to attempt to educate the public and humanize the face of mental illness, transforming the public's disdain of and aversion to people with mental illnesses into a posture of compassion – or at least of charity. The fact that stigma remains the number-one barrier to accessing care and recovery (Department of Health and Human Services, 1999) suggests that this strategy has not yet succeeded either.

How different this is from the recovery perspective, which, as we argued in the previous chapter, is grounded first and foremost in the civil rights movement. This is evident not only in the statement quoted above about a keystone of transformation involving honoring the rights of adults with serious mental illnesses but also in the basic message conveyed by the New Freedom Commission on Mental Health. This is 'the message that mental illnesses ... are treatable and that recovery is possible' (Department of Health and Human Services, 2005, p. 6). If recovery is already possible, then apparently it is not additional research into the causes or cures for mental illness that is being called for. The federal government does not appear to be tackling the problem of mental illness in the way it tackled polio or small pox, that is by accelerating research into the causes and cures of the disease and by disseminating new treatments or preventive interventions. According to the current *Action Agenda*, we already know 'how to enable people with mental illnesses to live, work, learn and participate fully in the community' (Department of Health and Human Services, 2005, p. 1). If we already know how to do so, what gets in our way? What needs to be different for us to achieve transformation?

What we appear to be dealing with is not so much an issue of science, not a breakthrough in understanding the nature of the disease or of its cure, but an issue of rights. Perhaps it is for this reason that the current *Action Agenda* frames the process of transformation as requiring 'nothing short of a revolution' (Department of Health and Human Services, 2005, p. 18). If all we were being asked to do was to hold out hope for clinical improvement in the people we treat and offer them the most effective care available for reducing symptoms and enhancing functioning, there would be no need for this kind of rhetoric; there would be no 'revolution'. The revolution appears, instead, to involve the ways in which we view and treat people with mental illnesses. It is no longer relevant whether people with mental illnesses are appealing or troublesome, whether they elicit compassion or charity; they are instead to be viewed as fellow citizens, entitled to the same rights and responsibilities of membership in society as everyone else. As succinctly stated in the National Council on Disability's (2000) report aptly entitled *From Privileges to Rights*: 'People with psychiatric disabilities are, first and foremost, citizens who have the right to expect that they will be treated according to the principles of law that apply to all other citizens' (p. 7).

Another major difference between the 1961 report and the current one is that the earlier report was written *by* mental health professionals *about* people with mental illnesses. The best that could be mustered through this approach was a consensus on the humanity of people with mental illness and the need to cultivate an appreciation of this in the public. What we have seen since the 1970s, however, has been a movement conceived and led by people with mental illnesses themselves who have advocated for and begun to secure their own rights to be afforded the same opportunities and responsibilities as everyone else. They have had to lobby for these rights, and the *Action Agenda* and National Council on Disability have felt it incumbent to join in lobbying for these same rights, because they have been denied in the past. People with mental illnesses have gone from being a misunderstood group suffering from debilitating illnesses in need of compassionate care to an oppressed minority group reclaiming their rights to full participation in the life of their communities. But how is it that their rights were denied in the first place? If we are speaking only of people with mental illnesses no longer being confined to hospitals against their will, this process began a half-century ago and has not yet been able to guarantee people 'a life in the community'. What more is required in order to ensure the 'protection and respect of the rights of adults with serious mental illnesses'?

Looking back to the civil rights and independent living movements which provided the main inspiration for the consumer/survivor/ex-patient movement offers a glimpse into the nature of this 'more'. The various civil rights movements established that people of color did not need to be white, women did not need to be men and lesbian/gay/bisexual/transgender people did not need to be limited to heterosexuality in order to be considered and treated as having, and accorded all of, the rights and responsibilities of citizenship. The independent living movement made a similar case for people with disabilities, insisting that it is in the presence of enduring disability that people most need to be guaranteed their rights to self-determination and full inclusion in community life (Deegan, 1996). Extrapolating to serious mental illnesses, the point would be that people living with these conditions do not need to be cured of their illnesses, do not need to become 'normal', in order to pursue their lives in the community alongside everyone else (Davidson *et al.*, 2001). In addition to no longer being confined to hospitals against their will, this means that people with mental illnesses can make their own decisions, follow their own dreams and pursue the activities they enjoy or find meaningful in the settings of their choice without first having to be cured of their illness. Similar to the decision a person with paraplegia makes not to wait to regain his or her mobility in order to resume his or her life, a person with a mental illness needs to be able to have a dignified, meaningful and gratifying life while continuing to have a psychiatric disability.

Despite appearances, such an argument does not contradict the emphasis of the New Freedom Commission on 'recovery'. This is because 'recovery', as defined by the consumer/survivor/ex-patient movement and the field of psychiatric rehabilitation, assumes ongoing disability rather than cure. As captured eloquently by Pat Deegan, this form of recovery 'refers to the ... real life experience of persons as they accept and overcome the challenge of the disability' (Deegan, 1988, p. 150). In order to reduce the considerable confusion which currently surrounds the various uses of this term in mental health, we have distinguished this form of recovery, which we have termed 'being in recovery' from the more conventional notion of recovery used in clinical research, which refers to the absence of symptoms and impairments and which we denote as recovery 'from' serious mental illness (Davidson and Roe, 2007; Davidson *et al.*, 2009). It is this relatively recent development of the notion of being 'in' recovery that we view as speaking most directly to the issue of rights, and which we view as the foundation for the current revolution in mental health care (Davidson *et al.*, 2006).

This is because the notion of being in recovery underscores the fact, as we noted above, that people are always already having to live their lives in the presence of mental illness. Incorporating the perspective of rights we have now described, it also reminds us that people with serious mental illnesses are active agents engaged in the process of living their lives, and legally entitled to make their own decisions, regardless of the degree to which they have achieved someone else's notion of 'normality'. For any conceptual framework to be up to the task of supporting such an approach, it will thus have to be founded upon an appreciation of the basic rights of individuals to act as agents in determining their own lives without their first having to satisfy any external criteria by which others will determine them capable of doing so. It is for this reason that we suggest adopting the capabilities approach, to which we now turn.

7.4 The capabilities approach of Amartya Sen

What is the 'capabilities approach' and how is it relevant to mental illness? The capabilities approach was initially developed by economic theorists and political philosophers to emphasize that any legitimate approach to social justice must begin with the recognition that human beings are agents who should be free to determine their own lives. The core aspects of human nature on which this approach to political and economic theory are built are those of the concepts of agency and the freedom to exercise that agency autonomously. In part due to its role in orienting the human development programme of the United Nations to promoting freedom around the world, this approach has been increasingly influential in recent years, earning Sen the Nobel Prize for Economics in 1998.

Stated in the reverse, the first priority of a capabilities approach is to liberate people from what Sen refers to as the 'substantive unfreedoms' currently constraining their exercise of agency, encouraging political leaders, policymakers and activists to look beyond their usual concerns with material deprivations (e.g. poverty or hunger) to social and political deprivations, such as oppression, prejudice and discrimination as well (Sen, 1999, p. 8). Expanding the scope to include freedom is essential, according to the capabilities approach, because the nature of human beings is such that what people can *do* and *be* is more important than what people can *have*. As Nussbaum, another proponent of the capabilities approach, describes it:

> The central question asked by the capabilities approach is not, 'How satisfied is Vasanti?' or even 'How much in the way of resources is she able to command?' It is, instead, 'What is Vasanti actually able to do and to be?' (Nussbaum, 2000, p. 71)

An economist by training, Sen pointed out that the capabilities approach does not disregard the role of material resources – or the other traditional preoccupations of economists with utility, income or satisfaction – it is rather that the capabilities approach adds to these a central focus on freedom. And for Sen, the relative importance of these different indicators and outcomes of development is clear, as he writes:

> Freedoms are not only the primary ends of development, they are also among its principal means ... Freedom is not only the basis of the evaluation of success and failure, but it is also a principal determinant of individual initiative and social effectiveness. Greater freedom enhances the ability of people to help themselves and also to influence the world, and these matters are central to the process of development. The concern here relates to what we may call ... the 'agency aspect' of the individual. (Sen, 1999, pp. 10, 18)

According to Sen, the primary ends of human development are first to establish (by reducing substantive unfreedoms) and then to enhance the freedoms people are able to enjoy. Also according to Sen, the primary means we have for undertaking this work are first to establish and then to enhance the freedoms people are able to enjoy. But does this equating of the ends of development with the means of development amount to circular reasoning? No, it does not, and three illustrations of the implications of this position will suffice both to demonstrate the non-circular nature of the reasoning involved and to suggest useful parallels between this perspective on development and the recovery-oriented approach to transformation.

As a first implication of this position, it would be inconsistent with the central value placed on freedom and agency for one group of people – regardless of how well-intentioned, well-resourced or experienced they may be – to attempt to 'develop' another group of people. While it may seem on the surface reasonable, if not noble, for one group to attempt to remove the substantive unfreedoms that another group is laboring under, there is no way for this second group to be made truly free other than for them to seize the reins and take control of their own situation. Otherwise, one oppressor has been replaced with another. The core focus on agency dictates that all parties be viewed as agents from the very first moment of the process, rather than one party's agency being viewed by another as contingent on the achievement of any material, social or political preconditions. We may recall here Harry Stack Sullivan's insistence that 'from the start' each of his patients was to be 'treated as a *person among persons*'. Sen makes this important point in relation to the approach of many development programmes which presume to know ahead of time what is in the best interest of a community without the members of the community in question being actively involved in the conversation. To be consistent, he writes:

> People have to be seen, in this perspective, as being actively involved – given the opportunity – in shaping their own destiny, and not just as passive recipients of the fruits of cunning development programs. (Sen, 1999, p. 53)

Rather than cunning developers from another country, he suggests earlier in this same text: 'It is the people directly involved who must have the opportunity to participate in deciding' their own fate (Sen, 1999, p. 31). This is not only because they will have the most intimate knowledge of their values, their challenges and the resources available to tackle these challenges but also because 'the *process* through which outcomes are generated has significance of its own. Indeed, "choosing" itself can be seen as a valuable functioning' (Sen, 1999, p. 76; italics in the original). If the freedom to exercise one's agency (i.e. to make one's own choices) is the desired outcome of the process of development, it can be brought about only by offering the people in question the opportunity to exercise their own agency (i.e. make their own choices). No amount of planning, or infusion of resources, by another party will be able to effect this transformation. It is only freedom that brings and enhances freedoms. It is for this reason that many previous revolutions have resulted in liberators turning into tyrants, and for this reason that the title of one of Sen's books was *Development as Freedom* (Sen, 1999).

How does this differ from other approaches to development, that is to what does this offer a more effective alternative? The second implication was implicit in the first, but given its parallels to recovery it is worth spelling out explicitly. As Sen describes, the capability approach:

> goes against – and to a great extent undermines – the belief that has been so dominant in many policy circles that 'human development' (as

> the process of expanding education, health care, and other conditions
> of human life is often called) is really a kind of luxury that only richer
> countries can afford. (Sen, 1999, p. 41)

The dominant approach to development has been to focus on economic growth
and stability first, for example to increase a country's gross national product
(GNP), with the other concerns of education, health care, quality of life and political
participation delayed to some point 'later' when the country has secured an adequate
resource (i.e. financial) base. Sen's empirical research has been instrumental in
demonstrating that this approach has not worked in the past; economic growth in
terms of GNP, income or utility – no matter on what scale – has not translated into or
effected political or social growth. The opposite, however, has worked. As he writes:

> The fact that education and health care are also productive in raising
> economic growth adds to the argument for putting major emphasis on
> these social arrangements in poor economies, *without* having to wait
> for 'getting rich' *first*. (Sen, 1999, p. 49; italics in the original)

Securing freedoms as a direct means of development, as quoted from Sen above,
is 'a principal determinant of individual initiative and social effectiveness' (Sen,
1999, p. 18). If afforded their freedoms, citizens of poor countries will be effective in
pursuing economic growth. No amount of wealth, however, can buy a population's
freedom from slavery or political oppression. The oppressors can always desire to
get still richer (one of the dangers of money is that 'one can never have enough of
it'), while a free citizenry will undoubtedly elect to act in their own collective best
interest, a process that typically involves generating an adequate resource base to
support the population. As one striking example of this, Sen points out that: 'no
famine has ever taken place in the history of the world in a functioning democracy',
regardless of a country's GNP or its level of food productivity or availability (Sen,
1999, pp. 16; see also Drèze and Sen, 1989).

A final illustration of this approach relates to the issue of diversity. Dominant
approaches either ignore the issue of diversity by identifying one measure as common
across all possible domains of choice – the best example here again being that of
wealth – or by relegating issues of diversity to a secondary status to be addressed
after the 'real' work of development has taken hold. This second possibility is
evident in theoretical approaches that stipulate that all people are fundamentally
or universally the same in their basic quest for X (e.g. safety, income), with all
possible markers of difference such as culture being seen as introducing only minor
or surface modifications. Sen is sensitive to the tendency on the part of adherents
of this approach to make 'freedom' simply the latest X in that equation, so he goes
to some length to reject the notion that freedom is just another commodity, to
reinforce the centrality of choice and to highlight the fact that choice necessarily
generates diversity, both between individuals and between countries and cultures. As
appears to be his own personal preference, he explains this point in relation to food:

> The capability perspective is inescapably pluralist ... to insist on the
> mechanical comfort of having just one homogeneous 'good thing'
> would be to deny our humanity ... It is like seeking to make the life
> of the chef easier by finding something which – and which alone – we
> all like (such as smoked salmon, or perhaps even French fries). (Sen,
> 1999, p. 77)

It is in the very nature of choice to result in variability, otherwise choice would
not really be free but would refer only to changes in the quantity of some basic
universal. While smoked salmon and French fries are, of course, both foods, to say
that a person who prefers smoked salmon to French fries has no real preference
because they are both foods is to miss the point of having preferences to begin with.
It is to gloss over the issue of choice, but this is precisely where our primary interest
lies. Without choice there is no freedom, and therefore no justice; but with choice
there inevitably will be differences and diversity. Sen concludes therefore that:

> Investigations of equality – theoretical as well as practical – that pro-
> ceed with the assumption of antecedent uniformity (including the
> presumption that 'all men are created equal') thus miss out on a major
> aspect of the problem. Human diversity is no secondary complication
> (to be ignored, or to be introduced 'later on'); it is a fundamental
> aspect of our interest in equality. (Sen, 1992, p. xi)

In anticipating the next section of this chapter, it may be useful to point out that
this is an insight which appears to have been grasped relatively infrequently in mental
health; a field in which various lifestyles or choices which were initially considered
pathological (e.g. 'run away slaves', 'homosexuals') are now considered legitimate.
Sen's point is reflected, in contrast, in D.W. Winnicott's bold assertion that 'with
human beings there is an infinite variety in normality or health' (Winnicott, 1986,
p. 45). We suggest that an approach to mental health that is based explicitly in
an appreciation of the basic and inevitable diversity inherent in human nature
is both a prerequisite for, and contributes significantly to, the transformation to
recovery-oriented care.

In summary, then, the capabilities approach diverts our attention away from the
usual concerns of political leaders and policymakers with the possession of *resources*
(e.g. utility, income) to the exercise of *freedoms*. This shift is not meant to deny the
crucial role resources play in social and political life, but rather places emphasis on
the fact that 'the usefulness of wealth lies in the things that it allows us to do – the
substantive freedoms it helps us to achieve' (Sen, 1999, p. 14). It is not effective to
view wealth as an end in itself, but only as a 'means for having more freedom to
lead the kind of lives we have reason to value' (Sen, 1999, p. 14). As suggested by
this last quotation, the focus of our efforts thereby shifts from what people, or a
population, have, to what they can do, to 'the *actual living* that people manage to
achieve' (Sen, 1999, p. 73; italics in the original). Given the centrality of freedom to

this view, it is important to understand that this 'actual living', also referred to as the person's 'capability', is necessarily a function of the person's free exercise of his or her own agency. The primary concern of this approach thus becomes the person's capabilities to function, to do or to be what he or she values and 'to take part in the life of the community' as he or she chooses (Sen, 1999, p. 73).

For our present purposes, there are two important corollaries to this basic position. One is that people should not be made to wait until certain material, social or political preconditions are in place in order to begin to choose, as people are active agents who are always already making choices in their lives on an everyday basis. In the same fashion, it does not work for people to wait until some mythical point, always 'later', at which another party will step in to provide whatever is needed or act in whatever ways are needed to restore to them their freedoms. As we saw in the last chapter, Martin Luther King, Jnr wrote in his classic 'Letter from Birmingham Jail' that 'freedom is never voluntarily given by the oppressor; it must be demanded by the oppressed' (King, 1981, p. 278). The capabilities approach goes one step further to explain how freedom *cannot* be given by one party to another; the most one party can do for a second party is not to continue to oppress or enslave them, and to offer them opportunities to determine their own lives. The second party will then have to take it from there, choosing freely to pursue those activities that they find valuable.

The second corollary that is a direct result of this first one is that choice necessarily involves and generates diversity, not as a secondary consideration or modification but as an essential aspect of the fact that choice is actually free. In other words, the second party must be able to pursue those activities which he or she values based on the fact that she or he values them, and not simply or strictly because they are valued by another (e.g. a dominant group). The very notion of equality presumes diversity and difference, and would be much less a relevant concern were everyone to choose the same thing (e.g. French fries). It therefore becomes impossible to determine, or predict, ahead of time what any one person, or group of people, will choose, as the very act of choice itself is partly constitutive of the outcome. While taking freedom seriously in this way obviously complicates the picture, and challenges our usual notions of science (which involve causality and prediction), the capabilities approach insists that freedom and self-determination are essential to what makes us human. Any approach that excludes or limits these considerations in the name of science or expediency (as in, we'll get around to those issues 'later', when the time is right), omits the very things with which it should be primarily concerned, and thus proves to be inadequate to the task in hand.

We suggested above that this was true of the conceptual framework implicit in the de-institutionalization movement, which failed to recognize and address the fact that people with serious mental illnesses remained active agents in their own lives and needed to be afforded the opportunity to live that life in a self-determined fashion, even in the presence of enduring disability. We now will consider how the capabilities approach, as an alternative conceptual framework, can be used to help mental health overcome this limitation.

7.5 Applying a capabilities approach to the work of transformation

How does adoption of a capabilities approach change the way we look at, and carry out the work of, transformation? The capabilities approach draws our attention to the fact that people with serious mental illnesses, as people first and foremost, are active agents and citizens of their communities, who – like other citizens – need to be able to exercise their agency freely and autonomously in order to function as fully human. Within the constraints of whatever substantive unfreedoms they may be subjected to based on historical legacies and current circumstances (e.g. stigma, discrimination), they are always already making choices in their day-to-day lives based on which capabilities they value and what choices may be available to them (based also on available resources, social structures, etc.). Affording people with serious mental illnesses 'a life in the community' thus no longer remains limited to community tenure, but shifts with this framework to focusing on the *actual living* that people manage to achieve. This makes sense as a logical extension or next step beyond de-institutionalization, if one considers that what is most problematic about long-term hospitalization or incarceration from the point of view of the person with mental illness is the loss of freedom and autonomy which results (Davidson *et al.*, 1996). What the capabilities approach adds is that more can be done in a positive way beyond releasing someone from an institution; in addition to no longer denying people's rights, constructive efforts can be made – and in some cases may need to be made – to promote and enhance their ability to choose freely those activities and lifestyles they have reason to value (Davidson *et al.*, in press).

While it is tempting to view the process of eradicating unfreedoms and promoting freedoms as something which a concerned and compassionate person or group of people may do for others less fortunate or less able than themselves (however that may be determined), it is crucially important within this framework to understand that freedom is not a 'thing' (i.e. a resource or possession) which one person can give *to* or establish *for* another. Rather, it becomes incumbent on the first party, morally and practically, to afford the second party *opportunities* to make his or her own choices (of what to do and be) and to determine his or her own fate (here we hear the echoes of Adolf Meyer). This is necessary not only because the second party has the most intimate familiarity with the activities he or she values, the challenges he or she faces in pursuing these activities and the resources he or she has available for tackling these challenges but also because it is only through achievement of this substantive freedom that the person will be able to generate additional freedoms for him- or herself. It is only by acting as an agent in determining his or her own life that he or she will be able to achieve the substantive freedom required to be an autonomous agent in the broader world.

How is the nature of mental illness understood within such a framework? According to Sen, all illnesses and disabilities can be viewed as 'deprivations', which either limit a person's opportunities or compromise his or her abilities to choose freely and achieve those 'functionings' that he or she values. Mental illness thus may pose an obstacle to the person's achievement of the kind of life he or she may wish to have, may make it more difficult for him or her to have that life and, at its most extreme, may even deprive the person of his or her life altogether. In none of these cases, however, does mental illness fundamentally alter the basic nature of human beings, which is that of being self-determined agents of their own lives, free to choose autonomously and pursue the kind of lives they value. Mental illness does not rob the person of his or her agency, nor does it deprive the person of his or her fundamental rights. Rather, given the obstacles mental illness often brings with it, this makes it all the more important that the person be enabled, and supported in his or her efforts, to exercise those freedoms and attain the kind of life he or she values to the greatest degree possible. Treatments, rehabilitation strategies and the provision of community supports may be essential to the person's ability to choose and pursue such a life, but their function is to be understood squarely within this context. Their function, in other words, is to support the person's own choices and pursuits, to be used by him or her as tools for his or her own recovery, rather than as prerequisites to or substitutes for the life he or she desires to lead.

There are, as we noted above, two additional dimensions to this picture relevant to our present interest. These points are cautionary in nature in highlighting some of the ways in which this framework may be compromised or undermined in practice, but the parallels to mental health are noteworthy. The first of these cautions is that people should not be made to wait until some point further down the road, at some mythical time 'later', when all of the necessary preconditions are in place for them to achieve and exercise their freedoms. There can be no material, social or political conditions required for people to be afforded the freedoms which are rightfully theirs as citizens of their communities. In mental health, as we noted earlier, the precondition held out for people with serious mental illnesses has been the need for them to be cured of their illnesses or to become 'normal' first before they can rejoin community life. A capabilities approach asserts to the contrary that it is only through participation in community life as self-determined agents that people with mental illnesses will acquire the capabilities needed to manage their conditions. As it is, we have no cure for mental illness, but we do have decades of experiences demonstrating that people cannot and will not learn how to manage their conditions effectively as long as they are viewed as defective and dependent and are confined to institutional settings.

The second, related, caution is that free choice presumes and necessarily involves and generates diversity. Material, social and political preconditions for the exercise of agency have typically been stipulated as safeguards to ensure that people will choose only certain things or in only certain ways, but this amounts only to the illusion of choice and is not truly free. In order to acknowledge that freedom necessarily results in difference and diversity, we must first accept Winnicott's (1986) assertion that 'with human beings, there is an infinite variety in normality or health'. Once this is accepted as a foundational principle for our science and practice, and we thereby reject any uni-vocal, static or predetermined notion of 'normality', it no longer makes sense to make people wait to rejoin community life until they first regain it.

This is because we have no way to know ahead of time what 'normal' will look like for any given individual, and he or she will only be able to determine this over time through the pursuit of those activities and lifestyles which he or she has reasons to value. There is no other way, other than trial and error, to figure out what 'normal' will look like for me. And this is as true of people with serious mental illnesses as it is for anyone, and everyone, else.

Based on these three core implications derived from a capabilities approach, we suggest that the transformation process will need to address the basic mission, vision and strategies utilized throughout the mental health field, changing dramatically our charge (our mission), the nature of the business we are in (our vision) and the major approaches we use to accomplish our charge (our strategies). In broad strokes, we suggest that transformation will take the following form at the level of a system of care (Davidson *et al.*, in press).

The major thrust of a capabilities-oriented system of care will be to increase the access of people with serious mental illnesses to opportunities and supports that will enable them to live a decent and self-determined quality life. A quality life comprises 'achieved functionings' in domains which the person values, incorporating but not limited to personal and social well-being. The core focus of the system will be on facilitating the process of development in which each person with a psychiatric disability actively engages, ensuring that a historically oppressed and presently vulnerable population has the resources, opportunities and ongoing supports it needs in order to function well in the environments and roles of its choice, with the eventual goal being that of its achieving the capability to live a dignified and fulfilling life despite the enduring presence of a disability.

An early component of transformation will involve identifying and removing obstacles and impediments to development that keep people with disabilities in circumstances of relative and real disadvantage. That is, system-level activities will critically assess and continue to act to reduce the myriad 'substantive unfreedoms' and layered aspects of disadvantage that are experienced everyday by many people with psychiatric disabilities, and which have catastrophic effects on their personal health (e.g. increased morbidity) as well as on their social lives (e.g. isolation). It is a tragic reality at the present time that people with serious mental illnesses are often discriminated against and, in comparison to the general public, achieve a lower level of education; experience more unemployment and impoverishment; are more often placed out of home as children and youth and more often homeless or ill-housed as adults; are more frequently the victims of early trauma and more likely to be re-traumatized through experiences of coercion within mental health systems; are more often victims of crime later in life; are disproportionately represented in jail and prison populations for non-violent, victimless and petty crimes; generally experience poorer physical health to the point of significant loss of lifespan and premature mortality; and are generally more socially disconnected than others. Redress of such inequalities and deprivations must occur so that people have increased chances 'to do' and 'to be' by engaging in activities and roles of their choice (Davidson *et al.*, in press).

In this respect, systemic efforts will focus on dismantling structural barriers, inequitable power arrangements, practices of social discrimination and unnecessarily constrained choices – including those embedded within a system of care – that serve to perpetuate social, economic, cultural and health disparities. Building capabilities of the people served, on the other hand, will reduce the vulnerabilities of these same people as well as increase their resiliencies and their substantive freedoms to do or to be as they choose. To build capabilities, systems will invest in creating, enriching and making more flexible and responsive the policies and opportunity sets available, expand the range of accessible and valued options and choices, and improve access to resources and supports so that people have the means necessary to engage in the activities they value. These directions of reducing substantive unfreedoms and expanding opportunities and supports are consistent with what people in recovery have advocated since the 1980s, when they have identified stigma, discrimination, coercion and lost opportunities, relationships and roles as binding them to a life of prolonged disability and dependency, proving to pose more formidable barriers to recovery than the serious mental illnesses themselves (Chamberlin, 1990; Deegan, 1992; Deegan, 1996).

This last comment reminds us of a crucially important principle of the capabilities approach that, in our experience, becomes easily lost or overshadowed by the multitude of political, financial and practical complexities impinging on transformational leaders at the system level. This is the principle we went to some length to reinforce in our earlier discussion, which suggests that one group of people, regardless of how well-intentioned, well-resourced or experienced they may be, cannot remove the substantive unfreedoms that another group labors under, nor can they pursue a development process for the benefit of others, without those others being actively and substantively involved in 'shaping their own destiny'. Bluntly stated, system leaders cannot view themselves as being more experienced and more capable of creating a vision, and setting an agenda, for transformation than people living with serious mental illnesses themselves, as this actually poses an additional obstacle to, rather than facilitates, transformation. People in recovery are not only the most intimately familiar with the realities of living with mental illness, the challenges this poses and the resources available to them to overcome these challenges but also, given the opportunity, their actions of creating a vision and setting an agenda for their own recovery will contribute importantly and directly to system change.

While adhering to this principle certainly poses formidable challenges of its own, there is no way for a system to become truly 'consumer-driven', as is mandated by the New Freedom Commission (Department of Health and Human Services, 2003), than for the recovery community to drive the transformation process itself. Consistent with Sen's concerns about countries waiting to become rich first or wanting to disregard issues of diversity in their own development efforts, system leaders are tempted to set pre-conditions for, or place parameters around, the involvement of people in recovery in their transformation initiatives. In our own work in pursuing transformation (Davidson *et al.*, 2007), and in consulting to other systems in their transformation initiatives (Davidson and White, 2007), this remains the most challenging, but also the most effective, lever for change. As a result, we remain convinced that if restoration of the rights of people in recovery to full citizenship, and their assumption of the responsibilities of this role, are not front and centre in transformation efforts, then this process will inevitably fall short of accomplishing its goals. If people in recovery are not allowed to, or do not step up to, lead the process, then we will surely fail once again to 'achieve the promise' of a life in the community first promised over half a century ago.

7.6 Human agency and mediation: the work of Lev Vygotsky

> Psychological processes have long been understood within a reactive context ... we must find a new methodology for psychological experimentation. (Vygotsky, 1978, pp. 59–60)

How are we to understand the nature of the agency and activity that people with mental illnesses will need to demonstrate in order to achieve transformation, and how can this agency and activity be best supported? For assistance with these questions, we turn finally to the work of the revolutionary psychologist Lev Vygotsky.

Vygotsky was born in Russia in 1896 (the same year as was Piaget) and died at the early age of 37 years old in 1934. In order to understand Vygotsky's work, it is essential to be aware of the social and historical context within which he lived and wrote. Vygotsky began his work in psychology around the time of the Russian Revolution, during which Marxist-Leninism became the dominant political, social and economic structure, replacing centuries of Tsarist rule. This violent revolution dramatically transformed Russian society. The new ethos stressed socialism, collectivism and the subordination of the individual to the social group and to society. Despite his explicit use of Marxist theory in grounding his intellectual work, Vygotsky's work was banned in the Soviet Union for 20 years during the Stalinist era, from 1936 to 1956, and was first translated into English in 1962. He remains little known in the United States, except among the community of social/critical psychologists and philosophers and psychologists of language.

Vygotsky integrates many of the elements of Marxist-Leninism into his theory of human development, as we noted above, producing what is considered a 'sociocultural' approach to psychology. The cornerstone of his model is that human development – meaning language, thought, reasoning, problem-solving and human relationships – results through social interaction (primarily with parents and other caregivers). In this fashion, the shared knowledge of one's culture is internalized as tools that mediate choices made and actions taken. Vygotsky writes:

> Every function in the child's cultural development appears twice:
> first, between people (interpsychological) and then inside the child

> (intrapsychological). This applies equally to voluntary attention, to logical memory, and to the formation of ideas, as the higher functions originate as actual relationships between individuals. (Vygotsky, 1978, p 57)

Development is therefore to be considered a process of 'internalization', whereby experiences of the world and of social relationships generate and deposit learning residues through which the person builds up an inner life. Thought, for example, is understood to be internalized speech, coming after and being produced by the person's incorporation of the language and thought processes encountered and learned through interactions with others. Vygotsky describes the process of internalization as consisting of:

> a series of transformations: a) An operation that initially represents an external activity is reconstructed and begins to occur internally; b) An interpersonal process is transformed into an intrapersonal one; and c) The transformation of an interpersonal process into an intrapersonal one is the result of a long series of developmental events. (Vygotsky, 1978, p. 57)

Based on this concept of internalization, Vygotsky suggested that human cognitive and emotional development could not follow a linear path, nor could it be understood as unfolding naturally through a series of pre-determined stages (as was being suggested at the time by Freud and Piaget). Instead, he believed that development was more about an ongoing, dynamic process rather than an end point. This process consisted of a series of qualitative transformations, dialectically involving a complex interplay of constant integration, disintegration and reintegration. This dialectical process was not universally the same for everyone, but would differ depending on sociocultural context and also would continue to evolve, unpredictably, over time. Central to this theory is the belief that culture is transmitted through the internalization of social signs and symbols – the major one, of course, being language – and that human cognitive development takes place through mediation by social, psychological and other tools, in particular through internalized cultural narratives. To illustrate this important point, Vygotsky offers the following example of the use of pointing as a tool:

> We call the internal reconstruction of an external operation *internalization*. A good example of this process may be found in the development of pointing. Initially, this gesture is nothing more than an unsuccessful attempt to grasp something, a movement aimed at a certain object which designates forthcoming activity. The child attempts to grasp an object placed beyond his reach; his hands, stretched toward that object, remain poised in the air. His fingers make grasping movements. At this initial stage pointing is represented by the child's movement, which seems to be pointing to an object – that and nothing more.

> When the mother comes to the child's aid and realizes his movement indicates something, the situation changes fundamentally. Pointing becomes a gesture for others. The child's unsuccessful attempt engenders a reaction not from the object he seeks but *from another person*. Consequently, the primary meaning of that unsuccessful grasping movement is established by others. Only later, when the child can link his unsuccessful grasping movement to the objective situation as a whole, does he begin to understand this movement as pointing. At this juncture there occurs a change in that movement's function: from an object-oriented movement it becomes a movement aimed at another person, a means of establishing relations. *The grasping movement changes to the act of pointing*. As a result of this change, the movement itself is then physically simplified, and what results is the form of pointing that we may call a true gesture. It becomes a true gesture only after it objectively manifests all the functions of pointing for others and is understood by others as such a gesture. (Vygotsky, 1978, p. 56; italics in the original)

The approach most appropriate to studying these phenomena would accordingly be a sociocultural one that would involve the following three components: (i) the use of a genetic, or developmental, method; (ii) the claim that higher mental functioning in the individual emerges out of social processes and (iii) the claim that human social and psychological processes are fundamentally shaped by cultural tools, or mediational means. As we will propose to bring these three components together in our approach to recovery-oriented research and practice, we dwell on each one briefly below.

The genetic method holds that mental processes can only be properly understood from the perspective of how and where they occur in human growth. In describing his approach, Vygotsky consistently emphasized that it was imperative to focus not on the product of development but on the process whereby higher forms are established. He posited that learning and development take place in society and in culturally shaped contexts; and, as historical conditions are constantly undergoing change, so do contexts and learning opportunities. Therefore, there can be no universal schema (à la Piaget) that can fully represent the changing dynamics between internal and external aspects of development.

Higher, or 'cultural', mental functions – including abstract reasoning, logical memory, language, voluntary attention, planning, decision-making and so on – have their origin in human interaction and appear gradually during the process of radical transformation of the lower functions. These are specific human functions that are formed and shaped gradually in a course of transformation of the lower functions, according to specific goals, practices and beliefs of the person's culture and social group (Vygotsky,1986). This transformation is made through what Vygotsky refers to as 'mediated activity' and 'psychological tools' (Vygotsky, 1986; Newman and Holzman, 1993), as noted above.

Wertsch (1985) suggests that there are four major differences between higher and lower mental functions. These are: (i) the shift of control from the environment to the individual, that is the emergence of voluntary regulation, (ii) the emergence of conscious realization of mental process, (iii) the social origins and social nature of higher mental functions and (iv) the use of signs to mediate higher mental functions.

Semiotic mediation, or mediation by signs, 'is defined here as the activity of relating a sign and its meaning, including the use of signs, the activity of investigating the relationship between sign and meaning, as well as improving the existing relationship between sign (or sign system) and meaning (or meaning system)' (Wertsch, 1985). Higher mental processes are mediated by tools, which can take one of three forms: symbols, material or another human being's behavior. They can include various systems for counting, mnemonic techniques, algebraic symbol systems, works of art, writing, schemes, diagrams, maps and technical drawings and all sorts of conventional signs such as internalized sociocultural and/or personal narratives, life stories and what Vygotsky (1986) refers to as 'voices of the mind'. Semiotic mediation in particular is central to all aspects of knowledge co-construction. Vygotsky regards semiotic mechanisms (including psychological tools) as mediating social and individual function, and connecting the external and the internal, the social and the individual. Wertsch elaborates on the centrality of this form of mediation in understanding Vygotsky's contributions to psychology and education:

> [Mediation] is the key in his approach to understanding how human mental functioning is tied to cultural, institutional, and historical settings since these settings shape and provide the cultural tools that are mastered by individuals to form this functioning. In this approach, the mediational means are what might be termed the 'carriers' of sociocultural patterns and knowledge. (Wertsch, 1994, p. viii)

Given the central role of mediation in both learning and subsequent behavior, this forms the focus for descriptive studies and analysis of experiences and behavior, which, for Vygotsky, are all considered sociocultural in nature. The unit of analysis for such a science is what Vygotsky (1986) refers to as a 'mediated action'. Wertsch offers the following description of how sociocultural analysis approaches mediated action:

> A starting point for the sort of sociocultural analysis I have in mind is the notion that it takes 'mediated action' as a unit of analysis. From this perspective, to be human is to use the cultural tools, or mediational means, that are provided by a particular sociocultural setting. The concrete use of these cultural tools involves an 'irreducible tension' (Wertsch, 1998) between active agents, on the one hand, and items such as computers, maps, and narratives, on the other. From this perspective, remembering is an active process that involves both sides of this tension. And because it involves socioculturally situated mediational means, remembering and the parties who carry it out are inherently situated in a cultural and social context.

As an illustration, consider the following episode. A colleague recently asked me to recommend a book on a particular topic. I knew the book I wanted to suggest, and could even 'see' it in my mind's eye in the sense that I could tell the colleague its color and approximate size. Furthermore, I could name the author. I was unable, however, to recall the book's title. I therefore used a cultural tool that has only emerged in a full-fledged form over the past few years, the Internet. I used my office computer to go to the bookseller Amazon.com, where I looked up the author of the book in question. Her list of books appeared on the screen, and I was able to recognize the correct title and recommend to my colleague the book I had intended.

Viewed in terms of mediated action, the question that arises here is, 'Who did the remembering?' On the one hand, I had to be involved as an active agent who had mastered the relevant cultural tool sufficiently well to conduct the appropriate search. On the other hand, this active agent, at least at that moment, was quite incapable of remembering the title of the book in question when operating in isolation – that is, without additional help from an external cultural tool. If I could have done so, I would not have turned to Amazon.com in the first place, an observation suggesting that perhaps Amazon.com should get the credit for remembering. But Amazon.com is not an agent in its own right – at least the same kind of active agent that I am (hopefully); it did not somehow speak up on its own to tell my colleague or me what we wanted to know.

From the perspective of mediated action there are good reasons for saying that neither I nor Amazon.com did the remembering in isolation. Instead, both of us were involved in a system of distributed memory and both were needed to get the job done. In short, an irreducible tension between active agent and cultural tool was involved. The nature of the cultural tool and the specific use made of it by the active agent may vary greatly, but both contribute to human action understood from this perspective. (Wertsch, 2002, pp. 37–38)

As suggested by this example, the framework for this kind of sociocultural analysis is that of the narrative flow found in stories. We are interested in mediation as the medium through which human 'action' takes form. Action always involves motion and change. In Vygotsky's psychology, as we saw in the quote that opened this section, human beings are not primarily reactive to their environments; they are not passive in their reception of stimulation. Rather, it is through their engagement in action that humans create the world that they encounter. As John-Steiner and Souberman comment in discussing Vygotsky's work: 'Humans are active, vigorous participants in their own existence' (John-Steiner and Souberman, 1978, p. 123). This is a view that is highly consistent with the ideas of King and Deleuze discussed in the previous chapter, viewing human action as having a constitutive function. It is because experience is constitutive that understanding experience requires the genetic, development method mentioned above, and described further by Cole and Scribner as follows:

> A central tenet of this method is that all phenomena be studied
> as processes in motion and change. In terms of the subject matter
> of psychology, the scientist's task is to reconstruct the origin and
> course of development of behavior and consciousness. Not only does
> every phenomenon have its history, but this history is characterized
> by changes both qualitative (changes in form and structure and
> basic characteristics) and quantitative ... The developmental method,
> in Vygotsky's view, is the central method of psychological science.
> (Vygotsky, 1978, pp. 6–7)

For help with fleshing out what such a narrative, genetic method entails, we turn
to the compatible work of the literary critic Kenneth Burke, who uses a 'dramatistic
method' to grapple with the complexities of human action (recall that Goffman
used a similar dramaturgical perspective). His approach to understanding human
action stresses the need to invoke multiple factors and perspectives as well as to
examine the ubiquitous dialectical tensions that exist among and between them. To
this end, he offers his pentad for analysing human motive and action, as follows:

> We shall use five terms as a generating principle of our investigation.
> They are: Act, Scene, Agent, Agency, Purpose. In a rounded statement
> about motives, you must have some word that names the *act* (names
> what took place, in thought or deed), and another that names the *scene*
> (the background of the act, the situation in which it occurred); also,
> you must indicate what person or kind of person (*agent*) performed
> the act, what means or instruments he used (*agency*), and the *purpose*.
> Men may violently disagree about the purposes behind a given act,
> or about the character of the person who did it, or how he did it,
> or in what kind of situation he acted; or they may even insist upon
> totally different words to name the act itself. But be that as it may, any
> complete statement about motives will *offer some kind of* answers to
> these five questions: what was done (*act*), when or where it was done
> (*scene*), who did it (*agent*), how he did it (*agency*), and why (*purpose*).
> (Burke, 1969, p. xv; italics in the original)

Burkes' pentad reflects an elegance of parsimony in that it addresses the basic
questions of: What? Where? Who? How? and Why? These are the essential issues
that every good reporter, criminal investigator and mental health consultant must
constantly elucidate. And yet, this grouping is wide ranging, complex and profound.
Take, for example, the elements of agent and scene. Often, these are viewed as static,
and independent in time and place. And yet Burke describes them in terms of an
'elastic container' (Wertsch, 1998) in time and place within which agents act and
acts occur.

> There is implicit in the quality of a scene the quality of the action that
> is to take place within it. This would be another way of saying that the
> act will be consistent with the scene ... Or, if you will, the stage-set

contains the action *ambiguously* (as regards the norms of action) – and in the course of the play's development this ambiguity is converted into a corresponding *articulacy*. The proportion would be: scene is to act as implicit is to explicit ...

[Moreover] one has a great variety of circumferences to select as characterizations of a given agent's scene. For a man is not only in the situation peculiar to his era or to his particular place in that era (even if we could agree on the traits that characterize his era). He is also in a situation extending through centuries; he is in a 'generically human' situation; and he is in a 'universal' situation. Who is to say, once and for all, which of these circumferences is to be selected as the motivation of his act, insofar as the act is to be defined in scenic terms? ... The contracting and expanding of scene is rooted in the very nature of linguistic placement. And a selection of circumference from among this range is in itself an act, an 'act of faith', with the definition or interpretation of the act taking shape accordingly. (Burke, 1969 pp. 6–7, 84; italics in the original)

An example of the pentad approach to exploring human motives and actions emerged when JR attended a small conference at MIT in 2002, titled 'Memories of War'. The meeting's organizer, the Professor of Political Science Roger Petersen, described having been in Lithuania in January 1991 when Soviet tanks attacked unarmed civilians, in some cases running them over. Petersen was in Vilnius with an old friend who was the son of Lithuanian refugees. This young man had been born and raised in Chicago. When the tanks began to attack, Petersen's friend had grabbed him by the arm and shouted: 'It's 1940! Let's go to the Parliament building and defend it from the tanks! Let's throw ourselves in front of the tanks!'

Of course, Petersen, an American, thought this a bizarre idea, and had no desire to do anything so foolhardy. For the young Lithuanian émigré, however, the 'elastic scene' was that it was 1940 again but that this time they would stand up to the tanks in a way that had not happened back then. Burke's pentad for this example may be as follows:

- **Act:** 'Let's throw ourselves in front of the tanks to protect the Parliament building!'

- **Scene:** Vilnius, January 1991, but 'It's 1940!'

- **Agent:** Young Lithuanian émigré from Chicago who was born in the United States long after 1940.

- **Agency:** Internalized memories of 1940, life stories, cultural narratives, memories of memories that serve as tools that mediate his choice of actions. In contrast, Petersen had no such urge to act.

- **Purpose:** Defend one's homeland (in a way that had not happened in 1940) and to free one's people from occupation and oppression.

Semiotic mediators are pre-programmed psychological tools. Symbols such as language are psychological tools that mediate an individual's psychological processes, material tools mediate between the individual and nature. We construct reality through language, we initiate our children into our culture and until they have the self-awareness and self-control to monitor their own actions we mediate the process for them. The mediation between individuals is the development of intra-mental abilities through inter-mental social interaction. How mediated action and tools can be useful for our own purposes will begin to become clear as we introduce two additional concepts of Vygotsky's that explain how learning occurs.

7.7 Action theory, the zone of proximal development and scaffolding

> All functions of consciousness ... originally arise from action.
> (Vygotsky, 1978, p. 93)

Vygotsky's work is one example of the application of the application of 'action theory' to psychology. As we have described elsewhere, action theory – or, more accurately, action theories, since there is not one theory of human action, but several – suggests that 'human agency creates as well as is created by ... environmental conditions and events, and that action can materially change, as well as be caused by, the world; it can, in effect, create a world different from that which preceded it' (Davidson *et al.*, 2006, p. 1144). This was the theory of human action implicit in our previous chapter, in our discussion of the work of Martin Luther King, Jnr, and Gilles Deleuze (as is described elsewhere; Davidson and Shahar, 2007), and is the theory at the heart of Vygotsky's approach to learning. In fact, we could say, metaphorically, of course, that for Vygotsky, each new act of learning creates a new world for the individual who internalizes the experience. Actions that that person takes in the future will be informed and shaped by all that that person has experienced and learned in the past, with parallels occurring at the interpersonal and societal/cultural level (i.e. the world we create today has been informed and shaped by the worlds created previously by our ancestors). How this process actually occurs, and how learning produces new understandings and new worlds, is explained by Vygotsky through the two interrelated concepts of the 'zone of proximal development' and 'scaffolding'.

To understand these concepts, it may be helpful first to contrast what an action theory of learning is to what it is not. For Vygotsky, this involved challenging the passive and receptive theory of learning that he had inherited from his German colleagues, and which had given rise to use of the term 'kindergarten' to describe the setting in which children had their first formal experience of learning. The first year of school was described as a 'kindergarten' because psychologists had what Vygotsky described as a botanical view of learning: children were to be metaphorically watered, fed and kept warm by their teachers so that they could grow naturally, as flowers do in a garden. But maturation, Vygotsky argues, is not solely a passive process of taking in nutrients from the outside world; it requires the person's active engagement with the world (Vygotsky, 1978, p. 20). The use of cultural tools for mediated action is thus not a mechanistic or botanical phenomenon. Instead, people as agents are always sorting through and actively making choices about which tools they will and will not use and for what purposes. There exists a ubiquitous, irreducible dynamic tension in terms of the mediated action process, between the cultural tools and the active agents. Mediated action and mediational means are cultural tools (e.g. historical narratives, language genres) that people employ during the flow and constant flux of ongoing human action, which of course is always situated in specific cultural contexts (cf. Wertsch, 1998). Even the kindergarten student is a curious and creative person who 'takes in' the world, not as a passive recipient but as a goal-directed and purposeful actor who is involved in the unfolding of a broader, longitudinal 'plot'.

One of the more important ways in which young children learn is by observing and modelling the actions of others. This fact cannot be considered so obvious as to be overlooked, but is instead one of the first things about learning that we need to account for in our science. How does this work, exactly? What mechanisms are at play when children observe and model the behaviors of another person and thereby internalize, or appropriate, the behaviors as their own? To account for the possibility of learning in this way, Vygotsky first suggests that people are not only to be described in terms of what they can do on their own but also, and perhaps even more importantly, in terms of what they can do with the assistance of someone else. In other words, learning is not so much about the product, or the content learned, as it is about the fact that people constantly remain open to incorporating new actions and behaviors to which they are exposed, should they find those actions or behaviors to be of use to them for some relevant purpose. Intelligence, ability and mental maturation are therefore determined not so much by what a person has already learned but rather by what he or she is capable of learning given a rich and stimulating environment, with present learning building on previous learning and providing a foundation for future learning. As Vygotsky suggests, this view was not nearly so obvious:

> Over a decade even the profoundest thinkers never questioned the assumption; they never entertained the notion that what children can do with the assistance of others might be in some sense even more indicative of their mental development than what they can do alone. (Vygotsky, 1978, p. 85)

It was to capture these interpersonal and dynamic characteristics of learning that he proposed the concept of the 'zone of proximal development', which he defined as follows:

> The zone of proximal development ... is the distance between the actual developmental level as determined by independent problem

solving and the level of potential development as determined through problem solving under adult guidance or in collaboration with more capable peers ... The zone of proximal development defines those functions that have not yet matured but are in the process of maturation, functions that will mature tomorrow but are currently in an embryonic state. These functions could be termed the 'buds' or 'flowers' of development rather than the 'fruits' of development. The actual developmental level characterizes mental development retrospectively, while the zone of proximal development characterizes mental development prospectively. (Vygotsky, 1978, pp. 86–87; italics in the original)

One of the many reasons why this concept can be so important and useful for our purposes is because it helps to ensure that people with serious mental illnesses will not be viewed as having reached a dead end, or considered as unteachable or unable to learn new skills, behaviors and habits. On the other hand, it does not suggest that anyone can learn anything at any given time, but that people can learn those things that are within 'proximal' reach of their current level of development. In other words, it does not suggest that a fifth-grade student can learn calculus without first learning algebra and geometry, but it does suggest that a fifth-grade student can learn many things that he or she has not yet mastered with appropriate guidance and modelling. While it may be obvious when couched this way, since most fifth-graders go on to become sixth-graders and so on, its obviousness wears off a bit when applied to adults in general (i.e. 'you can't teach an old dog new tricks'), and wears off altogether when applied specifically to adults with serious mental illnesses (owing to stigma and discrimination). As Vygotsky writes:

A full understanding of the concept of the zone of proximal development must result in re-evaluation of the role of imitation in learning ... a person can imitate only that which is within her developmental level ... Using imitation, children are capable of doing much more in collective activity or under the guidance of adults. This fact, which seems to be of little significance in itself, is of fundamental importance in that it demands a radical alteration of the entire doctrine concerning the relation between learning and development. (Vygotsky, 1978, p. 88)

This 'radical alteration' suggests that development takes place *through* learning at the same time that development provides the foundation, and parameters, *for* new learning; one of Vygotsky's several uses of the Marxian dialectic. Understanding the function of the zone of proximal development thus encourages practitioners to begin to identify what new behaviors, what new skills or habits, are within this person's 'proximity' in terms of what he or she already knows and can do and, equally importantly, what new actions which build on current knowledge will he or she view as useful in pursuing his or her own agenda. For as one among many human activities, learning is also determined in part by the person's ongoing pursuits of his or her own interests and aspirations. If an adult with a serious mental illness appears to be stuck, appears not to be learning anything new, then perhaps that is in part a result of the fact that no one is showing him or her how to do new things that he or she is interested in learning. Chances are, or until proven otherwise, if such an adult were shown new actions that interested him or her and that were within proximity to what he or she already knew, then he or she might be able to learn and internalize those actions. Within psychiatry, this process helps to account for the success of the psychiatric rehabilitation approaches of supported housing, supported employment, supported education and supported socialization. People with serious mental illnesses – who in the past were considered incapable of independent living, working and friendships – can learn how to be a responsible tenant, a productive employee, a successful student and a good friend by being shown the way by a credible and trustworthy role model.

The zone of proximal development is thus the concept underlying the clichéd proverb from the Taoist tradition: 'If you give a man a fish, you have fed him for a day, if you teach a man to fish, you have fed him for a lifetime.' What is so revolutionary about this insight for our purposes is that you cannot expect a person to fish until you show him or her how. While, again, this may be obvious in the case of fishing, it loses its sense of obviousness when applied to the activities of daily life in which people with serious mental illnesses wish to participate – unless you happen to be an occupational therapist (about which we say more in the next section). One example from our own experience is the story of a woman with a serious mental illness who had been homeless for an extended period and about whom her outreach team was becoming increasingly concerned as the New England winter approached. Given her age, her health status and the winter conditions that were expected, she would likely die of exposure were she still living on the streets come December. The team therefore started early in the year trying to persuade her to accept safe and affordable housing, something which, for a variety of reasons, she was reluctant to agree to. After several months of trust building, showing her numerous apartments in numerous neighborhoods, and patiently listening to and trying to address all of her concerns, some paranoid and some not, the woman finally agreed to move into an apartment that was situated in her old neighborhood. The team celebrated this decision and enthusiastically shopped for furniture with the woman and helped her to move into this sparse, but comfortable, studio apartment.

The team was therefore understandably distraught and frustrated the next morning when they encountered the woman back on the street and saw that she had once again slept outdoors in her sleeping bag. After calming themselves down, and with persistent and patient enquiries, the outreach workers were able to determine that the woman had stayed in the apartment all evening by herself and had attempted to sleep there as well. What had happened was that she found that she could not fall asleep in the new bed purchased for her new apartment because of the heat in the apartment. The landlord had turned the thermostat up the day before to warm up the vacant apartment for its new tenant, and it had occurred to neither he nor the outreach staff to turn the thermostat down before leaving. As a result, by 10 o'clock that night, the apartment was a toasty 85° and the woman found it unbearable. She had, therefore, returned to what she knew and what she had done for the previous few years to manage her situation; she found a heating grate on a sidewalk and slept beside it in her sleeping bag. Why had she not turned down the thermostat herself? She did not know what a thermostat was, or what it was used for. The outreach staff did not think to show it to her and explain its use to her when they oriented her to the rest of the apartment, and when they were helping to move her in it was a comfortable 75°. They learned, however, to include thermostats in their future apartment orientations for people who had been homeless.

This is only one example of many that illustrate the central importance of attending to and assisting people with serious mental illnesses to learn about and internalize those 'obvious' aspects of everyday life that many of the rest of us take for granted. Additional examples are provided in an earlier publication (Davidson, 2007b) and in the remaining sections of this chapter. Before turning to them, though, it is important to introduce and explain the last of Vygotsky's key concepts (for our purposes), which is that of 'scaffolding'.

Scaffolding is the process by which one person supports another person to acquire new behaviors, skills and habits through use of the zone of proximal development. The person who facilitates the new learning may be a parent, teacher, mentor, coach or simply a 'more capable peer' (from Vygotsky's original definition above), basically anyone who has already learned the particular action to be learned by the other. This person carries out two interrelated and essential functions that facilitate the other's learning. These include (i) providing non-intrusive instruction or demonstration while encouraging the learner to carry out those parts of the tasks that are within his or her capacity and, at the same (ii) carrying out the remaining parts of the task him- or herself. It is the other's presence and performance of those aspects of the task that the learner cannot yet do that is referred to as 'scaffolding' (Wood and Middleton, 1975; Wood, Bruner and Ross, 1976). While Vygotsky did not himself give the concept this name, Jerome Bruner introduced the term to capture what he saw as implicit in Vygotsky's theory.

For Bruner, the necessity of scaffolding grew out of the fundamental tension within the zone of proximal development, which he describes as follows:

> On the one hand the zone of proximal development has to do with achieving 'consciousness and control'. But consciousness and control come only after one has already got a function well and spontaneously mastered. So how could 'good learning' be that which is in advance of development and, as it were, bound initially to be unconscious since un-mastered? (Bruner, 1985, p. 106)

Bruner's solution to this apparent paradox was to highlight and flesh out the role of the more experienced person, describing how that person provides not only the required instruction or demonstration but also the external structure necessary for the learner to be able to complete the task. External structure is necessary at this point in the learning process, because the person has yet to internalize the structure required by the focal action, since that structure will only be internalized through the process of learning the focal action itself. As a result, the person needs to have a scaffold in place to support his or her efforts until the structure can be successfully internalized. Calling the process 'scaffolding' for obvious reasons, Bruner saw it as a structured, incremental and temporary process, whereby the degree of support given was determined by the learner's need at any given point in time. The scaffold was constructed when needed and as needed to enable the learner to achieve, by having had a task or skill that was within proximal reach of the learner modelled, broken down into simpler, more accessible elements that could be built upon existing strengths, keeping motivation and stimulation high and then by gradually dismantling and withdrawing the support as it was no longer required. Once the scaffold is no longer needed and has been withdrawn, the person can then transfer the newly learned skill to a different context. Only then can the knowledge gained be considered abstract or 'decontextualized'. The skills and knowledge initially gained as a result of learning that has been scaffolded are an example of what Vygotsky called 'inter-mental learning', whereas, when the individual internalizes the learning and can generalize and therefore decontextualize the learning, they have accomplished what he considered 'intra-mental learning'. It is through this process of appropriating and internalizing the knowledge that people are then able to use these new tools in novel contexts, further extending their learning to new situations and challenges.

There are two final lessons that Vygotsky and his students and followers have learned about scaffolding and the zone of proximal development that we also will find useful. One is that learning, especially in the case of complex tasks, requires not only breaking down activities into their constituent parts and scaffolding but also repeating over a long period the acquisition of the complex behavior (Vygotsky, 1978, p. 57); practitioners often underestimate how long the acquisition of new habits may take. Second, people have difficulty learning new actions that they do not know about or expect not to be accessible to them, with learning following after the person coming to imagine what is possible, even when he or she cannot see it per se. In children, this is considered one of the valuable functions served by play, through which, according to Vygotsky, 'the child begins to act independently of what he sees' (Vygotsky, 1978, p. 97). In adults, particularly in those adults who might have become stuck in a chronic illness, it may take a similar action of imagining the possible to be able to undertake learning tasks that one either is not aware of needing or considers impossible. Scaffolding can play an extremely useful function in such cases, as a way of helping the person initiate a new series of actions that are unfamiliar or may seem daunting or overwhelming. With incremental successes, the person can then accrue confidence incrementally as well, building up his or her capacities gradually over time. Such notions as the zone of proximal development and scaffolding provide the needed conceptual bridges that enable people to go from doing very little to doing more and more over time, without having to accelerate from 0 to 60 mph in a few seconds, days or weeks. And one thing we know about recovery in serious mental illnesses is that it seldom occurs in days, weeks or even months, but is more a matter of incremental changes evolving over a number of years.

7.8 Applying activity analysis: the case of fossilized behavior

We noted above, in Chapter 5, that, along with Adolf Meyer, Vygotsky is credited with founding the discipline of occupational science and therapy. While with Meyer, his contributions to this new field might have been primarily philosophical, theoretical or conceptual (e.g. the emphasis on opportunities), with Vygotsky, his contributions extended to the level of practice and method as well. Given the centrality of personal agency and action to his theory of learning and development, Vygotsky applied his genetic, development and sociocultural method to the actions of individual actors through an approach that has come to be called 'activity analysis' (Vygotsky, 1981). Activity analysis has and continues to represent a core approach for occupational science and therapy (Hersch, Lamport and Coffey, 2005), and, therefore, will be very familiar to people trained in this field. Unfortunately, while occupational therapy basically grew up within the context of (institutional) psychiatry, its presence within mental health more broadly has significantly diminished with the closing of hospitals and other institutional settings. As such, most mental health practitioners, even those in psychiatric rehabilitation, will be unfamiliar with the concepts and methods involved in activity analysis. There currently are glimmers of hope that the recovery movement may bring about a bit of a renaissance of occupational science and therapy within psychiatry, such as the recent special issue of the *Psychiatric Rehabilitation Journal* (a leading journal in the field) on this topic (Pitts, 2009). We would heartily welcome such a development, and suggest that the recovery movement would have much to learn from this discipline.

This section will be devoted to beginning to demonstrate how activity analysis can be used as a key tool in the recovery-oriented practitioner's toolbox. Not being trained as occupational therapists, we do not claim a high degree of fidelity for the use we are describing of activity analysis to the way it is understood within that field. It also is possible that modifications will need to be made as activity analysis is tailored specifically to the needs and interests of people with serious mental illnesses. Regardless, we offer the following discussion as an initial attempt to apply Vygotsky's teachings to the challenge of assisting people with serious mental illnesses to reclaim their everyday lives in the community. In addition to our own work and thinking in this area, we draw on the excellent article by our good friends Krupa *et al.* (2009) in the recent special issue mentioned above. Their article, entitled 'Doing daily life: how occupational therapy can inform psychiatric rehabilitation practice', provides key concepts and principles for practice at the levels of the individual, the environment and the community at large (reminiscent of Jane Addams' focus on multiple levels simultaneously), and is highly recommended for readers whose imagination is piqued by what they will read in this section.

The basic framework for activity analysis has already been provided for us by Goffman's dramaturgical or Burke's dramatistic perspective. We are interested in viewing human behaviors and experiences as parts of an ongoing narrative in which the person in question is viewed as the protagonist. While some individuals with prolonged psychiatric disabilities may no longer view themselves as being in this role (i.e. the protagonist of their own story), helping them to reclaim that status in their own lives can be a crucial early step in their recovery (Davidson, 2003). Regardless of how people may view the origins of their own experiences and behavior, the recovery-oriented practitioner begins with the assumption that each person is, in fact, the protagonist (and eventually, hopefully, the hero) in his or her own life story. The questions that remain regarding any particular activity in question, whether problematic or desired, are: 'What is the activity?' (the act), 'Where is it to be performed?' (the scene), 'How is it to be performed?' (agency) and 'Why is it to be performed?' (purpose).

Any activity can be dissected into these constituent elements, and doing so can serve two related purposes. Problematic behaviors or experiences can be traced to their origins in the previous experiences and situations from which they emerged, helping to liberate the person from their influence over the present (an insight of Meyer's couched in more 'common sense' language than Freud's is). Desired behaviors or experiences can likewise be deconstructed into their constituent parts so that people can begin to develop the repertoires of micro-decisions and micro-actions (Davidson and Strauss, 1995) that will be required for them to eventually carry out the complete series of action involved. We offer one example of each below.

A particularly useful concept of Vygotsky's when it comes to behaviors that a person considers problematic for him- or herself – but not necessarily behavior of one person that another person views as problematic – is that of what he describes as 'the problem of *fossilized* behavior' (Vygotsky, 1978, p. 63; italics in the original). As its name suggests, fossilized behaviors are behaviors that once were 'alive', once fulfilled an important function in the person's life, but which have since left merely a residue of what they once were. The person may continue the behavior even though he or she no longer actively wishes to, or despite the fact that it no longer fulfils any specific function, but because it has become habituated to the point of almost being reflexive. On the other hand, the person may continue a behavior without conscious awareness of why he or she is doing so, viewing the behavior perhaps *as* a fossil, while all the while the behavior continues to serve some undisclosed purpose of which the person is no longer aware.

Suggesting that a person may not be aware of his or her purpose in performing a given action does not necessarily require viewing the purpose or motivation of the behavior as being 'unconscious' in the psychodynamic sense. Vygotsky suggests, rather, that most of the purposes and motivations of our behaviors, as well as the tacit knowledge of how to carry them out, are not things we are necessarily aware of at the time that they are performed. Much of human life goes on outside of our conscious awareness, which can only process a few things at a time. Using cell phones while driving might have challenged our abilities to carry out too many cognitively intensive activities at the same time, but, short of that, it remains true that most of what we do we do *not* do consciously. Eating while reading the newspaper or talking to a friend, cooking while helping your children with their homework, reading or listening to music while exercising, planning what you will need for dinner while walking to the market, the list is endless, and this is not to mention those autonomic functions such as breathing, pumping blood through one's veins and so on.

One illustration of the utility of the concept of fossilized behavior is provided by a middle-aged man who had been diagnosed with schizophrenia around the age of 20 and who was being served by an outpatient clinic at a community mental health centre where we worked. The man was of African origin and was the only child in a single-parent family. He had graduated from high school but was unemployed, lived in his own apartment a few blocks from his mother, had few friends and spent most of his time alone. He heard angry, critical and threatening voices, often felt somewhat paranoid (afraid that the voices, or others, would hurt him in unspecified ways) and experienced some difficulty with concentration, attention and memory. He spoke slowly and softly and could appear to strangers (or mental health staff who did not know his history) to be developmentally disabled; he attributed his difficulties in conversations to the disruptive voices and his waxing and waning attention. He was a likeable and engaging man who appeared to be about 20 years younger than his 48 years and was otherwise considered by the staff who knew him to be rather unremarkable. In other words, he was considered at the time to be a 'chronic paranoid schizophrenic' who could expect little better out of life than what he had at the time. The staff had tried several different antipsychotic medications until they found one that he could tolerate relatively well (i.e. he did not complain), but it had a very limited impact on his symptoms. That done, the staff became resigned to providing ongoing maintenance care to see that he remained in his apartment, did not experience exacerbations of symptoms, took adequate care of his 'ADLs' (activities of daily living), and, most importantly, stayed out of the hospital. They didn't think there was much more they could do for him.

We will call this man Anthony. Anthony was unremarkable to the staff until he developed the problematic habit of frequenting the local hospital emergency room (ER) several nights a week. Not only was it burdensome for the staff to review the reports from the ER and have to place them in his medical record, but they were genuinely concerned about him and about what had happened that he now needed to visit the ER so frequently. In addition, the team leader was getting pressure from the agency's clinical director to stop Anthony from frequenting the ER, as it was both costly and he added to the burden of the already over-taxed ER staff, contributing to escalating wait times. The team leader passed this pressure on to Anthony's primary caregiver, his case manager, who tried her best to convince him that he did not need to visit the ER. Anthony did not report an increase in the severity, duration or intensity of his symptoms, and his case manager could not understand why all of a sudden he found these same symptoms to be too much to stand several nights a week. His psychiatrist was consulted, who recommended no changes in his medication, and the case manager implored Anthony not to go to the ER during the hours the clinic was closed. She would see him more regularly during clinic hours if that would help, but it did not. His frequent evening trips to the ER continued for several weeks more, at which time a consultant was brought in to try to address the situation.

In addition to getting to know him generally, the first thing the consultant did was to ask Anthony why he went to the ER. The case manager had, of course, asked Anthony this same question before, but she apparently had not pursued it further. Anthony's response was that he got scared of the voices and no longer felt safe alone in his apartment. The consultant probed further, asking what made Anthony think of the ER as the place to go when he no longer felt safe. There were, after all, other things Anthony could do in that situation, such as take a walk, call a friend or his mother, turn on the television, call the on-call clinician for the clinic and so on. What was it about the ER that made it seem like the best place to go? Anthony responded that that was where he felt safest. It was the same ER to which his mother had taken him 25 years earlier when he was first told what the voices were, and it was the same ER where he knew most of the staff and where they were nice to him and treated him well. They never told him to leave, they always allowed him to stay until he felt better, they chatted with him, offered him snacks, let him watch television and, in general, made him feel welcome. To Anthony, the ER was more like an extension of his living room than a costly health care unit designed and staffed to address trauma. Rather than being a deterrent, the noise level of the ER drowned out the voices and allowed him to relax, confident that there were people there who would look out for him and comfortable with his distant, but amiable, relationship with the staff there.

While painting this picture of Anthony's ER use – the what (act), the where (scene), the how (agency) and the why (purpose) of his presumably problematic behavior – was useful to the consultant, it didn't by itself suggest a course of corrective action. First of all, did Anthony see that there was any problem with this particular behavior? Was this a satisfactory solution for a way to handle the threatening voices and to feel safe, or might Anthony consider an alternative strategy? In respecting Anthony as an equal (a fellow human being), and in wishing to maintain transparency, the consultant shared with Anthony the staff's concerns about the behavior, its costs, the burden on the ER staff and so on; but the case manager had already found that these reasons were not sufficient to alter Anthony's behavior. Was there also a way in which this behavior was not totally satisfactory to Anthony? Was there a reason for him to change it as well? The key to understanding this aspect of the situation lay in why Anthony had started to frequent the ER now, as opposed to previously. If the symptoms were in fact the same as before, what had changed? Why had he started to visit the ER now, when he first went there 25 years ago and only infrequently since?

In pursuing these questions, the consultant discovered that, in the past, Anthony had spent several evenings a week at his mother's apartment watching television and drinking coffee with her. These visits had stopped recently, as his mother had 'taken up' with a man whom Anthony did not like, and who, at least according to Anthony, did not care for him either. As a result of his mother's budding relationship, Anthony was no longer welcome as often at his mother's place, especially in the evenings when her boyfriend had finished work and wanted to spend time with her. Anthony agreed that he would rather be at his mother's apartment than in the ER on these evenings, but this was no longer an option. The consultant asked Anthony if he would be interested in meeting with his mother and the consultant to discuss the situation, to which he readily agreed. He did not expect his mother to change her mind, but he responded favorably to the consultant's suggestion that there still might be other options to explore. His mother, the consultant suggested, might not have appreciated the impact this change was having on her son.

When they came together for the three-way meeting, it became apparent rather quickly that Anthony's mother did not, in fact, have any idea of the impact her relationship was having on her son. He had said nothing to her about it, and she had no idea he was spending several of his evenings a week in the ER of the local hospital. On the other hand, she complained about the fact that Anthony was now coming to her apartment in the middle of the day to have her do his laundry for him. She did not understand why a man his age could not do his own laundry. When the consultant asked both Anthony and his mother how his laundry had been done previously, Anthony's mother acknowledged that she had been doing it all along; it's just that in the past she had done it in the evenings while they were both watching television. Now that he was no longer coming around in the evenings, Anthony reasoned that the only way to get his laundry done was to bring it to his mother's during the day. Anthony's mother did not like this aspect of the new arrangement, and wanted Anthony to finally learn how to do his own laundry. This first meeting ended amicably, with both Anthony and his mother agreeing that they wanted to continue their close relationship despite her new boyfriend, but unsure of how best to do so. Meanwhile, Anthony's visits to the ER continued.

The following week, the consultant followed up with Anthony about the laundry issue, asking if he would be interested in learning how to do his own laundry. At first, Anthony complained that he had tried in the past but was unable to do so, just like he was unable to do so many other things. When the consultant asked Anthony how he knew that he was unable, he reported that he and his case manager had tried to tackle this problem before and had failed. The case manager had first explained to Anthony how to do his laundry, even drawing pictures for him in her office of where to put the quarters, which buttons to push and so on. Anthony had even taken these drawings with him to the Laundromat in his neighborhood, but the machines there didn't match the pictures and there were no instructions. He didn't feel like asking anybody, because then they would know that he was a 'mental patient' – everyone else just seemed to know what to do. Then his case manager had even gone with him to the Laundromat, showed him how to buy the soap, where to put the quarters and so on, but then she left and he felt uncomfortable being there by himself. What if something went wrong with the machines? He had seen things like that on television. What if he put in too much soap? He didn't want to be like Lucille Ball with the soap bubbles coming out of the washing machine. So he took his wet and dirty clothes and went home, and he hadn't been back since.

Would he go back to the Laundromat with the consultant, especially if he agreed to stay until the laundry was done? No, then people would think that he, Anthony, was gay (the consultant was male), and he didn't want that. Would he go back to the

Laundromat with the case manager, if she agreed to stay until the laundry was done? No, she'd already taken him once and he wasn't a child. He didn't need anyone to hold his hand. What was so wrong about his mother doing his laundry at her apartment? That way he didn't even have to pay for it. It was bad enough that he couldn't visit in the evenings any more, but not to be able to have his laundry done too, that seemed like too much to ask. Was she trying to get rid of him altogether? Did she want him roaming about town in dirty clothes? Was she too busy to do that one little thing for him?

In this train of questions, the consultant thought he heard some of the hurt that Anthony's mother's new relationship was undoubtedly causing him. The consultant wondered, out loud, if perhaps Anthony thought that if he didn't have dirty laundry for her to do perhaps he would have no reason, or perhaps no excuse, for being at his mother's apartment. If she weren't doing his laundry any more, would she do anything for him? If he weren't hanging around while his laundry was being cleaned, would he ever see his mother at all? These questions resonated with Anthony, who clearly was worried that he was losing his mother to her new boyfriend, and who saw his dirty laundry as one of the few connections he still had to her. At this point, the consultant suggested a second meeting with Anthony's mother to explore options for their continued relationship. In preparation for this meeting, the consultant asked Anthony if perhaps he would prefer that his mother be the one to teach him how to do his own laundry. Perhaps she didn't mind his being in the apartment; perhaps she would even like his being in the apartment, as long as she didn't have to do his laundry. Anthony thought this an idea worth pursuing.

In the second meeting, Anthony proposed his plan of having his mother teach him how to do his own laundry, asking also if she would allow him to continue to do the laundry in her place as long as he did it himself. She thought this a splendid idea and was happy to show him how to do it, and happy for his company. She was surprised to hear that Anthony was afraid of losing her to her boyfriend, reassuring him of her love for him and the fact that this budding romance did not change in any way her feelings about or commitment to him. This brought Anthony back to the evenings he used to spend with her watching television and drinking coffee. She agreed that she missed seeing him more often also and was happy to consider other activities they could do together. Since her boyfriend worked during the day, and since Anthony was not currently working, there was no reason why they could not spend more time together during the day. She reiterated that what she was not interested in was doing his laundry, but she was interested in doing other things with him, like going shopping, going to the movies or simply watching television and drinking coffee while *he* did his own laundry. This appeared to be an alternative he could accept.

But what did any of this have to do with Anthony's frequent ER visits? On the surface, it seemed like Anthony was going to the ER when he felt unsafe and threatened by the auditory hallucinations that were part of a mental illness. Were this the whole story, then a solution might be found in helping Anthony to identify other ways of dealing with the voices and his feelings of being unsafe alone in his apartment, such as calling a friend, taking a walk or perhaps even participating in cognitive-behavioral psychotherapy through which he would learn how to manage these voices more effectively. And all of these options were worth considering. In Anthony's case, however – as is true in much of human experience – this one action of frequenting the ER was multidetermined and not nearly so simple. The voices had not changed after all; what had changed was his way of dealing with the voices. Understanding that this was the activity of interest (i.e. handling the voices by going to the ER) opened up possibilities for a richer and more intricate narrative to evolve, out of which the consultant and Anthony were both able to identify several new options to pursue in addressing his multiple purposes (e.g. spending time with his mother as well as feeling safe).

The consultant's main role was to identify what Anthony was trying to achieve (a continued relationship with his mother) and to identify or create new opportunities for Anthony to take advantage of, should he decide to do so. While real life is seldom this straightforward, it did turn out that by spending a few afternoons a week with his mother, either at her apartment or doing activities with her, Anthony then felt less lonely in the evenings and no longer found it necessary to go to the ER for company. The underlying story that was elicited did, in fact, have everything to do with Anthony's problematic use of the ER. This story would not have been elicited, however, were Anthony not viewed as actively making decisions, actively pursuing his own purposes and falling back on fossilized behaviors in the face of adversity in the process.

7.9 Applying activity analysis: using the zone of proximal development

> Play creates a zone of proximal development. (Lev Vygotsky, 1978, p. 102)

Mental health staff working with individuals with serious mental illnesses may be frustrated just as much by their perceived failure to 'motivate' their patients or to convince their patients to try new things as they are by such 'problematic' behaviors as frequenting ERs (or refusing to take medication, or not showing up for appointments, or being unwilling to take care of themselves in ways staff think appropriate, etc.). Especially now that mental health practitioners are attempting to shift their practice to a recovery orientation, we often hear complaints that their patients don't want to try new things, don't want to take risks, don't have goals or aspirations and so on. In response to this common perception and frustration, we choose to close this chapter with one such example in which a practitioner was frustrated with her patient's apparent unwillingness to do something that the practitioner knew to be extremely important. This example was suggested by a participant in a training seminar on recovery-oriented practice, and seemed to be useful to her and her colleagues, and so we use it here as well.

The following story provides, of course, only one example of how activity analysis can be useful in helping people with serious mental illnesses take part in new activities, occupy new roles and develop new habits. Any action can be subjected to this same analytic approach, and many will generate an equally impressive array of micro-decisions and micro-actions involved in what otherwise looks like a simple or trivial task. One of the main things we think we have learned about recovery thus far, however, is that much of the process involves learning how to do precisely those things that other people, who do not have a mental illness, take for granted in their everyday lives (Borg and Davidson, 2007; Davidson, 2007b).

In this case, a young woman of Hispanic origin, whom we will call Mira, desperately needed a pair of glasses, but refused to go to the eyeglass store in order to be fitted for them. Owing to Mira's increasing difficulties with her vision, her case manager had arranged for the eye examination and for Mira's mother to accompany her to the ophthalmologist's office. Now that Mira had the prescription for the glasses, the case manager initially assumed that Mira would follow through with getting the glasses so that she could once again see clearly. In the case manager's experience, that was simply what one does when one needs glasses – one goes and gets them so that one can once again see clearly, vision being highly valued in most cultures. In Mira's case, there also was the added complication that the doctor had encouraged Mira both to get and to wear the glasses every day, all the time, as she was concerned that Mira's vision appeared to be deteriorating. Were the problem not corrected, and were Mira not to begin to use her eyes again and exercise the appropriate muscles, she could very well lose her vision altogether. This concern was conveyed both to Mira and to Mira's mother, and made her case manager's insistence that Mira get the glasses and wear them all the more urgent. Perhaps Mira did not understand the significance of what the doctor had told her, the case manager at first reasoned; she did, after all, have a major mental illness. But then her mother surely should understand and should insist on her getting the glasses. No progress was made over a period of several months, and the case manager did not know what else she could do.

In this case, it was helpful for the case manager to take a breath and step back from the frustrating situation in order to consider what might be involved in Mira getting her new glasses. In other words, why might Mira *not* get the glasses? What does this do for her? What is she doing when she is not going to get the glasses, and what function does that serve? What would she have to change in her life in order to go and get and wear new glasses, and what might keep her from wanting to make such a change? All of these are ways of raising the dramaturgical question of what is the story behind this one particular activity, an activity which in this case is the focus of the practitioner's interest not because the patient is doing it but precisely because the patient is not doing it (when the practitioner thinks he or she *should* be doing it). Once again, this approach is not sufficient when the activity in question is something that only one person wants another person to do, when the second person is not interested him- or herself. That would bring us into the even more complex territory of interpersonal relationships (beyond that between the practitioner and the patient). So, for the sake of this example, let us assume that Mira agrees with the case manager that she does in fact need the glasses and that getting the glasses is something that she would like to do. What gets in her way?

In order to answer this central question, the case manager will need to take a microscope to the phenomenon of interest and dissect it into its constituent parts. For example, if we work backwards from buying the glasses, the first thing that Mira would need to do would be to pay for them. Does Mira know how she is going to pay for the glasses? Are they covered by her health insurance (in this case Medicaid), and if they are, does Mira know that? Does she know how to pay for the glasses using her Medicaid card? Will she have to pay out of pocket and then get reimbursed, and, if so, does she have the money to do so? If not, will showing her Medicaid card suffice for payment, or are there only certain glasses that Medicaid will pay for and others that it will not (i.e. is there a pre-determined limit for eyeglass coverage)? If Mira's Medicaid covers only certain glasses, how will she know which ones they are? And how will she figure out how much the glasses will cost when the lenses and frames each have their own price? If she asks the salesperson about what Medicaid will cover, will that tip everyone off in the store that Mira is poor and/or mentally ill? Will they even accept Medicaid patients? Will they ask her to leave, or escort her out of the store, as the manager did of that one apparel store she was in a few years ago when the woman told her that she couldn't 'loiter', whatever that meant.

Let's assume, for the sake of this argument, that Mira understands Medicaid and what it will pay for and is not concerned about being kicked out of the store. Backing up from actually purchasing the glasses, what else is involved? Once Mira picks out a frame that she likes, which may itself feel like an overwhelming task – being confronted with wall after wall of frames and being able to choose only one – she will then have to be fitted for the glasses by the salesperson. When was the last time Mira was that close to a stranger? When was the last time Mira allowed anyone, other than her own family, to touch her face or hair? What if she had to look in the mirror in order to see how the glasses looked? She didn't like looking in the mirror, didn't like what she saw when she did – and now to have to do that in front of a stranger!

The salesperson would undoubtedly ask Mira questions. Would she be able to answer the questions? Would she understand the questions to begin with? What if she took her mother with her? Would her mother be able to answer the questions? Her mother had never worn glasses, what could she know? And would people wonder why a woman her age needed her mother to go with her to buy glasses? Would that tip people off to the fact that she had a mental illness? Would they ask her to leave the store because she had a mental illness? The woman at the apparel store had no other reason to ask her to leave that she could think of; what would keep that from happening again? Even if she could answer the questions, how could she pick out the frames to begin with? The reason that she needed glasses was that she couldn't see; so how could she see to pick out the glasses? The doctor is the crazy one if she thinks that I can see well enough to pick out glasses. If I could, then I wouldn't need them. What didn't she just give me a pair when I was in her office? That would have been much better than just giving me this slip of paper with scribbles on it. What makes her think that the salesperson will be able to read her scribbles? They may kick me out just for that, for having a scribbly doctor.

Assuming Mira could manage picking out and being fitted for glasses, how would she first manage to get to the store? Does Mira drive? If not, does she have transportation to the glasses store? Where is the store? If the store is in the mall, how does Mira feel about going to the mall? Mira used to hang out with her friends in this mall before her illness started. Would she be comfortable going back to the mall now, under these circumstances? Does she go to the mall already, or has she not been back since she dropped out of high school because of her illness? What if she ran into her old friends at the mall, would she know what to do? Would she be comfortable running into people she used to know? The mall has security guards in uniform posted at entry ways; how does Mira feel about being around men in uniforms? Has Mira had prior experiences with the police that would make her afraid of the security guards? Would Mira know how to find the glasses store in the mall? Does Mira have clothes that she would consider appropriate to wear to the mall? What will she say when she walks into the store and a salesperson approaches her and asks: 'How are you today?' or 'How may I help you?' or 'Are you looking for anything in particular today?' and so on (or whatever glasses salespeople say when you walk into their store)?

Prior to embarking on what is appearing now to be an adventure fraught with some risk, what is involved in Mira's decisions of whether to go to the glasses store? What would having to wear glasses say about, or mean to, Mira? What has been her experience with glasses in the past? Has she ever worn them before? If not, has she known people who have? If so, who were they? Were they people she admired, or perhaps people who were made fun of at school? What would she use the glasses for? Currently, in part because her vision is so poor, Mira does not leave the house very often and when she does she is often accompanied by her mother – or, more accurately, she accompanies her mother on her mother's own errands and activities. Her family does not currently expect much from Mira, because of her mental illness and her poor vision. If her vision were corrected, would they start to expect more? What would that more be? Would they start expecting her to go out by herself? Or, on the contrary, would her father start to put more limits on what she could do if she started to become more independent? What would people at church think of her? God is supposed to heal the sick, and they've been praying for Him to correct her vision, the way Jesus did in the Bible. Would wearing glasses mean that she had turned her back on God? That she had given up? Does she see anybody else wearing glasses at church? Only the little old ladies who are hunched over. Would wearing glasses make her one of them? Would she ever get a boyfriend if she wore glasses? She has trouble keeping track of things already, would she be able to keep track of a pair of glasses? And what would happen if she lost the glasses? She remembers how angry her father got when she flushed her medication down the toilet, not because she wasn't taking them but because of how much they cost. What if she lost, or broke, a $200 pair of glasses? How angry would he be then?

As the reader might have surmised, this list of questions could go on for several more pages, as we take more and more of Mira's life story into account and the role that a pair of glasses may or may not play within that context. It is obviously not reasonable, or required, for a practitioner to go through all of these, and many other related, questions in any one instance. These are only examples of the kinds of questions that are raised by a psychiatric use of activity analysis, incorporating personal, interpersonal and social dimensions as well as the traditional focus on functional capacities and material resources. What is most crucial about the generation of such questions is that they place us more in Mira's shoes, give us more of a sense of her own perspective on the situation, than a mere objective or task analysis might. There are, of course, other ways to empathically join with Mira and her struggles. Some approaches may be taken from the psychotherapy tradition and others, perhaps, from acting (Andres-Hyman, Strauss and Davidson, 2007). The advantage of this type of activity analysis for psychiatric rehabilitation is that it opens up and situates the focal activity within Vygotsky's 'zone of proximal development'. Buying glasses is apparently something Mira cannot do on her own. Is it perhaps something she can do with 'guidance or in collaboration with more capable peers' (Vygotsky, 1978, pp. 86–87)?

This use of the zone of proximal development as a way to facilitate the learning of new skills through supported participation in new activities gives additional theoretical weight to the notion and use of peer support in recovery-oriented practice. As we noted above, it also helps to account for the effectiveness of such psychiatric rehabilitation interventions as supported housing, supported employment, supported education and supported socialization. People with serious mental illnesses can learn how to be responsible tenants, productive employees, successful students and good friends by being shown the way by credible role models. Who better to accompany Mira to the glasses store than someone else who has had a mental illness and has tackled many of the same concerns that we imagine Mira to have? Peer staff may not need to generate the same kind of list of micro-concerns, micro-decisions and micro-actions that we have just done because they have had similar first-hand experiences. They know what it's like to be approached by a stranger when you're not sure you'll know how to respond, how to tolerate having a stranger touch your face and hair for the first time in many years and, perhaps most importantly, how to negotiate the Medicaid system without feeling embarrassed or humiliated. Offering this type of experiential expertise, whether through their own practice or by sensitizing non-peer staff to the importance of these issues, may be one of the most important contributions peer services make to our systems of mental health care as they transform to a recovery orientation.

7.10 Summary of lessons learned

From this review of the work of Sen and Vygotsky, we suggest the following lessons:

- Now that most people with serious mental illnesses are no longer living their lives within the confines of institutions, it is important to recognize that they are always already making choices and decisions as they go about living their lives with mental illnesses in the community. Human beings are active agents in their own lives.

- The freedom and autonomous agency that are the birthrights of citizens of democratic societies extend to individuals with serious mental illnesses unless extreme circumstances have led to these rights being temporarily suspended in the case of serious, imminent risk or curtailed by a judge in the case of incapacity.

- For choice to be free people have to have the latitude to decide what they want based on their own values, preferences, interests and life history, as well as based on available resources.

- Free choice necessarily generates diversity as a primary, rather than secondary, aspect of human nature. Diversity cannot be attended to later, but must be part and parcel of the nature of our work from the very beginning.

- In adopting a capabilities framework, the focus of our efforts shifts from what people have to what they can do, to the *actual living* that people manage to achieve.

- Transformation efforts need to be led by the recovery community if one form of oppression is not simply to be replaced by another.

- Learning is an active process that can be facilitated by other people through the use of 'scaffolding' within the 'zone of proximal development'.

- People with serious mental illnesses may need to, and can, learn how to perform actions that other people take for granted as 'obvious' aspects of everyday life. In such cases, learning can occur incrementally through modelling and may require an extended period to be consolidated into new habits.

Lessons to avoid repeating:

- Time in the community is not the same as a life in the community. There is more to recovery than staying out of hospitals and jails.

- Active participation in community life as a contributing citizen cannot be viewed as, or reserved for, the reward of recovery, but rather provides the foundation for recovery.

- One person cannot give freedom to another person, nor can one person set the criteria for another person's freedom (unless sanctioned by law).

- People cannot be required to have a certain amount of normalcy, resources or skills in order to take up and pursue recovery. Just as no country is too poor for democracy, no person is too ill or disabled to be in recovery. The question is: 'What supports does this person require in order to be able to *do* what he or she wants to do?'

- What a person can do is not as limited by what he or she is currently doing as by the nature of the environment and opportunities the person has to pursue his or her interests.

8
Conclusion

The Meeting of the Minds was a US television show that ran from 1977 to 1981. In this show, the host, Steve Allen, would have chosen several historical figures, had actors dress up in costumes representing the periods and cultures from which they had come and have them seated around an oval table. He would have written the script based on writings of and about these figures, and he would have them engage in an imaginary dialogue that would highlight the unique contributions and accomplishments of each. To a budding young intellectual (LD), this provided much grist for the reflective mill and was a far better source of mental stimulation than trying to read the original works of these masters, some of which dated back to antiquity. There never seemed to be much order or reason to the selections for a given week, as Benjamin Franklin might be talking about electricity and/or democracy to St Thomas Aquinas and Cleopatra, for example. But the conversations were invariably interesting as well as entertaining, and it seemed a good way for young people to be introduced to the history of ideas. Apparently, not many young people took advantage of this particular opportunity, though, as it was a short-lived show, and Steve Allen went on to bigger and better projects.

The show left quite an impression on at least one of us (LD), however, and we have resurrected the format for our concluding chapter. In our case, of course, there is a consistency to our selection of key figures, as they are the people with whose work we have been concerned in the previous seven chapters, and our common topic is recovery from and in relation to serious mental illnesses. Aside from that difference, and the fact that there is no interlocutor or facilitator for the discussion (i.e. the role played by Allen), we have borrowed from Allen the essential ingredients of this venue for expressing and exploring the ideas of our great thinkers and doers.

We chose this format not only out of sentimentality for the golden days of childhood but also because we think it premature to try to integrate all of the concepts and approaches of these diverse people into one, single model for recovery-oriented practice. As we suggested in our introductory chapter, there is an inevitable tension between some of these approaches. These tensions are not only the result of obvious sources of disagreement between people, such as the clear

The Roots of the Recovery Movement in Psychiatry   Larry Davidson, Jaak Rakfeldt, John Strauss
© 2010 John Wiley & Sons, Ltd

difference in opinion about the role of the state hospital, retreat or asylum between Dorothea Dix and Franco Basaglia. The tensions are also evident between two individuals whose thoughts are for the most part highly compatible, and at times even within one thinker's perspective. One such tension is that between the rights and responsibilities of citizenship, exemplified perhaps by Gilles Deleuze on the side of rights and Jane Addams on the side of social responsibilities. A similar tension can be found between the development of personal identity (Vygotsky and Sen) and the cultivation of social relationships (Meyer and Sullivan). Neither can exist without the other, but neither can be reduced to the other either. It is for this reason that we have chosen an interactive and dynamic format for our conclusion, as we do not yet see a way of bringing all of these themes and concepts together into one static snapshot. Life is full of tensions and apparent contradictions, and so is our conclusion. Perhaps recovery-oriented care can be characterized, in part, by the degree to which it preserves, or avoids coming to premature closure on, these very tensions.

Our suggestion to the reader in terms of this chapter comes from something we think we learned from Adolf Meyer. In his spirit of pragmatism, we suggest that you take the parts of the following dialogue that work for you, that make sense of some aspect of your experience, and leave the rest. This dialogue could go on for many more pages, but it had to end somewhere. The reader is welcome to pick it up where we leave off and take it in his or her own direction.

DIX: I appreciate being invited back to witness the state of affairs at the end of this first decade of the twenty-first century, but I must say it is depressing to see so many people with serious mental illnesses languishing, once again, in jails, prisons and what you now call 'board and care homes'. This was the travesty we tried to correct a century and a half ago, and look how little progress has been made! Part of me thinks I may just need to start over and go through the whole thing again. It looks as though I failed.

GOFFMAN: With all due respect, Ms Dix, before you start advocating for re-opening the hospitals, you might stop to consider that that strategy didn't work very well the first time. No one questions your intentions, of course, but the hospitals you helped to create never offered the respite and recuperation you had planned, nor did they offer the kind of treatment which you advocated. Even if they did at first, the care you had wanted them to provide was quickly outstripped by the dumping of thousands of people into them whom society did not want. That just wasn't a workable solution to the problem of mental illness.

DIX: It would have been had President Pierce signed the legislation which I fought so hard to pass. If only Congress had acted sooner, when Millard Fillmore had still been president, all of that wouldn't have happened. The federal government would have provided adequate funds for mental health care and the hospitals would not have become warehouses.

PINEL: I'm afraid that it would have taken more than adequate funding to
            create truly therapeutic hospitals, though. It seems to me that you
            folks lost sight of what you were trying to do. You were supposed to
            be offering comfort and solace to people in distress, involvement in
            meaningful activity to people who had become unmoored from their
            everyday lives and companionship to people who had found the harsh
            realities of the world to be too much for their exquisitely developed
            sensitivity. Your hospitals weren't doing any of those things!

TUKE: We tried to do those things, and some other extremely important
            things besides, like bring people back into conversation with their
            Maker, cultivate their spirit and instil them with healthy self-discipline.
            We tried to offer them another chance to become fully human by
            promoting their use of reason and enhancing their self-mastery.

SULLIVAN: What made you think that that was what people with serious mental
            illnesses needed? What made you think that they were less human
            to begin with? That attitude just made things worse for them. You
            took a vulnerable, distressed and highly sensitive population and
            just stamped on their feet, on their heads and all over their souls.
            They didn't need you to be their parents; they already had their own
            parents, and, believe me, once was probably already too much. If
            anything, they suffered from other people's efforts to shape them
            in their own likeness, and you made that your institutional mission.
            There was nothing therapeutic about your retreats.

TUKE: That is not a fair criticism, Dr Sullivan, and ignores the fact that we
            had an 80–90% recovery rate for the people in our care, when they had
            been ill for less than a year at admission. How can you say that what we
            did didn't work when it so clearly did? The proof was in the pudding.

STRAUSS: Unfortunately, I think you did not factor in the rate of spontaneous
            recovery during the first year after onset of a psychotic disorder.
            It is quite possible that the people you admitted so early after the
            onset of their disorder would have improved anyway, without your
            assistance. The rates at which people improve seem to have more to
            do with factors outside of treatment than with treatment itself. Maybe
            you provided a supportive environment in which it became possible
            for people to find their own ways out of psychosis. That would be
            worthwhile also, even if some aspects of your approach weren't that
            effective in and of themselves.

SULLIVAN: Yes, well, we know that it is the relationship between the patient
            and the doctor that is the most important treatment-related factor
            in promoting recovery. Maybe the willingness you showed to accept
            people and to treat them as worthwhile and capable of civilized

company made a difference. Maybe they felt loved and valued with you, when they hadn't before.

DELEUZE: What makes you think that they hadn't been loved and valued before? The only reason they were referred to your hospitals was because they didn't respect and honor your parochial version of bourgeois society and the demands it placed on their desire. It's just as likely that they were loved and valued too much, if there can be such a thing, so much that they didn't feel beholden to you and your authority and refused to become part of the anonymous mass of producers. Then you took them in and re-engineered them so that they would fit the mould, the mould that should have been thrown away to begin with. Why did they have to learn manners and etiquette? Surely not because of mummy and daddy's failures to love them?

BASAGLIA: I agree. And as long as we have mental hospitals, we will continue to fill them with people who don't fit the mould. That way society can at least justify the existence of such people based on the fact that their re-engineering offers employment opportunities for others. How can keeping someone in an institution help to restore their sanity, or mental health, when it denies the very capacity they need to be exercising in order to be healthy: their autonomous agency? Your grandfather, Mr Tuke, did not help people to feel loved, or to recover, as much as he did to help them learn how to get by in the workaday world of industrial capitalism.

KING: Even so, these were people in distress and people who, like most of us, wanted to fit in and to have a decent life. Not everyone wants to be on his or her own; we all want to be part of something bigger than ourselves. That's part of what makes us human. What concerns me more is what people may have to give up or tolerate in order *to* fit in. Our job shouldn't be to fix them, but rather to fix us. We can create a society in which people already fit in, and already fill the mould, just by being human, by being who they already are. That was one of the mistakes your field made early in its history: assuming that if someone didn't fit in then it must be that person's fault, or that person who needs to be changed, when in reality it was the country that needed to change. We still have a long way to go in learning how to respect people for who they are and accept them on their own terms.

MEYER: While I certainly do not disagree with a word of what you have said, Reverend, I am afraid that we are losing sight of the properly psychiatric dimension of this problem. Society, culture, community, capitalism, all of these are certainly important as providing the context for what we consider to be 'mental disorders', but they alone do not provide a complete picture. The people we are talking about are having significant difficulties negotiating their everyday lives in our shared world. They want what we want, no more and no less, but they have difficulty in achieving such an ordinary life. I agree that there appears to be something going on between the individual and his or her environment that produces a poor fit, but I don't think that society, capitalism, industrialism or any widespread cultural issue can be the answer. If it were, then why wouldn't everyone appear to be 'mentally ill'? The fact is that we just don't know yet why some people develop so-called mental disorders and others do not. The best we can do is to help them make the most of the life that they have, while we are tying to figure out how to implement your noble vision.

GOFFMAN: While you are doing that, Dr Meyer, I hope that you are not advocating opening more hospitals or sending people away to some artificial setting in order to help them out. We have learned repeatedly that when they come back they are no better off than when they left. Rescuing them from the situation in which they encounter such a poor fit doesn't change the situation or the fact that they eventually return to it, and the problems come back as well.

PINEL: What do you propose then? These are people in pain we are talking about, at times terrible and immobilizing pain. Do you not think that they need intervention?

ADDAMS: They certainly can benefit from intervention; I don't think anyone would disagree with that notion. The questions are: what kind of intervention, by whom and to what ends. I agree that sending people off to some faraway place that doesn't resemble their everyday lives will have little utility in addressing their difficulties. While the situation is definitely part of the problem, the answer is to be found in changing the situation rather than escaping from it. We have had much success *in bringing the help to the person rather than trying to bring the person to the help*. Without having to change the entire society, we can intervene and help the person to change his or her situation on an individual basis. And it is key that the person be the one to identify the situation and to decide how best to alter it. We can't know ahead of time what will be best for that person, only he or she can know. Our job is to support the person in making those decisions and implementing them. They have to do the hard work themselves.

BASAGLIA: On the individual level, I would agree with you, Ms Addams. But I would think from your own life's work that you would also have to agree that the society as a whole could be changed as well. We had much success in changing people's attitudes towards mental illness and in creating a welcoming and accepting culture in northern Italy. People were accepted for who they were and not forced to change to suit anyone else. And you, of all people, can attest to the power of social change to reduce human misery and resolve myriad problems that people can face in difficult circumstances.

ADDAMS: Yes, of course, Doctor, I would agree with that as well. I think you have to begin with individuals, however, and from there and them you can learn what the solutions will be. One mistake we often make is to try to fix problematic situations *for* people, viewing them as incapable of doing so on their own or with a modicum of help. Not knowing much about the situation from their perspective, and now knowing what their range of options are, we then often make things worse for them rather than better. Reform of any kind and at any level has to begin with the people most directly affected, and the best solutions will come from them. They are our teachers and our guides, not only the other way around. Reciprocity is essential.

SEN: I couldn't agree more, Ms Addams, and I would add to that that there are no shortcuts that would allow us to bypass the diligence, attention and persistence required to do the very work you describe. The road to Hell could certainly be paved with these kinds of good intentions gone astray. There is no way to substitute for first-person experience and insider knowledge of an issue, and no way to liberate a population of people without their playing a leading and active role. Otherwise, we simply substitute one form of oppression with another.

VYGOTSKY: I appreciate the emphasis on individual activity; that is, after all, the only way we learn. I would suggest, though, that this is not an either/or matter. In fact, individual effort and social change are dialectical in nature, and each requires the other to exist. Creative activity may be carried out by individuals, but it changes the world. And changes in the world likewise bring about changes in individuals. My question, if you'll forgive me, is what does any of this have to do with mental illness and recovery?

MEYER: What you call 'mental illnesses' are learned strategies or habits that are maladaptive in present circumstances, or they result from the disintegration of those habits because of changes in the person's circumstances. There may be a biological component to this picture, as far as we know, that may make the habits either less hardy or more brittle than ordinary, but, regardless, the person has to be helped to establish new behaviors that can constitute new and more adaptive habits. This is best done, to return to our earlier argument, within the context of the person's everyday life, rather than in some distant hospital.

SULLIVAN: And this is also best done, if I can add to Dr Meyer's excellent explanation, within the context of a fully genuine, human interaction between two equals. I can't be of help to you if I put you down or make you feel inferior to me. I have to help you identify those aspects of yourself that are most valuable to you, most effective in the world and most appealing to others. Once you feel secure in your own abilities, you will then be able to figure out yourself what to do to change your situation for the better. I am just a human bridge.

VYGOTSKY: I assume you would couple this with effective action in the world, no? This can't just happen in your office. It has to bring about material changes in the world.

BASAGLIA: Yes, I agree. Offices may be useful in getting to know someone and earning their trust, which I agree with Dr Sullivan is necessary for any progress to be made, but the actions the person undertakes have to be in the world, as difficult as that is. The person has to learn to relate to other 'real' people, not just mental health staff, and to engage in meaningful and gratifying activities that will benefit others, not just make crafts or work in a sheltered workshop. This became a primary focus of the work we did once we closed the hospital in Trieste. We joined with people, encountered the same barriers to integration that they encountered and worked in partnership with them to come up with creative solutions to address those barriers. We mediated between them and their landlords, their employers, their family members; anywhere that a problem was encountered, that's where you would find us. So a human bridge to the community, yes, but of course one with tremendous flexibility, creativity and skill.

MEYER: Before you disparage making crafts, Dr Basaglia, consider that some people who have been seriously disabled or immobilized by their difficulties may need to make small, incremental steps towards the kinds of efforts you're talking about. They may not feel up to, or may not be able to do, those things in what you call the 'real world', at least not initially. For some people, being able to complete a project like a craft, and having something tangible to show for their effort, may represent an extremely important early step in their recovery. Don't be dismissive of the importance of these small steps.

BASAGLIA: On the contrary, rather than belittling such efforts I am arguing that they should be regarded as equally valuable and as contributions to the greater good, even if they do not generate a capitalistic profit, even if they do not produce a good that can be sold. People can contribute to the world without necessarily being materially productive, and they can do it outside of hospital settings, without being segregated. That, Dr Meyer, was my point.

ADDAMS: I believe that that is a hard point to keep foremost in our minds, given the world we live in. There is such pressure on all of us, not just those people whom you regard as your 'patients', to bend their will and their labor to the aim of amassing more and more material wealth that at times I despair of making real progress. People should be valued for their gifts, their talents, their love, their companionship, their creativity, their passion and their compassion, and not for how much they can be exploited to generate profits for others. Do you think there would be mental illnesses if the world we lived in were a fully just and fully compassionate world? The people I see have been so beaten down, so demoralized and felt so abandoned and alone that it is hard to see what remains of a so-called mental illness when all of these layers have been stripped away. I don't see illness as much as I see trauma and its after-effects.

PINEL: Trauma is certainly important, but there are many, many people who suffer from horrific trauma who do not develop mental illnesses. I believe that the illnesses, or at least the underlying vulnerabilities to illness, are there before the trauma and the trauma brings it out.

BASAGLIA: And then, perhaps in the dialectical way Professor Vygotsky described, the illness and the trauma become intertwined in mutually detrimental ways. What you refer to, Ms Addams, we have thought of as the secondary illness: the constellation of passivity, apathy, withdrawal and despair that results especially from institutionalization. But there is still a primary illness as well. It is just impossible to determine what that primary illness is when it is so encrusted over by trauma and abuse.

STRAUSS: Unfortunately, that constellation of passivity, apathy and isolation occurs outside of institutions as well. That same constellation is seen in individuals who have had prolonged and involuntary unemployment, which is the trauma that is heaped on top of the illness these days. Even though most people are outside of hospitals now, we still can't tell what the illness truly looks like without all of those negative factors covering it over.

GOFFMAN: And yet you remain convinced that there is a primary illness nonetheless? What if that secondary illness is all there is, with nothing else underneath?

SULLIVAN: I can tell you first-hand that there is something else underneath. It's difficult to describe, but I've seen it myself and in the young men I used to treat in Baltimore. They hadn't become demoralized and apathetic yet. They were isolated and terribly lonely, that's for sure, but that was primarily because they were convinced that no one else would be able to understand what they were going through. Meeting someone who could and did, that had a powerful effect, and in most cases they didn't develop that hard outer crust you're talking about.

MEYER: But was it an illness, Harry?

SULLIVAN: I don't know if it was an illness or not. What I can tell you is that it wasn't anything that any one of you couldn't experience also. It wasn't that different from everyday experience in most respects, just by a matter of degree.

STRAUSS: That's certainly what we found in our research. Many people hear voices, for example, and these experiences aren't always distressing or pathological. They can be comforting, and helpful, as with Socrates, or they can be syntonic with a person's cultural or religious background, like in Native American culture and in Confucianism. And as people start to improve, they report that the voices become more muted, or recede into the background, before disappearing altogether. The same kind of continuum can be found with delusions.

SULLIVAN: Precisely, Dr Strauss. And if people can be helped to understand and integrate those kinds of experiences, they can recover without ever developing that secondary crust of chronicity. I've seen it many, many times.

STRAUSS: Are you suggesting, then, that we shouldn't tell people that they have an illness? Do you think a label like that reifies their experiences? For me, the most important thing is to try to put together the idea that this person has a problem with an understanding of where that problem fits in the person's overall life. Employing medical terms and concepts can be useful, but that needs to be combined with trying to understand how the problems and the person's life context are experienced from his or her point of view so that we can understand the processes that are involved and be of maximum help. Understanding the person's experience is where I think the arts and especially the theatre can help us and why they should be a part of our training and research. Actors spend their lives trying to grasp another person's experience and gain an understanding of his or her world. We psychiatrists often think we're good at that but very often underestimate the skill and training it takes to get there.

ADDAMS: I must say that I have seldom found it useful to place an abstract label on people's experiences. It introduces a distance not only between them and me but also between them and their own experiences. Usually, it has the effect of objectifying them into a category that only suits the purposes of politicians or policemen; it does little to help them per se and makes it even more difficult for us to achieve the kind of understanding Dr Strauss is arguing for.

DELEUZE: That has been the tragic history of your whole field of psychiatry, has it not? It certainly has not been to the benefit of the so-called patients.

PINEL: I have to disagree in one respect. When I first proposed that mental illnesses were illnesses like physical illnesses, my purposes were just as medicinal as they were scientific. I thought of diagnosing and treating mental illnesses the same way we diagnose and treat illnesses like the flu or bacterial infections. When you have a fever, it helps to know what the cause of the fever is and, when possible, to treat the fever effectively so that both the symptoms and their underlying cause, the illness, go away. That's what I had in mind. I had no idea how such an approach to mental illness could go so far astray. I still think it has merit. People are relieved when you can diagnose and label, as you say, their condition, especially when that leads to effective care and cure. Even in cases where there is no cure, it can still be reassuring to know what you are dealing with. Don't you think it important that people be offered that information?

KING: I think it's always important that people be offered accurate information, at least as accurate as we have at any given time. It matters, though, how that information is given. It can be used as a putdown, as a discussion ender, as a way to dismiss the person and his or her concerns. It's been used as a way to keep marginalized populations on the margins for centuries. On the other hand, it can be offered with respect, as one person to another, both being equals. It can be more like, 'Hey, this is what I think you're dealing with. What do you think you can do about that? And, is there a way I can help you?' That leaves it open to the person to decide.

SEN: Deciding for yourself is very important. That's the only way the person will be able to develop more self-confidence.

VYGOTSKY: It's also the only way the person can learn what kind of person he or she is, by seeing what kinds of decisions he or she makes.

DIX: But that brings us back to where we started. People with serious mental illnesses make bad decisions all the time; their judgement is impaired by the illness. We can't just stand by and let them ruin their lives, and the lives of other people around them. What kind of compassion is that? If they knew how to make their own decisions, we wouldn't have these problems to begin with. That answer makes no sense to me.

PINEL: I don't believe that we have any data to support your thesis, Ms Dix. In my experience and observation, people with serious mental illnesses make decisions as well as anyone else does, or at least no worse than anyone else does. It is just that sometimes the premises of their judgements are faulty. It is their perceptions and beliefs that are problematic, not their judgement.

TUKE: How can you possibly separate the two? Perceptions and beliefs are products of judgement as well as the premises for judgement. If the reason is affected, then it is all of the rational faculties that have become distorted. You can't pick and choose.

MEYER: Oh, yes, Mr Tuke, I'm afraid that it is much more complicated than you suggest. After all, your retreat would not have been able to function had you not assumed that your patients at least retained the rational wish to be approved of and valued by others. That was your own sort of secret weapon, was it not?

TUKE: But even children want the approval and affection of others. I don't see how that can be taken as a sign of rational judgement.

VYGOTSKY: Do you not see children as rational beings, Mr Tuke? Why, I find children to be supremely rational beings, no more or less than their parents, or ourselves, for that matter. The only difference is the accumulated experience and what has been learned and internalized by that body of experience as the child grows into an adult. As Dr Pinel suggested, and with which I must agree, it is not the reason that is distorted or lacking in mental illness. It is that people are making rational judgements based on anomalous, or at least unusual, experiences. This, I believe, was Dr Sullivan's belief as well, yes?

SULLIVAN: Yes, precisely, Professor. Anomalous, or perhaps extreme, experiences can generate seemingly bizarre or extravagant gestures. If you perceive the gestures to be irrational, or even incomprehensible, then that merely represents *your* failure to empathize and to imagine whence such gestures might have arisen. Obviously, the gestures come from somewhere and have some aim. It is our job as clinicians to strive to understand what sense is being made and what aims are being pursued through these gestures. It is easy, as you have shown, to simply dismiss or diagnose the gestures away as being 'irrational'; but what have you gained thereby? You haven't learned anything about the person. You have only learned about the limits of your own intellect and imagination. No offence intended, of course.

DELEUZE: One important point that I think you are making implicitly, that is worth explicating, Doctor, is that no one person has a monopoly on truth or reason, no one stands at an Archimedean point from which to be able to judge what is truly, purely or objectively rational and what is not. To be of any real help to the person, you have to be able to accept the reality that his or her perspective is just as valid as your own. That requires having a fairly loose grasp on your own sense of reality; otherwise, you will be just as stuck as the person you're trying to help. It's a bit of a tricky business, you know, having one foot in each universe.

SULLIVAN: It's only tricky if you'd been tricking yourself into believing that you owned the truth in the first place. As for me, I was disabused of that notion very early on in life, which made me particularly well suited to this work. That's why I chose from among my recovered patients to hire the staff for my unit. They also had an appreciation for the tenuousness of truth. Anyone who thinks they already know everything there is to know about the world, in its infinite diversity, should choose another field to work in.

BASAGLIA: Fair enough, but I think we are losing the gist of the concern raised by Ms Dix. In our work, we found it very possible, and extremely effective, to join with, to stand alongside of, someone who was making what seemed like bad decisions without having to use coercion, much less to place that person in a hospital. What is essential is to first have gained that person's trust. Once the person believes that you are looking out for his or her best interest, he or she is much more likely to listen to what you have to say, to follow your lead or at least to consider a compromise, as long as you are trying to help the person get what he or she wants, and not just what you want. If you can suggest an easier, straighter or more scenic route to where they are trying to go, they'll be more likely to try it out, and even to be appreciative.

VYGOTSKY: Yes, having the other person there, that is essential. That way the other person can better understand what you're trying to do and will be in a position to actually show you how to do it. Otherwise, how could you possibly know what to do? Dr Meyer might suggest that it would be 'common sense', but I'm not impressed by what typically passes for common sense. Only if you are yourself in the same situation, facing the same obstacles and opportunities, will you be able to figure out what to do and how to do it. Then the person can learn from you. How else can we expect them to learn new responses to old situations? It's really not that much different from learning how to tie knots, is it? You Americans, you do that I believe in something called the Boy Scouts? Scout leaders, or better yet older boys, show younger boys how to tie knots. Then they learn to do it themselves. We would never expect them to be able to do it by themselves, would we? And it's much harder to learn how to do it by sitting in a room and looking at diagrams without a piece of rope in your hand. You learn by watching others and by others encouraging you and helping you along. Then you can help other people. If psychiatry hasn't tried that model yet, perhaps it should.

SULLIVAN: As long as we don't forget that we're talking about how to live one's life and not how to tie knots.

VYGOTSKY: Yes, of course, but life is lived through such activities, some more complex than others. In general, the focus should be on activity and on how to assist people in participating, and being successful, in the activities they want to participate in. What else is there?

References

Addams, J. (1910) *Twenty Years at Hull-house with Autobiographical Notes*, The Macmillan Company, New York.

Alport, G. (1937) *Personality: A Psychological Interpretation*, Holt, Rinehart, & Winston, New York.

American Psychiatric Association (1980) *Diagnostic and Statistical Manual of Mental Disorders*, 3rd edn, American Psychiatric Association, Washington.

American Psychiatric Association (1994) *Diagnostic and Statistical Manual of Mental Disorders*, 4th edn, American Psychiatric Association, Washington.

American Psychiatric Association (2000) *Diagnostic and Statistical Manual of Mental Disorders*, 4th edn (Text Revision), American Psychiatric Association, Washington.

American Psychiatric Association Committee on Nomenclature (1952) *Diagnostic and Statistical Manual of Mental Disorders*, American Psychiatric Association Committee on Nomenclature, Washington.

Andreasen, N. (1982) *The Broken Brain: The Biological Revolution in Psychiatry*, Harper & Row, New York.

Andres-Hyman, R., Strauss, J.S. and Davidson, L. (2007) Beyond parallel play: science befriending the art of Method Acting in pursuit of a healing relationship. *Psychotherapy: Theory, Research, Practice, Training*, **44** (1), 78–89.

Anthony, W.A. (2004) The principle of personhood: the field's transcendent principle. *Psychiatric Rehabilitation Journal*, **27** (3), 205.

Arieti, S. (ed.) (1959) *The American Handbook of Psychiatry*, Basic Books, New York.

Basaglia, F. (1964) The destruction of the mental hospital as a place of institutionalization. Presentation delivered to the First International Congress of Social Psychiatry, London.

Basaglia, F. (1979) The therapeutic vocation, in *Scritti*, Einaudi, Torino.

Basaglia, F. (1980a) Breaking the circuit of control, in *Critical Psychiatry: The Politics of Mental Health* (ed. D. Ingleby), Pantheon Books, New York, pp. 184–192.

Basaglia, F. (1980b) Crisis intervention, treatment, and rehabilitation. *World Hospitals*, **16** (4), 26–27.

Basaglia, F. (1980c) Problems of law and psychiatry: the Italian experience. *International Journal of Law and Psychiatry*, **3**, 17–37.

Basaglia, F. (1985) What is psychiatry? *International Journal of Mental Health*, **14**, 42–51.

Basaglia, F. (1987) Institutions of violence (Shtob, T., trans.), in *Psychiatry Inside Out: Selected Writings of Franco Basaglia* (eds N. Scheper-Hughes and A.M. Lovell), Columbia University Press, New York, pp. 59–85.

Beers, C. (1908) *A Mind that Found Itself: An Autobiography*, Longman, New York.

Berger, M. (1978) *Beyond the Double Bind*, Bruner/Mazel Publishers, New York.

Bernard, C. (1865) *Introduction à l'étude de la Médicine Expérimentale*, Champs/Flammarion, Paris.

de Biran, M. (1805) Académie de Berlin Programme, in *Dans De L'aperception Immédiate*. Le Livre de Poche, Paris.

Bleuler, E. (1950) *Dementia Praecox or the Group of Schizophrenias*, International Universities Press, New York.

Bockoven, J.S. (1956) Moral treatment in American psychiatry. *Journal of Nervous and Mental Disease*, **124**, 292–321.

Borg, M. and Davidson, L. (2007) The nature of recovery as lived in everyday experience. *Journal of Mental Health*, **16** (4), 1–12.

Borthwick, A., Holman, C., Kennard, D. *et al.* (2001) The relevance of moral treatment to contemporary mental health care. *Journal of Mental Health*, **10** (4), 427–439.

Breier, A. and Strauss, J.S. (1983) Self-control in psychotic disorders. *Archives of General Psychiatry*, **40** (10), 1141–1145.

Brown, T.J. (1998) *Dorothea Dix: New England Reformer*, Harvard University Press, Boston.

Browne, W.J. (1969) A psychiatric study of the life and work of Dorothea Dix. *American Journal of Psychiatry*, **126** (3), 335–341.

Bruner, J. (1985) Vygotsky: an historical and conceptual perspective, in *Culture, Communication, and Cognition: Vygotskian Perspectives* (ed. J. Wertsch), Cambridge University Press, London, pp. 21–34.

Burke, K. (1969) *A Rhetoric of Motives*, University of California Press, Berkeley, CA.

Burti, L. (2001) Italian psychiatric reform 20 plus years after, *Acta Psychiatrica Scandinavica*, **104**, (Suppl. 410), 41–46.

Canguilhem, G. (1966) *Le Normal et le Pathologique*, Quadrige/PUF, Paris.

Care Services Improvement Partnership (2006) Pathways to Recovery Paper 1. Core Vision and Values for a Modern Mental Health System, Department of Health, London.

Chadwick, P., Birchwood, M. and Trower, P. (1996) *Cognitive Therapy for Delusions, Voices, and Paranoia*, John Wiley & Sons, Ltd, London.

Chamberlin, J. (1990) The ex-patients' movement: where we've been and where we're going. *Journal of Mind and Behavior*, **11**, 323–336.

Cohen, N.L. and Marcos, L.R. (1992) Outreach intervention models for the homeless mentally ill, in *Treating the Homeless Mentally Ill* (eds H.R. Lamb, L.L. Bachrach and F.I. Kass), American Psychiatric Association, Washington, pp. 141–158.

Cohen, N.L. and Tsemberis, S. (1991) Emergency psychiatric intervention on the street. *New Directions for Mental Health Services*, **52**, 3–16.

Colton, C.W. and Manderscheid, R.W. (2006) Congruencies in increased mortality rates, years of potential life lost, and causes of death among public mental health clients in eight states. *Preventing Chronic Disease*, **3** (2), Downloaded from: http://www.cdc.gov/pcd/issues/2006/apr/05_0180.htm.

Cooper, J. and Sartorius, N. (1977) Cultural and temporal variations in schizophrenia: a speculation on the importance of industrialization. *British Journal of Psychiatry*, **130**, 50–55.

Corin, E. and Lauzon, G. (1992) Positive withdrawal and the quest for meaning: the reconstruction of experience among schizophrenics. *Psychiatry*, **55** (3), 266–281.

Corrigan, P.W., Mueser, K.T., Bond, G.R. *et al.* (2008) *Principles and Practice of Psychiatric Rehabilitation: An Empirical Approach*, Guilford Press, New York.

Davidson, L. (1988) Psychologism in psychology: the case of schizophrenia. *Practice: A Journal of Psychology and Political Economy*, **6**, 2–20.

Davidson, L. (2003) *Living Outside Mental Illness: Qualitative Studies of Recovery in Schizophrenia*, New York University Press, New York.

Davidson, L. (2006) What happened to civil rights? *Psychiatric Rehabilitation Journal*, **30** (1), 11–14.

Davidson, L. (2007a) At issue: a basic criterion for transformation. *Psychiatric Services*, **58** (8), 1029.

Davidson, L. (2007b) Habits and other anchors of everyday life people with psychiatric disabilities may not take for granted. *Journal of Occupational Therapy Research*, **27** (S), 1–9.

Davidson, L. and Roe, D. (2007) Recovery from versus recovery in serious mental illness: one strategy for lessening confusion plaguing recovery. *Journal of Mental Health*, **16** (4), 1–12.

Davidson, L. and Shahar, G. (2007) From deficit to desire: a philosophical reconsideration of action models of psychopathology. *Philosophy, Psychiatry and Psychology*, **14** (3), 215–232.

Davidson, L. and Strauss, J.S. (1995) Beyond the biopsychosocial model: integrating disorder, health and recovery. *Psychiatry: Interpersonal and Biological Processes*, **58**, 44–55.

Davidson, L. and White, W. (2007) The concept of recovery as an organizing principle for integrating mental health and addiction services. *Journal of Behavioral Health Services and Research*, **34**, 109–120.

Davidson, L., Borg, M., Marin, I. *et al.* (2005) Processes of recovery in psychosis: findings from a multi-national study. *American Journal of Psychiatric Rehabilitation*, **8** (3), 177–201.

Davidson, L., Flanagan, E., Roe, D. and Styron, T. (2006) Leading a horse to water: an action perspective on mental health policy. *Journal of Clinical Psychology*, **62** (9), 1141–1155.

Davidson, L., Harding, C.M. and Spaniol, L. (2005) *Recovery from Severe Mental Illnesses: Research Evidence and Implications for Practice*, vol. 1, Center for Psychiatric Rehabilitation of Boston University, Boston.

Davidson, L., Harding, C.M. and Spaniol, L. (2006) *Recovery from Severe Mental Illnesses: Research Evidence and Implications for Practice*, vol. 2, Center for Psychiatric Rehabilitation of Boston University, Boston.

Davidson, L., Hoge, M.A., Godleski, L. *et al.* (1996) Hospital or community living? Examining consumer perspectives on deinstitutionalization. *Psychiatric Rehabilitation Journal*, **19**, 49–58.

Davidson, L., Kirk, T., Rockholz, P. *et al.* (2007) Creating a recovery-oriented system of behavioral health care: moving from concept to reality. *Psychiatric Rehabilitation Journal*, **31** (1), 23–31.

Davidson, L., O'Connell, M.J., Tondora, J. *et al.* (2006) The top ten concerns about recovery encountered in mental health system transformation. *Psychiatric Services*, **57** (5), 640–645.

Davidson, L., Ridgway, P., Wieland, M. and O'Connell, M. A capabilities approach to mental health transformation: a conceptual framework for the recovery era. *Canadian Journal of Community Mental Health*, in press.

Davidson, L., Stayner, D.A., Lambert, S. *et al.* (1997) Phenomenological and participatory research on schizophrenia: recovering the person in theory and practice. *Journal of Social Issues*, **53**, 767–784.

Davidson, L., Stayner, D.A., Nickou, C. *et al.* (2001) 'Simply to be let in': inclusion as a basis for recovery from mental illness. *Psychiatric Rehabilitation Journal*, **24**, 375–388.

Davidson, L., Tondora, J. and O'Connell, M.J. (2006) In reply. *Psychiatric Services*, **57** (10), 1510–1511

Davidson, L., Tondora, J., O'Connell, M.J. *et al.* (2009) *A Practical Guide to Recovery-oriented Practice: Tools for Transforming Mental Health Care*, Oxford University Press, New York.

Deegan, P.E. (1988) Recovery: the lived experience of rehabilitation. *Psychosocial Rehabilitation Journal*, **11** (4), 11–19.

Deegan, P.E. (1992) The independent living movement and people with psychiatric disabilities: taking back control over our own lives. *Psychosocial Rehabilitation Journal*, **15**, 3–19.

Deegan, P.E. (1993) Recovering our sense of value after being labeled mentally ill. *Journal of Psychosocial Nursing*, **31** (4), 7–11.

Deegan, P.E. (1996) Recovery as a journey of the heart. *Psychiatric Rehabilitation Journal*, **19**, 91–97.

Deegan, P.E. (2007) The lived experience of using psychiatric medication in the recovery process and a shared decision-making program to support it. *Psychiatric Rehabilitation Journal*, **31** (1), 62–69.

Deleuze, G. (1983) *Nietzsche and Philosophy* (Tomlinson, H., trans.), Columbia University Press, New York.

Deleuze, G. and Guattari, F. (1982) *Capitalism and Schizophrenia: Anti-Oedipus* (Massumi, B., trans.), University of Minnesota Press, Minneapolis.

Department of Health and Human Services (1999) Mental Health: A Report of the Surgeon General, Department of Health and Human Services, US Public Health Service, Rockville, MD.

Department of Health and Human Services (2003) Achieving the Promise: Transforming Mental Health Care in America, President's New Freedom Commission on Mental Health. Final Report (DHHS Pub. No. SMA-03-3832), Department of Health and Human Services, US Public Health Service, Rockville, MD.

Department of Health and Human Services (2005) Transforming Mental Health Care in America. Federal Action Agenda: First Steps, Substance Abuse and Mental Health Services Administration, US Public Health Service, Rockville, MD.

Dilthey, W. (1977) *Descriptive Psychology and Historical Understanding* (Zaner, R.M. and Heiges, K.L., trans), Martinus Nijhoff, The Hague.

Drake, R.E., Becker, D.R., Biesanz, J.C. *et al.* (1994) Rehabilitative day treatment vs. supported employment: I. Vocational outcomes. *Community Mental Health Journal*, **30**, 519–532.

Drake, R.E., Becker, D.R., Clark, R.E. and Mueser, K.T. (1999) Research on the individual placement and support model of supported employment. *Psychiatric Quarterly*, **70**, 289–301.

Drèze, J. and Sen, A. (1989) *Hunger and Public Action*, Clarendon Press, Oxford.

Dumont, J. and Jones, K. (2002) Findings from a consumer/survivor defined alternative to psychiatric hospitalization. *Outlook: Practice, Evaluation, Research*, Spring, 4–6.

Engel, G. (1977) The need for a new medical model: a challenge for biomedicine. *Science*, **196**, 129–136.

Erikson, E. (1950) *Childhood and Society*, Norton, New York.

Flanagan, E. and Davidson, L. (2007) 'Schizophrenics,' 'borderlines,' and the lingering legacy of misplaced concreteness: does the DSM-IV-TR classify people or disorders? *Psychiatry*, **70** (2), 100–112.

Flanagan, E., Davidson, L. and Strauss, J.S. (2007) Incorporating patients' subjective experiences into the DSM-V. *American Journal of Psychiatry*, **164** (3), 391–392.

Flanagan, E., Miller, R.M. and Davidson, L. (2009) 'Unfortunately, we treat the chart': stigma in mental health settings. *Psychiatric Quarterly*, **80**, 55–64.

Floersch, J. (2002) *Meds, Money, and Manners: The Case Management of Severe Mental Illness*, Columbia University Press, New York.

Foucault, M. (1965) *Madness and Civilization* (Howard, R., trans.), Random House, New York.

Fowler, D. and Garety, P.A. (1995) *Cognitive Behaviour Therapy for Psychosis: Theory and Practice*, John Wiley & Sons, Ltd, London.

Freud, S. (1907) *Le délire et les rêvees dans la Gradiva de W. Jensen: Traduit de L'allemand par Paule Arbex et Rose-Marie Zeitlin*, Gallimard, Paris.

Fromm, E. (1941) *Escape from Freedom*, Rinehart, New York.

Giannichedda, M.G. (1988) Crisis and identity: extracts from the theory of Franco Basaglia, in *Psychiatry in Transition: British and Italian Experiences*, Pluto, London, pp. 252–260.

Goffman, E. (1959) *The Presentation of Self in Everyday Life*, Anchor Books, New York.

Goffman, E. (1961) *Asylums: Essays on the Social Situation of Mental Patients and Other Inmates*, Doubleday, New York.

Goffman, E. (1963) *Stigma: Notes on the Management of Spoiled Identity*, Prentice Hall, New York.

Gollaher, D. (1995) *Voice for the Mad: The Life of Dorothea Dix*, Free Press, New York.

Greenstone, J.D. (1979) Dorothea Dix and Jane Addams: from transcendentalism to pragmatism in American social reform. *Social Service Review*, **53** (4), 527–559.

Griesinger, W. (1882) *Mental Pathology and Therapeutics*, Wood's Library of Standard Medical Authors, New York.

Harding, C.M., Zubin, J. and Strauss, J.S. (1987) Chronicity in schizophrenia: fact, partial fact, or artifact? *Hospital and Community Psychiatry*, **38**, 477–486.

Harrow, M. and Quinlan, D. (1977) Is disordered thinking unique to schizophrenia? *Archives of General Psychiatry*, **34**, 15–21.

Hersch, G.I., Lamport, N.K. and Coffey, M.S. (2005) *Activity Analysis: Application to Occupation*, 5th edn, Slack, Inc., Thorofare, NJ.

Hoge, M.A., Davidson, L., Griffith, E.E.H. and Jacobs, S. (1998) The crisis of managed care in the public sector. *International Journal of Mental Health*, **27**, 52–71.

Horney, K. (1937) *The Neurotic Personality of Our Time*, Norton, New York.

Interagency Council on the Homeless (1991) *Reaching Out: A Guide for Service Providers*, Department of Housing and Urban Development, Washington.

Jackson, J.H. (1958) in *Selected Writings of John Hughlings Jackson*, vols 1 and 2 (ed. J. Taylor), Staples Press, London.

Johnson, A.B. (1990) *Out of Bedlam: The Truth About Deinstitutionalization*, Basic Books, New York.

John-Steiner, V. and Souberman, E. (1978) Afterward, in *Mind in Society: The Development of Higher Psychological Processes* (eds L.S. Vygotsky, M. Cole, V. John-Steiner *et al.*), Harvard University Press, Cambridge MA, pp. 121–134.

Joint Commission on Mental Illness and Health (1961) *Action for Mental Health: Final Report*, Basic Books, New York.

Karon, B. (2008) An "incurable" schizophrenic: the case of Mr. X. *Pragmatic Case Studies in Psychotherapy*, **4** (1), 1–24.

King, M.L. (1981) Letter from Birmingham Jail, reprinted in *King Remembered* (eds F. Schulke and P. McPhee), Norton, New York, pp. 276–284.

Kingdon, D.G. and Turkington, D. (1994) *Cognitive-behavioral Therapy of Schizophrenia*, Bassetlaw Hospital, Bassetlaw.

Kraepelin, E. (1904) *Clinical Psychiatry*, Macmillan, New York.

Kraepelin, E. (1921) *Clinical Psychiatry: A Textbook for Students and Physicians* (Diefendorf, A.R., trans.), Macmillan, New York.

Krupa, T., Fossey, E., Anthony, W.A. *et al.* (2009) Doing daily life: how occupational therapy can inform psychiatric rehabilitation practice. *Psychiatric Rehabilitation Journal*, **32** (3), 155–161.

Laine, C. and Davidoff, F. (1996) Patient-centred medicine: a professional evolution. *Journal of the American Medical Association*, **275** (22), 152–156.

Laing, R.D. (1967) *The Politics of Experience*, Ballantine, New York.

Leff, J. and Warner, R. (2006) *Social Inclusion of People with Mental Illness*, Cambridge University Press, Cambridge.

Leighton, A. (1959) *My Name is Legion: The Sterling County Study of Psychiatric Disorder and Sociocultural Environment*, vol. 1, Basic Books, New York.

Lidz, T. (1966) Adolf Meyer and the development of American psychiatry. *American Journal of Psychiatry*, **123**, 320–332.

Lief, A. (ed.) (1948) *The Commonsense Psychiatry of Dr. Adolf Meyer: Fifty-two Selected Papers*, McGraw-Hill, New York.

Lilleleht, E. (2002) Power: exploring the disciplinary connections between moral treatment and psychiatric rehabilitation. *Philosophy, Psychiatry, and Psychology*, **9** (2), 167–182.

Marrone, J., Hoff, D. and Helm, D. (1997) Person-centred planning for the millennium: we're old enough to remember when PCP was just a drug. *Journal of Vocational Rehabilitation*, **8**, 285–297.

Marshall, H.E. (1937) *Dorothea Dix: Forgotten Samaritan*, University of North Carolina Press, Chapel Hill , NC.

Maslow, A. (1966) *The Psychology of Science: A Reconnaissance*, Harper & Row, New York.

McCarrick, A.K., Manderscheid, R.W., Bertolucci, D.E. *et al.* (1986) Chronic medical problems in the chronic mentally ill. *Hospital and Community Psychiatry*, **37** (3), 289–291.

McCormack, B. and McCance, T.V. (2006) Development of a framework for person-centred nursing. *Journal of Advanced Nursing*, **56** (5), 472–479.

Meehl, P. (1973) Schizotaxia, schizotypy, schizophrenia, in *Psychodiagnosis: Selected Papers* (ed. P. Meehl), W.W. Norton & Company, New York, pp. 135–155.

Mental Health Commission (1998) Blueprint for Mental Health Services in New Zealand, Mental Health Commission, Wellington.

Meyer, A. (1910) The dynamic interpretation of *dementia praecox*. *American Journal of Psychology*, **21** (3), 385–403.

Meyer, A. (1919) The life chart and the obligation of specifying positive data in psychopathological diagnosis, in *Contributions to Medical and Biological Research*, vol. 2, Paul Hoeber, New York, pp. 1128–1133.

Meyer, A. (1922) The philosophy of occupation therapy. *Archives of Occupational Therapy*, **1** (1), 1–10.

Meyer, A. (1928) Presidential address: thirty-five years of psychiatry in the United States and our present outlook. *American Journal of Psychiatry*, **8** (1), 1–31.

Minkoff, K. (1987) Beyond deinstitutionalization: a new ideology for the post-institutional era. *Hospital and Community Psychiatry*, **38**, 945–950.

National Council on Disability (2000) From Privileges to Rights: People Labeled with Psychiatric Disabilities Speak for Themselves, accessed 20 August 2005, from http://www.ncd.gov/newsroom/publications/privileges.html.

Newman, F. and Holzman, L. (1993) *Lev Vygotsky: Revolutionary Scientist*, Routledge, London.

Nussbaum, M.C. (2000) *Women and Human Development: The Capabilities Approach*, Cambridge University Press, New York.

O'Brien, J. (1987) A guide to life-style planning: using the activities catalogue to integrate services and natural support systems, in *A Comprehensive Guide to the Activities Catalogue* (eds B. Wilcox and G.T. Bellamy), Paul Brookes, Baltimore.

O'Brien, J. (2002) Person-centred planning as a contributing factor in organizational and social change. *Research and Practice in Persistent and Severe Disability*, **27** (4), 261–264.

O'Brien, J. and Lovett, H. (1992) Finding a Way Toward Everyday Lives: The Contribution of Person-centred Planning, PA Office of Mental Retardation, Harrisburg.

O'Brien, C. and O'Brien, J. (2000) *The Origins of Person-centred Planning: A Community of Practice Perspective*, Responsive Systems Associates, Inc., Syracuse, NY.

Parrish, J. (1989) The long journey home: accomplishing the mission of the community support movement. *Psychosocial Rehabilitation Journal*, **12** (3), 107–124.

Parry-Jones, W.L. (1971) *The Trade in Lunacy: A Study of Private Madhouses in England and Wales in the Eighteenth and Nineteenth Centuries*, Routledge & Kegan Paul, London.

Perry, H.S. (1982) *Psychiatrist of America: The Life of Harry Stack Sullivan*, The Belknap Press, Cambridge.

Pinel, P. (1806) *A Treatise on Insanity* (Davis, D.D., trans.), W. Todd, Sheffield.

Pitts, D.B. (2009) Introduction to special section on occupational therapy. *Psychiatric Rehabilitation Journal*, **32** (3), 151–154.

Rakfeldt, J. and Strauss, J.S. (1989) The low turning point: a control mechanism in the course of mental disorder. *Journal of Nervous and Mental Disease*, **177** (1), 32–37.

Redlich, F. and Freedman, D. (1966) *The Theory and Practice of Psychiatry*, Basic Books, New York.

Reilly, F., Harrow, M. and Tucker, G. (1975) Looseness of association in acute schizophrenia. *British Journal of Psychiatry*, **127**, 240–246.

Rosenberg, S. and Tucker, G. (1979) Verbal behavior and schizophrenia. *Archives of General Psychiatry*, **36**, 1331–1337.

Rowe, M. (1999) *Crossing the Border: Encounters Between Homeless People and Outreach Workers*, University of California Press, Berkeley, CA.

Salyers, M. and Tsemberis, S. (2007) ACT and recovery: integrating evidence-based practice and recovery orientation on assertive community treatment. *Community Mental Health Journal*, **43** (6), 619–641.

Sartre, J.P. (1956). *Being and Nothingness* (Barnes, H., trans.), Washington Square Press, New York.

Scheper-Hughes, N. and Lovell, A.M. (1986) Breaking the circuit of social control: lessons in public psychiatry from Italy and Franco Basaglia. *Social Science and Medicine*, **23** (2), 159–178.

Scheper-Hughes, N. and Lovell, A.M. (1987) *Psychiatry Inside Out: Selected Writings of Franco Basaglia*, Columbia University Press, New York.

Scull, A. (1981) *Madhouses, Mad-doctors, and Madmen: The Social History of Psychiatry in the Victorian Era*, University of Pennsylvania Press, Philadelphia.

Sen, A. (1992) *Inequality Re-examined*, Clarendon Press, Oxford.

Sen, A. (1999) *Development as Freedom*, Anchor Books, New York.

Silverstein, S. (1976) *The Missing Piece*, HarperCollins, New York.

Snow, D.L. and Newton, P.M. (1976) Task, social structure, and social process in the Community Mental Health Center Movement. *American Psychologist*, **31**, 582–594.

Snow, D.L. and Swift, C.F. (1985) Consultation and education in community mental health: a historical analysis. *Journal of Primary Prevention*, **6**, 3–30.

Spiegel, J. and Bell, N. (1959) The family of the psychiatric patient, in *The American Handbook of Psychiatry* (ed. S. Arieti), Basic Books, New York, p. 115.

Standing Senate Committee on Social Affairs, Science and Technology (2006) Out of the Shadows at Last: Transforming Mental Health, Mental Illness, and Addiction Services in Canada, from http://www.parl.gc.ca (accessed 21 June 2006).

Stein, L.I. and Test, M.A. (eds) (1978) *Alternatives to Mental Hospital Treatment*, Plenum Press, New York.

Stein, L.I. and Test, M.A. (1980) Alternative to mental hospital treatment: I. Conceptual model, treatment program, and clinical evaluation. *Archives of General Psychiatry*, **37**, 392–397.

Strauss, J.S. (1969) Hallucinations and delusions as points on continua function: rating scale evidence. *Archives of General Psychiatry*, **21**, 581–586.

Strauss, J.S. (1994a) Is biological psychiatry building on an adequate base? in *Schizophrenia: from Mind to Molecule* (ed. N. Andreasen), American Psychiatric Association Press, Washington, pp. 31–44.

Strauss, J.S. (1994b) The person with schizophrenia as a person: II. Approaches to the subjective and complex. *British Journal of Psychiatry*, **164** (Suppl. 23): 107–109.

Strauss, J.S. (2007) La réalité et le concept de maladie mentale. *Psychiatrie, Sciences Humaines, et Neurosciences*, **5**, 125–130.

Strauss, J.S. and Carpenter, W.T. Jr (1972) Prediction of outcome in schizophrenia: I. Characteristics of outcome. *Archives of General Psychiatry*, **27**, 739–746.

Strauss, J.S., Hafez, H., Lieberman, P. and Harding, C.M. (1985) The course of psychiatric disorder: III. Longitudinal principles. *American Journal of Psychiatry*, **142** (3), 289–296.

Strauss, J.S., Staeheli-Lawless, M. and Sells, D. Becoming an expert. *Psychiatry*, in press.

Sullivan, H.S. (1940) *Conceptions of Modern Psychiatry*, Norton, New York.

Sullivan, H.S. (1953) *The Interpersonal Theory of Psychiatry*, Norton, New York.

Sullivan, H.S. (1962) *Schizophrenia as a Human Process* (ed. H.S. Perry), Norton, New York.

Szasz, T. (1961, 1974) *The Myth of Mental Illness: Foundations of a Theory of Personal Conduct*, Harper & Row, New York.

Tiffany, F. (1890) *Life of Dorothea Lynde Dix*, Houghton, Mifflin, & Company, Boston.

Tondora, J., Pocklington, S., Gorges, A. *et al.* (2005) Implementation of Person-centred Care and Planning. From Policy to Practice to Evaluation, Substance Abuse and Mental Health Services Administration, Washington.

Torrey, E. (1983) *Surviving Schizophrenia: A Family Manual*, Harper & Row, New York.

Tuke, S. (1813) *A Description of the Retreat, An Institution Near York, for Insane Persons of the Society of Friends*, W. Alexander, York.

Turner, J.C. and TenHoor, W.J. (1978) The NIMH community support program: pilot approach to a needed social reform. *Schizophrenia Bulletin*, **4**, 319–348.

Tyson, A. (1989) The interaction between developmental striving and the course of mental disorder. Unpublished medical school thesis, Yale University.

Vaccaro, J.V., Liberman, R.P., Friedlob, S. and Dempsay, S. (1992) Challenge and opportunity: rehabilitating the homeless mentally ill, in *Treating the Homeless Mentally Ill: A Report of the Task Force on the Homeless Mentally Ill* (eds R.H. Lamb, L.L. Bachrach and F.I. Kass), American Psychiatric Association, Washington, pp. 279–297.

Vygotsky, L.S. (1978) *Mind in Society: The Development of Higher Psychological Processes* (eds M. Cole, V. John-Steiner, S. Scribner and E. Souberman), Harvard University Press, Cambridge, MA.

Vygotsky, L.S. (1981) The instrumental method in psychology, in *The Concept of Activity in Soviet Psychology* (ed. J.V. Wertsch), Sharpe, Armonk, NY.

Vygotsky, L (1986) *Thought and Language*, (ed. and trans., Kozulin, A), MIT Press, Cambridge, MA.

Warner, R. (1983) Recovery from schizophrenia in the Third World. *Psychiatry*, **46**, 197–212.

Warner, R. (1985) *Recovery from Schizophrenia: Psychiatry and Political Economy*, Routledge & Kegan Paul, Boston.

Waxler, N. (1979) Is outcome for schizophrenia better in non-industrial societies? *Journal of Nervous and Mental Disease*, **167**, 144–158.

Weiner, D.B. (1979) The apprenticeship of Philippe Pine: a new document, 'Observations of Citizen Pussin on the Insane'. *American Journal of Psychiatry*, **36** (9), 1128–1134.

Weiner, D.B. (1992) Pinel's 'Memoir on Madness' of December 11, 1794: a fundamental text of modern psychiatry. *American Journal of Psychiatry*, **149**, 725–732.

Wertsch, J.V. (1985) *Vygotsky and the Social Formation of Mind*, Harvard University Press, Cambridge , MA.

Wertsch, J.V. (1994) Mediated action in sociocultural studies. *Mind, Culture, and Activity*, **1**, 202–208.

Wertsch, J.V. (1998) *Mind as Action*, Oxford University Press, New York.

Wertsch, J.V. (2002) *Voices of Collective Remembering*, Cambridge University Press, Cambridge.

Wexler, B., Davidson, L., Styron, T. and Strauss, J.S. (2008) Severe and persistent mental illness, in *40 Years of Academic Public Psychiatry* (eds S. Jacobs and E.E.H. Griffith), John Wiley & Sons, Ltd, London, pp. 1–20.

Wing, J.K. and Brown, G.W. (1970) *Institutionalism and Schizophrenia*, Cambridge University Press, London.

Winnicott, D.W. (1986) *Home is Where We Start From: Essays by a Psychoanalyst*, (compiled and edited by C. Winnicott, R. Shepherd, M. Davis) W.W. Norton, New York.

Wood, D., Bruner, J.S. and Ross, G. (1976) The role of tutoring in problem solving. *Journal of Child Psychology and Child Psychiatry*, **17**, 89–100.

Woods, E.A. and Carlson, E.T. (1961) The psychiatry of Philippe Pinel. *Bulletin of the History of Medicine*, **35**, 14–25.

Wood, D. and Middleton, D. (1975) A study of assisted problem-solving. *British Journal of Psychology*, **66**, 181–191.

Index

The Roots of the Recovery Movement in Psychiatry   Larry Davidson, Jaak Rakfeldt, John Strauss
© 2010 John Wiley & Sons, Ltd

Printed and bound by CPI Group (UK) Ltd, Croydon, CR0 4YY